DRUGS
IN THE CLASSROOM

A conceptual model for
school programs

Remember when HIPPIE meant big in the hips,
and a TRIP involved travel in cars, planes or ships?
When POT was a vessel for cooking things in,
and HOOKED was what grandmother's rug may have been?
When FIXED was a verb that meant mend or repair,
and NEAT meant well organized, tidy and clean,
and GRASS was a ground cover, normally green?
When lights and not people were SWITCHED ON and off,
and THE PILL might have been what you took for a cough?

When GROOVY meant furrowed with channels and hollows,
and BIRDS were winged creatures like robins and swallows?
When FUZZ was a substance, fluffy like lint,
and BREAD came from bakeries and not from the mint?
When ROLL meant a bun and ROCK was a stone,
and HANGUP was something you did with the 'phone?
When CHICKEN was poultry, and BAG meant a sack,
and JUNK trashy cast-offs and old bric-a-brac?

When CAT was a feline, a kitten grown up,
and TEA was a liquid you drank from a cup?
When a SWINGER was someone who swings in a swing,
and a PAD was a sort of cushiony thing?
When WAY OUT meant distant, and far, far away,
and a man wouldn't sue you for calling him GAY?

Words once so sensible, sober and serious
are making the freak-scene like psycho-delirious.

It's groovy, man, groovy, but English it's not.
Methinks that the language has gone straight to pot.

TSR
(Source unknown)

DRUGS
IN THE CLASSROOM
A conceptual model for
school programs

HAROLD J. CORNACCHIA, Ed.D.

Professor of Health Education, San Francisco University,
San Francisco, California

DAVID E. SMITH, M.D.

Associate Clinical Professor of Toxicology, Department of
Pharmacology, University of California Medical Center;
Founder and Medical Director, Haight-Ashbury Free
Medical Clinic, San Francisco, California

DAVID J. BENTEL, D.Crim.

Assistant Professor of Sociology, California State
University, Fresno, California

SECOND EDITION

THE C. V. MOSBY COMPANY
SAINT LOUIS   1978

The C. V. Mosby Company
11830 Westline Industrial Drive, St. Louis, Missouri 63141

Library of Congress Cataloging in Publication Data

Cornacchia, Harold J
    Drugs in the classroom.

    Includes bibliographies and index.
    1. Drug abuse—Study and teaching—United
States. 2. Alcoholism—Study and teaching—United
States. I. Bentel, David J., joint author.
II. Smith, David Elvin, 1939-   joint author.
III. Title. [DNLM: 1. Drug abuse—In infancy
and childhood. 2. Drug abuse—Prevention and
control. 3. Health education. 4. School
health. WM270 C812d]
HV5808.C6 1977   375′.362′290973   77-22968
ISBN 0-8016-1043-5

GW/CB/CB 9 8 7 6 5 4 3 2 1

Preface

Schools continue to be expected to help resolve the youth drug problem that exists in the United States today despite indications that drug use may be leveling off, although it is not diminishing. It is estimated that approximately 60% to 90% of young people have used alcoholic beverages; 32% to 72%, tobacco (a million new teen-age smokers yearly); 14% to 64%, marijuana; 3% to 21%, LSD; and 2% to 6%, heroin. Drugs are being used at earlier ages by young people. In addition, 750 aspirin pills are used and $225 is spent each year on legal drugs for every man, woman, and child.

The beneficial effects of drug education in schools at the present time are unknown. This conclusion is supported by evidence from a variety of sources including an unpublished survey of state drug education coordinators we conducted in 1976. Although many programs have introduced a variety of approaches that show promise of student impact, including values clarification and mental health or affective education that focuses on self-concept, decision-making, and communication skills, the evidence in their support is not clearly defined or conclusive. Actually, education has been considered in disrepute by a variety of individuals. Several studies have revealed that cognitive or knowledge program emphasis may lead to increased drug use.

Helen Nowlis, Office of Education, one of the national leaders in the drug field, has stated that drug education has not been given a fair chance to be successful in the nations' schools. We agree with her statement. We believe that the failure is due to numerous reasons, some of which have been identified by the Education Research Service (1975) to be lack of (1) definition of drug education, (2) reasonable and achievable goals, (3) functional and model approaches, and (4) use of evaluation procedures. This book has been prepared to assist with the resolution of such problems.

Schools have been faced with the dilemma of trying to provide viable programs with limited funds (which appear to be diminishing in both federal and state support), uncreative approaches, and inadequate guidelines and models for use in determining appropriateness, adequacy, or impact. Our identification of these needs led to the discovery of the existence of numerous difficulties in the development, organization, implementation, and evaluation of drug programs. Recognition of these problems resulted in the writing of this book the purpose of which is to introduce a *conceptual model of a multidimensional, differential, school drug program* designed to meet the needs of the variety of student drug users and abusers as well as nonusers. It is an approach that should prove useful to all school personnel in their attempt to attack the youth drug problem. Since the first edition was produced, many of its suggestions have been utilized in schools. However, programs continue to be partial, incomplete, and inadequately funded and frequently do not meet student needs. Greater attention to the *conceptual model* outlined herein must be given consideration.

The focus in this text is on preventive aspects (advocated by the National Institute on Drug Abuse) of the drug problem for kindergarten through grade 12 and includes behavioral objectives for drug education. The

v

guidelines introduced are threefold in nature: education, identification and assistance for drug misusers and abusers, and suggested ways to modify the school atmosphere to make it more conducive to learning. This volume should help schools to resolve the dilemma they are now facing by providing desperately needed directions.

Many activities and changes in drug education in recent years at national, state, and local levels have not resulted in preventive programs. Thus, we have synthesized and organized the most promising demonstrations, approaches, and information to provide functional solutions to school problems. This book is an effort to provide a total approach to drugs, a *conceptual model*. The information is usable for preservice and inservice teachers, administrators, counselors, nurses, and other school personnel at all grade levels. The guidelines that have emerged come from a comprehensive review of the latest data available in the literature, an array of school programs in operation, the vast experiences of federal, state, and local leaders, and our own extensive exposure to an involvement in the drug scene.

This second edition has been completely updated with current statistical data, new program illustrations, references and materials, and additional approaches being used in schools. It includes attention to the increasing alcoholism problem as well as to mental health or affective education, alternative education and activities, and peer and cross-age counseling and tutoring.

In addition to school use, this book should be valuable for community organizations, including parents. It will help them understand the school drug program and encourage them to initiate action for the development of such programs. School programs should not be developed in isolation from community programs, since drugs affect and are used by all people in varying ways and degrees. The greatest impact on students will undoubtedly be achieved through coordinated efforts of the school and the community.

Teachers, nurses, or other school personnel will find this text a valuable resource to have available for use in the instructional program and in other ways. Counselors will find it helpful in dealing with drug abusers. Administrators will find it useful in handling numerous administrative problems in conjunction with drug problems of youth. Curriculum directors will find guidelines for the development of curriculums and teaching units. Some additional features of the text include the following:

1. Utilization of current curriculum ideology, including the concept, needs, and behavior approaches
2. Identification of clearly defined, achievable, and measurable behavioral goals at the primary, intermediate, junior high, and senior high school levels as categorized in the cognitive, attitude, and action domains
3. Over 400 teaching techniques gathered from the review of more than 60 curriculum guides and other sources and grouped under these four headings: alcohol, drugs, tobacco, and psychic-social-spiritual
4. More than 100 sources of education materials including 15 newsletters, 17 professional journals, and a variety of textbooks usable in grades 1 to 12
5. Films and filmstrips recommended for use by the National Coordinating Council on Drug Education and other audiovisual materials
6. A variety of illustrative evaluative instruments that may be used, or adapted, for local situations, including a quantitative-qualitative device to assess the total school drug program
7. Physical and behavioral signs and symptoms of drug abusers and suggested procedures for aiding these young people
8. Guidelines for the development of policies and procedures in terms of sale, use, and possession of drugs in schools

Although the main emphasis in the volume is on the *conceptual model* of a school drug program and its implementation, the early chapters provide fundamental information about the school dilemma and the drug scene. Such background is necessary to better understand the program that has been introduced. It is also useful for the classroom teacher.

Part one covers the dilemma faced by the

schools. Part two discusses the drug scene: a current synthesis of pharmacological, psychological, and sociological aspects of drugs; rehabilitation and treatment resources; and the law and law enforcement procedures. In Part three is found a *conceptual model* of the school drug program, which includes (1) formal and informal drug education with specific suggestions for curriculum development and practical ideas (values clarification, decision-making, mental health) for use by classroom teachers, (2) drug services to identify drug abusers and procedures for helping these students, (3) school atmosphere needed to understand student unrest, what to do about the physical and emotional needs of students, and provision for humanism in the school, and (4) coordination of the school drug program necessary for an administrative structure to develop policies and procedures, to conduct in-service programs, and for other purposes. Part four provides evaluation guidelines and suggestions for use by teachers, administrators, and others, with illustrative procedures.

The reader must be aware that drugs are a problem of people and not of substances. Therefore, understanding of the individual as an organismic and integrated whole—his physical, psychological, social, and spiritual aspects—must receive consideration in any proposed attempt to resolve the problem. This book focuses on these factors, providing a unique approach that offers unusual potential for use in school drug and drug education programs.

Harold J. Cornacchia
David E. Smith

Contents

PART ONE

INTRODUCTION

1 The dilemma, 3

Recent developments in school drug programs, 5
School problems, 6
Contributing factors in the school dilemma, 8
  Nature of drug use in society, 8
  Preventive approach, 11
  Classification and numbers of drug users and abusers, 13
  Polydrug abuse, 18
  The meaning of drug education, 18
  Formal education, 20
  Informal education, 21
  Behavioral approach, 21

PART TWO

THE DRUG SCENE

2 Society and drugs, 27

What is the drug problem? 28
Conflicts of reality: different ways we think about drugs, 28
  Conceptual views of drug abuse, 28
  Factors affecting drug use and abuse, 32
  Basic definitions of drugs and drug abuse, 33
Summary of drug terms, 35
Commonly abused drugs, 36
  Central nervous system stimulant drugs, 36
  Central nervous system depressant (sedative-hypnotic) drugs, 37
  Psychedelic (hallucinogenic) drugs, 38
  Narcotic drugs, 40
  Over-the-counter or nonprescription drugs, 41
Summary, 43

3 Psychosocial factors and the adolescent, 45

Patterns of drug abuse, 45
The world of the adolescent, 48
  Two views of adolescence, 48
  Rationales for drug abuse, 50
  Psychological motivations, 51
  Search for identity, 52
  Values, 53
  Rejection of the culture, 53

Affluence and permissiveness, 54
Summary of motives for drug use, 55
The "cop-out" from society, 55
The school environment, 56
Rejection of the school culture, 57
Development of a school program responsive to human needs, 58
Alternatives to drugs, 59

4   Pharmacological aspects of drug abuse, 63

Physiological action of drugs, 63
The nervous system, 63
Drug effects, 64
Categorizing drugs, 66
Central nervous system stimulant drugs, 69
Amphetamines, 69
Cocaine: new uses of an old drug, 71
Cigarettes and tobacco, 72
Caffeine, 79
Central nervous system depressant (sedative-hypnotic) drugs, 80
Barbiturates, 80
Alcohol, 82
Inhalants—volatile hydrocarbons, 85
Marijuana, 86
Psychedelic drugs (hallucinogens), 90
LSD, 90
Narcotic drugs, 92
Opium and heroin, 92
Methadone—a chemical approach to heroin addiction, 95
Narcotic antagonists, 96
Nonchemical treatment approaches to addiction, 96
Tranquilizers and antidepressant drugs, 96
Over-the-counter drugs, 97
General pharmacological classification of drugs, 97

5   The role of the community in the drug problem, 100

Treatment and rehabilitation, 100
Multimodality concept, 100
Procedures, 102
Crisis intervention, 102
Detoxification, 104
Aftercare, 104
Government programs and resources, 111
National programs, 111
State level, 112
Local level, 113
Legal perspective, 113
Federal laws regarding narcotics and drugs, 113
State laws, 118
Community action, 127
Objectives, 128
Coordination by a drug abuse council, 128
Role of law enforcement, 130
Community programs and facilities, 130
Summary, 134

PART THREE

THE ROLE OF THE SCHOOL

6 The school drug program, 139

Principles, 140
The program, 142

7 Drug education, 144

Drug education for students, 145
  Student formal education, 145
    Patterns of instruction, 146
    Curriculum, 149
    Methods of teaching, 163
    Drug education resource materials, 202
    Evaluation, 217
    Mini-courses, 217
  Student informal education, 218
  Resource centers, 220
  Roles of school and community resource personnel, 221
Drug education for parents, 222
  Parent formal education, 223
  Parent informal education, 224
Categorical references, 226

8 Drug services, 228

Identification of drugs of abuse, 228
Identification of drug users and abusers, 229
  Observable signs and symptoms, 229
  Taking prescribed medicines at school, 232
  Peer identification, 233
  Self-identification of drug abusers, 233
  Clinical tests, 234
What to do for abusers, 234
Follow-up procedures, 236
  Counseling and guidance, 236
  Use of community resources, 239
  Adjustment of school programs, 240
    Alternative school movement, 240
Summary, 242

9 School atmosphere, 244

Student alienation and unrest, 245
Physical and psychological needs, 247
Creating humaneness in schools, 249

10 Coordination of the school drug program, 254

Administrative problems, 254
Administrative organization, 256
Policies and procedures, 257
  Guidelines, 258
  Suggested areas to include in policies, 259
Illustrations of school district policies and procedures, 262
Role of school personnel, 266
Financing, 266
In-service preparation, 269

PART FOUR

CONCLUSION

11   Evaluation, 277

Scope, 278
Principles of evaluation, 279
   How to evaluate, 279
   Who evaluates, 279
   When to evaluate, 280
   Problems in evaluation, 280
Illustrative evaluation instruments, 281
   Total program evaluation instrument, 281
   Education program evaluation instruments, 281
      Objectives, 281
         Knowledge instruments, 282
         Attitude instruments, 282
         Practice survey form, 282
         Knowledge-attitude instrument, 282
      In-service, 282
      Resource materials, 283
Sources and resources of instruments, 321

APPENDIX   Drug abuse in sports, 323

PART ONE

INTRODUCTION

. . . we have not won the war on drugs. By 1975, it was clear that drug use was increasing. . . . Today, drug abuse constitutes a clear and present threat to the health and future of our nation.

PRESIDENT GERALD R. FORD
A Message to the Congress of
the United States: Drug Abuse
April 27, 1976

1
The dilemma

Within the past several years, education . . . selected information . . . has fallen into disrepute. It has been judged ineffective if not counterproductive in many instances . . . all education has been questioned as effective strategies for prevention. Neither information nor education . . . with the best principles of behavioral science has been given a fair test.

HELEN H. NOWLIS
1975

We should stop raising unrealistic expectations of total elimination of drug abuse from our society . . . we probably always will have a drug problem of some proportion . . . education and prevention should play a more important role in the national program than they have in the past.

White House Paper on Drug Abuse
1975

. . . is need for better formal alcohol education in the schools and more informal education in the home . . .

PARKER MARDEN and
KENNETH KOLODNER
1976

Every major group in the population, by overwhelming majorities would require students to attend a program on the effects of drugs and alcohol . . .

Seventh Annual Gallup Poll
1975

Parents, legislators, and the community have expected schools to help in the resolution of the drug problem among young persons in the United States. Although this stress may be lessening, laws have been passed, funds have been authorized, and pressures have been applied for appropriate action. Schools and school districts have made sincere efforts to comply by developing programs with unclear guidelines and models needed for direction, and without qualified leadership, despite efforts in the training of teachers over the past 3 or more years. Bland best describes the action of schools when she says, "In the rush to teach about drug abuse, we resemble Stephen Leacock's mythical character who 'flung himself from the room, flung himself on his horse, and rode off in all directions!'"[5] The result has been that numerous fragmented, piecemeal, "crash," poorly planned, misguided, and frequently uncoordinated pro-

3

grams have been developed. Is it any wonder that schools have been ineffective? Is it any wonder that schools have not had much impact on the young? When you realize the complexity of the drug problem, which by itself does not have simple answers, the community expectations for action have created a dilemma for the schools. Therefore the variety of criticisms that have been advanced regarding the ineffectiveness of programs needs further examination despite well-meaning efforts by schools and their dedicated personnel.

Numerous authorities in 1971 said they believed that educational programs had little if any impact on students. The evidence revealed this to be true. It was stated that, although such programs may have provided an increase in drug information, they encouraged student experimentation and use of mind-altering chemicals. Studies in Pennsylvania and California indicated that drug use, rather than diminishing, tended to increase after students were exposed to limited information-centered drug education programs. Some schools, parents, and communities proceeded cautiously or had failed to take any action along educational lines because of this possible hazard. Drug education programs have been greatly expanded since 1970. However, they continue to have limited impact on young people. Table 1-1 provides data obtained from a survey we conducted in 1976. Opinions of forty-four of the fifty state drug educators in the United States tend to support the apparent ineffectiveness of programs' conclusion. In the junior and senior high schools, 41 to 43% of the leaders stated that some educational

efforts had impact, while 39 to 43% said the effects were unknown.

The school problem is the result of a variety of factors. One important matter is the failure to define adequately the precise objectives of the educational program. Dr. Warner from Pennsylvania State University conducted a study of eighth grade, eleventh grade, and college student programs and discovered that: "You're not going to stop kids from taking drugs. If that's our goal we'd better reexamine it. . . . All education can do is maybe make them examine their motivations, steer them away from bad drugs, let them know what the risks are, unless you have a real alternative for them in terms of something to really absorb their energies."[64] Thus the question must be asked as to what educational goals have been established by the schools. Today, despite the variety of curricula that have been written and introduced into schools, the need for greater clarity of goals still exists. Should not youths also be encouraged to avoid legal drugs? Should values clarification also include values identification? What about student help with self-concept, alternatives to drugs, and decision-making?

However important the establishment of educational objectives is, other questions must be raised. What are the frames of reference from which the critics are making judgments? What should be the nature and type of drug program to be conducted? There are no model programs, although some constructive patterns have developed. There are no clear standards nor have guidelines been prepared. Add these difficulties to the lack of generally acceptable, identifiable, educa-

TABLE 1-1. State drug educators' opinions of effectiveness of school drug programs (N = 44)

| | Percentages | | | | | |
Grades	All	Most	Many	Some	None	Unknown
Primary	2	20	30	36	7	5
Intermediate	0	9	15	36	2	38
Upper and junior high	0	7	11	43	0	39
Senior high	0	7	5	41	4	43

tional goals and much confusion exists over the following: (1) the nature of the school drug program: is it more than, or solely, educational? (2) the differentiation and the interrelationships between school and community drug educational programs, (3) the distinction between formal and informal education and the place of each in the school program, (4) the definition of prevention and its application within the school, (5) the types of student users and abusers of drugs and the application of this information to the school program, and (6) whether provisions for multiple programs to meet the needs of differing students should be made in schools.

In summary, the problem is one of defining the role of the school in helping to resolve the drug problem among youth. Therefore, however appropriate and necessary they are, the criticisms that have appeared must be given consideration only in the light of the factors just presented.

RECENT DEVELOPMENTS IN SCHOOL DRUG PROGRAMS

Further understanding of the school dilemma can be obtained by a review of some recent developments and problems related to drug programs.

Prior to 1970 many school drug programs, including drug education, were being conducted in various parts of the United States, with minimal financial support provided by the federal government, by state legislatures, by local school districts, and by other sources. In 1969 the federal funds available for drug education amounted to approximately $2.5 million. In addition to these funds, schools received limited personnel, cooperation, and materials from a variety of community sources. School programs, although relatively numerous in some states, were sporadic, limited, or nonexistent in many other states. The nature and support of the programs differed greatly. Overall they were not extensive and occurred with inconsistent frequency.

In March 1970 a massive, nationwide effort to reach all schools was made when former President Nixon released $3.5 million

for the development and implementation of educational programs. This money was distributed to all states in the form of grants-in-aid in proportion to the number of youths in each state's schools, with the amounts ranging from $40,000 to $200,000 per state. The grants awarded were determined in accordance with state populations. For many states this was the only money available. However, numerous state legislatures, local districts, and communities provided additional funds; in other states the previous level of financial aid was maintained. Each state was permitted to develop its own proposal for the use of the federally allocated funds under broadly defined guidelines established by the Office of Education, but the financial support was primarily earmarked for the stimulation of drug education programs in all schools throughout the United States.

A portion of the federal funds authorized by former President Nixon in 1970 was set aside to establish four national training centers in New York, Wisconsin, Texas, and California. We directed the California center at San Francisco State College. In the summer of 1970, administrators, teachers, students, parents, and community leaders representing a variety of racial and ethnic minorities from each state were sent to the centers for training. These individuals were to be prepared to assume leadership roles in drug education and were expected to train other leaders within their states, who, in turn, would prepare still other drug educators.

The Comprehensive Drug Abuse Prevention and Control Act of 1970, which provided state grant-in-aid funds, was extended through 1973, with $5.4 million provided in 1971, $13 million in 1972, and $11.9 million in 1973. However, half of these moneys was given to states, and the remaining half was distributed to agencies and organizations for community education programs.

In 1972 the Office of Education established a number of regional training centers in various parts of the country. Their purpose was to train a team of teachers, administrators, and students. School districts could apply for $10,000 direct grants (called mini-grants) to pay for the training of the team and to permit the expenditure of up to $6000 to release a person to serve as a project coordinator in the school district.

In 1974, formula grants to states were discontinued; only the regional training centers and the mini-grants for teacher-training exist at this writing. The Office of Education had its appropriated moneys curtailed as follows: 1974, $5.7 million; 1975, $4 million; 1976, $2 million; in 1977 it was anticipated that $2 to 3 million would be available (see Chapter 10).

Numerous governmental agencies that have been and continue to be involved in drug education programs in recent years include the Office of Education (OE), the National Institute of Mental Health (NIMH), the National Institute on Drug Abuse (NIDA), the National Institute on Alcohol Abuse and Alcoholism (NIAAA), and the Drug Enforcement Agency (DEA). It is estimated that approximately $42 million has been spent since 1971 by the Office of Education for drug education programs and activities. This represents an average of 1.5%, the total federal budget for drug abuse for each year. Law enforcement and treatment services received the lion's share of the almost $3 billion appropriated over the years.

The National Institute on Drug Abuse, Prevention Branch, has received $3.7 million each year from 1974 to 1977 for community education programs. It is supporting a Multicultural Resource Center to produce a series of prevention resource booklets for Asian-American, black, Indian, and Spanish-speaking minorities.

Many states have allocated moneys since 1971 in support of drug education programs. At one time every state had a person designated as a drug educator. Duties included a variety of services to schools and school districts. Recent evidence indicates that a number of states have abandoned such positions. There are no data to indicate the amounts of funds received by states; it is estimated in any 1 year they ranged from

$25,000 to $2 million. It appears that such allocations are lessening and in some cases programs and activities are diminishing. Legislators apparently are less prone to appropriate funds for the ever-increasing drug problem. New funds from both federal and state levels in the past few years through the NIAAA are being designated for use against the problems of alcohol abuse and alcoholism.

It should be obvious that school drug and other drug education activities and programs have been growing and developing in recent years. Numerous school districts have designated or employed individuals to administer and provide leadership to their programs. Despite the need for greatly improved coordination between agencies and organizations, numerous creative and innovative methods, ideas, and materials have been developed and prepared, many of which are being piloted, or are now in use in schools throughout the country. These new approaches include "drop-in" centers, "hotlines," values clarification, use of peer teaching, coping with stress, developing self-concept, decision-making, use of cross-age tutoring, use of ex-addicts, multicultural programs, improved school and community relationships, alternative education, greater involvement of parents and students in planning and conducting programs, crisis intervention procedures, policies for handling drug users and abusers, "rap" sessions, and publication of numerous books, pamphlets, curricula, and visual materials.

SCHOOL PROBLEMS

Despite the variety of efforts now taking place to cope with the tremendous drug problem in schools, many programs have not been very effective and some show that recipients use more drugs. Dupont reported in a survey of 1500 students that their attitudes toward existing information programs indicated that they were outdated and should be abolished.[11] There is still much to be done and these are the problems in need of attention:

1. Lack of understanding of the nature of the total school drug program in which education is but one important phase
2. Numerous educational programs with goals that primarily emphasize the acquisition of pharmacological or physiological information without consideration of the psychological, sociological, and spiritual aspects associated with drug use
3. Unclear understanding of the independent roles of the school and the community as well as the importance of cooperation and coordination of these programs at federal, state, and local levels with police departments and other community agencies and organizations
4. Lack of communication procedures for alerting the community regarding the drug problem and for gaining support for school drug programs
5. Failure to design adequate programs to meet the special needs of students in low-income areas and to be relevant to minorities
6. Inadequate consideration of the involvement of students, parents, and community representatives, including minorities, in drug programs together with insufficient understanding of effective ways of utilizing such persons
7. Fragmented, piecemeal, uncoordinated, and frequently ineffective programs in schools and school systems
8. Lack of adequate, continuous, and dedicated leadership in some areas of the nation (Considerable change has taken place, especially on the state and local school district levels. However, in 1970 and 1971 the state drug leadership personnel changed in approximately half of the western states. This practice has continued at a lessened pace, yet many local school districts have no administrative leadership. Limitations of funds available for education, reduction of federal and state allocations, and a belief that the drug problem has been reduced or resolved are some of the contributing reasons for this action.)
9. Unfamiliarity with the distinction between formal and informal education, especially on the part of community people
10. Failure to recognize the need for differing types of school drug programs and drug education to meet the variety of types of student users and abusers found in schools
11. Inadequate consideration and emphasis in school drug programs of the behavioral and humanistic relationships
12. Lack of understanding and development of more effective communication with students, especially drug users
13. Need for clear and realistic objectives; turning off young people from drugs may be impossible to achieve
14. Use of "scare" tactics, sensationalism, assembly programs, and speakers as the main, or sole, approach to educational programs
15. Need to clarify the roles of administrators, teachers, nurses, counselors, and other school personnel
16. Apathetic attitude toward change and toward attempts to develop creative and innovative approaches to the drug problem by administrators, teachers, community leaders, and others
17. Insufficient recognition of and inadequate attention to important administrative concerns related to the drug program such as the curriculum, the place of education in the curriculum, the objectives to be achieved, teacher qualifications, inservice preparation of personnel, methodology, the financial support and cost of programs, and the establishment of policies and procedures for handling drug users and abusers
18. Lack of or limited procedures to assess the effectiveness of programs quantitatively and qualitatively

CONTRIBUTING FACTORS IN THE SCHOOL DILEMMA

How to best attack the drug problem in society has not been determined. It is a difficult problem to resolve because drugs are not the cause but rather the effect. That is to say that the legal and illegal use and abuse of drugs is more symptomatic of a people's problem than of a drug problem. As one pharmacist has noted, "Drugs have been on my shelves for years and never caused anybody any problem. It's the people that cause the problems." It is certain that a variety of approaches must be made, including involvement of the schools. There is an acute need for a coordinated and cooperative effort on the part of every American community to face the current epidemic of youthful drug abuse and to deal with it compassionately and maturely, involving the home, the school, and the community organizations and agencies.

Presently much confusion exists regarding the proper role of the school in handling the increasing drug problem. Despite a number of fine efforts and the expenditure of funds in recent years, the massive amount of literature addressed to this matter does not adequately deal with this problem or with the alternatives open to schools in preventing or handling drug abuse. It is not surprising that many schools have in desperation initiated fragmentary, superficial, incomplete, and uncoordinated programs that have done little to resolve the problem.

Although schools and teachers cannot solve all humanity's ills, they have a special role to play in drug misuse and abuse.* They can be instrumental in helping to reduce the drug problem through preventive action.

The difficulty of role identification is compounded by a number of contributing factors that add to the school dilemma. Confusion continues to exist about the nature of drug use in society, especially among youth, the meaning of prevention or preventive action,

*Drug use = consumption of a drug; drug misuse = periodic or occasional improper or inappropriate use; drug abuse and polydrug abuse (use of one or more psychoactive drugs, including heroin and alcohol) = interference with the individual's health or his economic or social adjustment (Chapter 2).

the types and numbers of drug users and abusers in schools, and the conflicting views about drug education.

There are, of course, no simple answers or simple solutions. That is why the problem has not been resolved. But there are useful alternatives that may need modification to fit the particular needs of every community. The situation is far from hopeless. Perhaps this book will provide some of the needed guidelines for schools.

Nature of drug use in society

People use drugs to awaken in the morning, to keep awake or to sustain themselves throughout the day, to lose weight, to flush out the bowels, to enhance social and religious experiences, for pleasure and relaxation, to escape from reality, to go to sleep, to treat disease and medical conditions, before and after dinner, and for a variety of other purposes. People have used a variety of drugs for centuries and probably will continue to use them for thousands of years in the future. Lipscomb says:

> The United States is a drug-using culture. On any given day an American adult is likely to ingest 4-5 identifiable chemical compounds that are pharmaceutical in nature. Consider the individual who arises in the morning, brushes his teeth with toothpaste containing fluoride, downs a Bromo-Seltzer, has two cups of coffee containing caffeine, takes a dexedrine to help him with his weight problem, lights his post-coffee cigarette containing nicotine and heads for a round of events in the business or professional world which may include cocktails and wine with meals followed by brandy and a good cigar—this individual is more likely to be typical than unusual. While for the most part individual adults do not get into trouble through their use of drugs, some unfortunates do experience complications—social and medical.*

Pharmacologically, drugs are generally grouped into a variety of categories, among which are stimulants, depressants, psychedelics, and narcotics (Chapter 4). Drugs may also be classified as legal and illegal. Legal drugs refer to those that may be purchased in two ways—over the counter or by prescription. A person may buy such drugs as alcohol, tobacco, aspirin, laxatives, and cough syrups

*Lipscomb, W. R.: An epidemiology of drug use-abuse, J. Public Health **61:**1794-1800, 1971.

whenever desired in any drug store, supermarket, or liquor store by paying the requested over-the-counter price. A person may also acquire legal drugs such as pep, sleeping, and relaxing pills when they are prescribed by a physician for some personal ailment that is in need of treatment or cure. Illegal drugs such as marijuana, heroin, and cocaine, however, are considered narcotics by law and may not be purchased through the usual legal channels. Some legal drugs such as pep and sleeping pills may be considered illegal because they are obtainable and sold through unlawful channels.

We live in a drug-oriented society. Many persons throughout the United States are using, misusing, and abusing numerous legal and illegal drugs. The drug problem is not one involving only youth and the military. It is one that may affect the life of every individual to a greater or lesser degree. There are many individuals at all social and economic levels, in homes and in business, who are using drugs and who are creating problems. Although drug abuse in rural areas is increasing, it is not as severe and still behind that in metropolitan sections. Drug use is more sophisticated and polydrug patterns predominate, with opiate use being slower to emerge in the less populated sections of the country.[3]

Why is the focus only on illegal drugs? The drug problem is one in which not only illegal drugs but also the readily available legal drugs are involved. The prevalence of drug misuse and abuse continues to grow at alarming rates in all of society, with the legal drug problem being far greater than the illegal one.

Numerous persons are engaged in the self-diagnosis of physical, mental, and emotional ailments; they attempt to treat or cure these conditions with readily available legal drugs and possibly through the use of illegal drugs. Nowlis identifies this problem when she says, "Relying more on medication than on the physician, the person medicates himself excessively and indiscriminately. He uses medication as a kind of magical protector and depends on medication rather than people to handle certain emotional drives

and needs."[45] The magnitude of the drug problem is identified by Lennard, who reports:

Although most of the current voluminous writing about the misuse of drugs concerns the misuse of psychoactive agents by young people, and especially the use of drugs obtained illegally, it seems no use to decry the use and misuse of drugs by young people while paying so little attention to the growing use and misuse of psychoactive agents in general, both those prescribed by physicians and those obtained over the counter without prescription, is highly misleading and unproductive.*

The steady and marked increase of the legal psychoactive drugs has gone unnoticed. Louria states, ". . . it is reasonable to estimate that half of the sedatives and tranquilizers prescribed by physicians are given unnecessarily."[33]

Alcohol, cigarettes, cough syrups, laxatives, sleeping aids, vitamins, aspirin, and other nonprescription items are readily obtainable. Billions of dollars are spent yearly on prescription drugs alone. In 1970, 202 million legal prescriptions for psychoactive drugs—stimulants, sedatives, tranquilizers, and antidepressants—were filled in pharmacies for patients of physicians. Table 1-2 shows that 3 to 9% of the population has used these drugs.

Alcohol is perhaps the most popular social drug used in the United States. About two-thirds of the population over 15 years of age, or over 70 million people, drink alcoholic beverages.[40] About 90% drink in moderation and are not adversely affected by their drinking practices. Thus approximately 7 to 10 million do have problems. About 15 billion aspirin tablets (27.2 million pounds) are consumed yearly by Americans.[7] This amounts to about 750 pills for every person per year (approximately two daily). Some 8 billion amphetamine tablets are produced yearly and 50% of these get into illegal traffic—35 doses of 5 milligrams each for every man, woman, and child in the United States.[56] It is estimated that there are 70 million smokers in this country, with 1 million new teenage smokers each year.[29] Despite the millions of

---

*Lennard, H. L., and others: Mystification and drug misuse, San Francisco, 1971, Jossey-Bass, Inc., Publishers.

Table 1-2. Regular use of dangerous drugs (% of population aged 14 or over)*

	Ever used	Regular use	Regular nonmedical use	Regular nonmedical multiple drugs	Number of users in trouble
Sedatives	5.7%	2.3%	0.3%	0.2%	270,000-300,000
Stimulants	3.1	1.8	0.7%	0.3	400,000-490,000
Tranquilizers	9.1	4.9	1.6%	0.3	400,000-490,000

*From U.S. Department of Health, Education and Welfare, National Institute of Drug Abuse, Domestic Council on Drug Abuse Task Force: White paper on drug abuse, September, 1975, Washington, D.C., 1975, U.S. Government Printing Office.

people who have stopped smoking, the sale of cigarettes is at its highest level. Women and young people are smoking more.

Food and Drug Administration Commissioner Dr. Edwards[18] as well as Halleck[25] indicates that the so-called "legal" drugs are at least as great a societal problem as the abuse of illegal drugs.

The public is constantly being encouraged to purchase and use drugs through the mass communication media; television has contributed extensively to bringing the medicine man into every household. Thus individuals may be more prone to self-diagnosis of bodily ailments and self-medication of their problems, as a result of the media influence.

An indication of the possible extent of legal drug use may be obtained from these data, which represent approximations of the funds expended for the purchase of selected legal drugs and drug products in the United States in 1975[55]:

Alcoholic beverages	$19,502,110,000*
Tobacco and accessories	15,570,000,000*
Prescriptions	8,145,940,000
Cough and cold items	735,220,000
Acne preparations	71,000,000
Internal analgesics, including aspirin	719,270,000
Vitamin concentrates (nonprescription)	342,430,000
Dentifrices	493,540,000
Laxatives and other elimination aids	241,820,000
Diet aids	149,020,000
Antacids	141,340,000
Sleeping aids (nonprescription)	34,710,000
Motion sickness preparations	22,890,000
Tonics and alteratives	121,790,000
	$46,291,080,000

*Telephone conversation with Litton Publications, Inc., Oradell, N. J.

It may be generalized from this information that approximately $225 ($170 for alcoholic beverages and tobacco accessories) for each man, woman, and child was spent for selected legal drugs in 1975.

A variety of drugs such as sleeping and pep pills, marijuana, heroin, and LSD are readily available on the illegal market despite police surveillance and control. The Federal Food and Drug Administration estimates that 10 billion barbiturate and amphetamine pills are produced yearly, and that half of these are bootlegged through illegal channels. In recent years the increase in the use of amphetamines, barbiturates, hallucinogens (including LSD), and sedative-hypnotics (including marijuana), has been extensive.

Marijuana is the most popular illicit drug; its use has significantly increased among Americans in recent years, with some 30 million (20% above 11 years of age) or more involved. Heroin has shown a dramatic rise in use. There has been a 30 to 50% increase in the number of addicts, so that daily users are now estimated to be 300,000 to 400,000 people, and 2 to 4 million are classified as occasional users. Cocaine is the new "in" drug; it is estimated that 3% of adults have tried the substance at least once. Hallucinogens are still popular but addiction and extended use are rare occurrences.

The White House Paper on Drug Abuse[62] in 1975 identified the extent of the use of a variety of drugs in the United States (Fig. 1).

Robert L. DuPont, Director of the National Institute on Drug Abuse, recently reported that findings of two national studies reflect a stability in drug usage by Americans when compared with the sharp increases that occurred in the 1960s and early 1970s.[16]

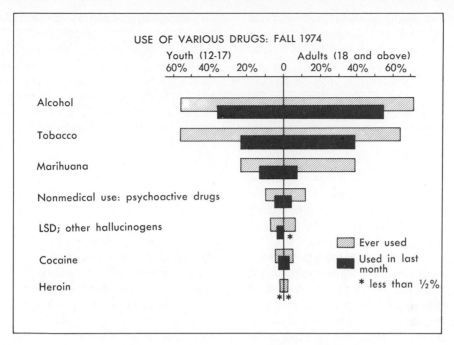

FIG. 1. Use of various drugs: Fall, 1974. (From U.S. Department of Health, Education and Welfare, National Institute on Drug Abuse, Domestic Council on Drug Abuse Task Force: White paper on drug abuse, September, 1975, Washington, D.C., 1975, U.S. Government Printing Office.)

DuPont also reported that a recent study showed that the use of marijuana continues to rise among high school students. Approximately 53% of high school seniors had ever used the drug, and 32% are actively using it.[16]

The extensive use of legal and illegal drugs provides documentation that society is faced with an extensive, difficult, and complex problem if it hopes to curtail or reduce the use, misuse, and abuse of drugs. Drugs have become deeply ingrained in people's lifestyles despite the adverse effects they may have on the life, health, and welfare of many people, both young and old. The drug problem has grown in recent years because of the involvement of a large percentage of young people, the experimentation with drugs by the so-called middle class, the advent of television, and more recently, the participation of military personnel. Sixty percent of the mayors of cities with 100,000 to 200,000 population ranked drug abuse among their five most serious problems.[43] Drugs may now be found in the classroom and on school campuses. They are creating a tremendous dilemma for parents, teachers, administrators, and other school personnel. A recent Gallup poll[22] ranked the use of drugs by students as the sixth leading problem facing schools today.

Preventive approach

Prevention has many meanings for many people. Although a precise definition is not readily available and may be difficult to clearly identify, it is necessary to provide a frame of reference for a better understanding of the purpose of this book. Literally, to prevent is to keep from happening or occurring. More specifically, in medicine it refers to a prophylactic or procedure that arrests the threatened onset of a disease or condition. Application of these statements to the drug problem leads to the conclusion that education, laws, and law enforcement as well as rehabilitation and treatment are preventive procedures. All of these elements have features with which schools must be concerned and involved. However, the role of the school is primarily an instructional one and it is in this context that prevention will be defined.

Prevention involves primary, secondary, and tertiary aspects. Their application to the drug scene will be interpreted in the descriptions that follow.

Primary prevention

Primary prevention is a poorly understood and very neglected area. It has both negative and positive aspects. It refers to action taken to prevent something from happening or measures to stop something before it starts. Specifically, it is the attempt to encourage and help students, or other people, primarily through education, either (1) to refrain from or reduce the misuse and abuse of drugs, or (2) to make more intelligent use of drugs. Nonspecifically, it deals with individual behavior unrelated to drugs such as values clarification, development of self-image, decision-making, and alternative activities. This type of prevention may take place inside the school or in the community. Within the school, the education may be formal or informal and may be provided for students, parents, school personnel, and members of the community.

Recently the National Institute for Drug Abuse identified a definition of primary prevention that Dr. John Olsen, Chief, Prevention Branch, says, brings attention to the "whole human being." It is one that deemphasizes the role of drugs and broadens the attack on all self-destructive behavior.

Primary drug abuse prevention is a constructive process designed to promote personal and social growth of the individual toward full human potential and thereby inhibit or reduce physical, mental, emotional or social impairment which results in or from the abuse of chemical substances.[42]

Secondary prevention

Procedures taken after something has occurred to forestall the condition from growing worse or from becoming more advanced constitute secondary prevention. It is the steps or actions taken to provide help or service to individuals who are using, misusing, or abusing drugs and who are present in schools. It includes early detection or case-finding, with prompt treatment following, to prevent disorders from becoming more serious. These pupils may attend school under the influence of drugs or the use of drugs outside the school may affect their ability to learn effectively. The services rendered may include crisis intervention, information on alternatives to drug use, understandings toward more intelligent use of drugs, guidance to a community agency, or therapy. This aid may come in the form of counseling, education, or treatment.

Since schools are not expected to provide treatment services that are preventive, this assistance must take place outside the school; it is similar to that provided in medical clinics with outpatient services by physicians, psychiatrists, and others. In the school the nontreatment assistance may be analogous to the health services phase of the school health program, whereby student health deviants are identified and follow-up procedures are initiated to provide the help needed to enable the student to learn better. Such services may include informal education, guidance and counseling, diagnostic examinations or procedures, observations or symptomatic behavior, first aid, referral to community agencies, adjustment of programs, and improvement of teacher-pupil relationships. The assistance may be rendered by counselors, nurses, physicians, psychologists, and others, and may include rap sessions, dropin centers, and hot-lines. Such services may be located inside, outside, or adjacent to the school. They may or may not be conducted by school personnel.

Secondary prevention is generally of short-term duration and may occur within the school or elsewhere in the community.

Tertiary prevention

Tertiary prevention is an extension of secondary prevention wherein action is taken to ward off the development of more serious conditions resulting from drug misuse and abuse. It refers to long-term, extensive, technical health, rehabilitation, and educational services rendered by such persons as physicians and psychiatrists to save lives, prevent serious personality damage, provide crisis intervention, and aid in the adjustment of individuals to society. Services may vary from inpatient therapeutic communities, such as Synanon in California or Daytop in New York, to outpatient community-based projects such as the Haight-Ashbury Free Medical Clinic. Extended care may also be given in programs such as those established in the methadone maintenance programs. Tertiary prevention takes place outside the school.

• • •

The school setting can provide primary and secondary prevention to the extent previously defined. This will be discussed more fully later in the text. Justification for the services identified as secondary prevention is based on the premise that, although parents are primarily responsible for the medical and health care of their children and youth, they (1) often do not recognize problems, (2) frequently do not know what to do when a health deviation occurs and may look to the school for guidance, and (3) often ignore their responsibilities and continue to send pupils with drug problems to school to be educated. Children and youth who are physically, mentally, or socially ill will have trouble learning under the best environmental conditions. Thus schools must have available educational services that will inform, guide, encourage, and direct parents and students to action, thereby enabling pupils to attain the highest levels of wellness.

School-community coordination in prevention

The school and community must coordinate their efforts in drug prevention to render the best possible service to students. Children and youth with drug problems who are attending school may need to be referred to resources outside the school for assistance. Such help may be available from a physician, psychiatrist, guidance clinic, drop-in center, or other agency or organization. However, if such services are in short supply, the school may need to become active in trying to promote their development. By the same token, if schools are not attending to students with drug problems, the community organizations may find it necessary to encourage schools to take action. In addition, community educational programs may be transmitting information that is in conflict with that presented in the school. For example, the school may be teaching that marijuana use is always injurious to health. Community representatives may be indicating that marijuana use may cause little or no danger to humans physiologically. These differing views may create unnecessary difficulty between students and parents as well as between students, teachers, and the school. Such differences, if they exist, must be recognized by the teachers and the school; measures must be taken to resolve them.

These illustrations should make it apparent that schools and communities, each with their independent programs, cannot act in isolation but must function cooperatively to satisfactorily attack the drug problem. The need for clear identification of the roles of the school and of the community, including their relationships, should be evident. Such clarity and cooperation does not often exist with any degree of regularity in the United States, although there is growing evidence of improvement in these relationships.

Classification and numbers of drug users and abusers

Most if not all adolescents use drugs in some form at some time in their lives. However, not all young persons who use drugs are problems, nor do many who use drugs develop problems. This is especially true when consideration is given to such legal drugs as alcohol and tobacco, but it is also applicable to the illegal drugs. Marin and Cohen state, "Hard narcotics are always destructive and their spread is frightening, but the soft drugs—marijuana, the psychedelics—are more variable. Some of them give some trouble to some adolescents at some time; but not always, not even most of the time."[31] The World Health Organization

TABLE 1-3. Percentage of drug use reported by San Mateo County, California, in *male* junior and senior high school students*

Drug	Grades	Any use during past year					Ten times+ during past year					50+ use				
		Date of survey					Date of survey					Date of survey				
		1972	1973	1974	1975	1976	1972	1973	1974	1975	1976	1972	1973	1974	1975	1976
Alcoholic beverages	7	58.5	72.8	73.0	70.0	67.9	19.8	25.3	24.9	21.0	18.2	NA	10.5	10.4	8.0	6.7
	9	75.8	82.4	84.4	82.7	81.9	39.1	47.5	45.9	44.5	39.0	17.6	23.4	23.3	20.8	17.7
	10	81.7	85.6	84.9	87.0	85.9	50.0	54.5	56.1	54.7	49.8	28.3	31.3	29.4	27.2	25.2
	12	87.5	86.4	89.5	89.3	87.1	66.0	63.0	66.4	68.8	64.1	39.8	39.9	44.8	41.8	37.6
Amphetamines	7	5.2	3.6	3.4	2.7	2.6	1.4	1.1	0.7	0.6	0.7	NA	0.8	0.5	0.4	0.5
	9	16.9	14.6	11.1	11.0	8.8	5.3	5.3	3.6	3.8	2.5	2.3	2.7	1.8	1.7	1.2
	10	22.8	20.3	17.7	14.1	13.6	8.5	7.1	6.1	4.8	4.0	3.6	3.1	2.4	2.1	1.9
	12	25.8	21.1	22.2	21.2	18.4	10.9	7.8	8.0	8.7	6.8	5.4	4.4	3.5	3.8	3.3
Barbiturates	7	5.1	5.3	5.0	3.8	3.3	1.2	1.4	1.2	0.6	1.0	NA	0.8	0.7	0.3	0.5
	9	11.9	13.7	11.5	10.5	10.0	3.2	5.3	2.6	2.8	2.3	1.4	1.9	1.4	1.1	1.1
	10	16.0	15.4	14.6	11.1	12.1	5.5	4.4	4.5	2.7	2.7	2.8	2.3	1.9	1.6	1.2
	12	15.4	14.3	14.7	13.1	12.2	5.8	5.4	3.8	3.9	3.2	2.8	2.1	1.3	1.8	2.2
Heroin	7	NA	NA	NA	NA	2.2	NA	NA	NA	NA	0.8	NA	NA	NA	NA	0.6
	9	2.7	3.4	3.3	2.7	4.0	1.1	1.7	1.9	1.4	1.2	0.7	1.4	1.7	1.0	0.8
	10	4.0	4.2	5.9	3.2	2.8	1.7	1.8	1.8	1.7	1.3	1.2	1.2	1.4	1.2	1.0
	12	4.6	4.3	4.2	4.3	3.8	1.6	2.0	1.7	1.6	1.4	1.2	1.8	1.4	1.4	1.1
LSD	7	2.7	4.0	4.2	2.9	3.5	0.8	3.7	6.0	7.2	1.0	NA	1.3	2.3	2.8	0.6
	9	12.2	14.6	12.9	12.4	9.8	1.0	4.8	5.5	6.2	2.2	0.6	2.2	2.2	2.6	0.9
	10	17.6	18.8	18.4	15.2	14.1	1.2	3.7	5.6	5.3	2.8	0.8	1.8	2.1	1.8	1.0
	12	21.2	20.0	20.1	19.6	17.8	0.7	3.1	4.5	5.2	4.6	0.2	1.4	1.8	2.4	1.9
Marijuana	7	17.2	20.0	22.7	21.1	21.7	5.8	6.7	8.4	6.9	7.2	NA	3.3	4.0	3.3	3.9
	9	43.9	51.2	48.6	49.2	47.8	26.8	31.9	29.9	29.5	27.0	15.9	20.3	19.6	19.9	17.0
	10	51.9	56.1	57.3	56.5	57.8	36.8	39.6	39.1	36.9	36.7	25.5	27.9	26.3	24.0	24.3
	12	60.8	61.0	61.9	63.6	61.1	45.0	45.4	47.0	45.0	41.8	31.7	32.4	34.2	30.7	30.0
Tobacco	7	42.2	50.4	48.2	45.8	42.2	16.1	17.9	16.0	14.4	12.7	NA	10.3	9.2	7.4	7.3
	9	55.5	61.1	58.0	58.5	51.6	31.7	33.7	30.4	29.8	25.6	22.9	24.3	19.8	20.6	18.1
	10	54.4	58.8	56.1	56.7	54.1	34.8	34.8	33.3	33.1	28.4	27.8	26.3	23.9	23.2	21.1
	12	54.5	57.2	56.9	54.7	49.6	37.1	37.6	35.3	33.1	30.0	31.3	30.1	28.1	24.7	23.3

*From a report prepared by Mrs. Lillian Blackford, San Mateo County, California, Department of Public Health: Alcohol-Amphetamines-Barbiturates-Heroin-LSD-Marijuana-Tobacco: Student Drug Use Surveys, 1968-1976.

TABLE 1-4. Percentage of drug use reported by San Mateo County, California, in relation to junior and senior high school students

Drug	Grades	Any use during past year					Ten times+ during past year					50+ use				
		Date of survey					Date of survey					Date of survey				
		1972	1973	1974	1975	1976	1972	1973	1974	1975	1976	1972	1973	1974	1975	1976
Alcoholic beverages	7	48.6	67.2	70.7	63.7	60.4	13.9	18.3	19.7	14.8	12.8	NA	8.0	8.1	5.2	4.8
	9	73.7	80.3	82.2	82.2	80.3	35.5	40.4	42.2	40.8	36.6	14.5	17.8	20.2	17.1	14.5
	10	79.5	84.5	84.8	86.2	84.6	44.0	46.8	50.0	49.0	49.3	19.3	21.2	22.9	21.0	23.6
	12	83.2	86.8	88.3	87.6	88.4	52.5	58.1	59.0	59.5	56.4	25.1	28.8	30.6	30.0	26.2
Amphetamines	7	6.1	2.7	3.4	2.8	2.0	1.4	0.6	0.9	0.7	0.2	NA	0.4	0.4	0.5	0.2
	9	21.7	16.6	15.3	12.6	9.8	8.5	5.6	5.2	4.0	2.8	3.1	2.3	2.0	1.9	0.9
	10	27.4	21.4	20.1	18.8	15.4	11.1	8.5	7.4	6.8	6.4	4.5	3.5	3.0	2.5	2.1
	12	24.4	20.8	23.8	22.3	18.6	11.4	9.9	10.2	10.4	9.0	4.9	4.1	5.0	4.4	3.9
Barbiturates	7	4.8	4.7	4.7	3.4	2.7	0.8	0.6	0.9	0.9	0.5	NA	0.3	0.5	0.5	0.1
	9	13.7	14.0	15.8	12.5	10.0	3.5	4.5	3.4	3.3	2.3	1.3	1.7	1.3	1.3	0.8
	10	17.2	15.5	13.9	14.4	15.1	5.3	4.1	3.3	3.4	4.4	1.9	1.4	1.4	1.1	1.4
	12	14.1	11.8	14.7	14.1	11.8	4.0	5.4	3.4	3.5	4.3	1.4	2.2	1.3	1.3	1.0
Heroin	7	NA	NA	NA	NA	1.0	NA	NA	NA	NA	0.2	NA	NA	NA	NA	0.2
	9	2.3	2.3	2.3	2.5	2.2	0.9	0.9	0.6	1.2	0.4	0.7	0.7	0.4	0.8	0.2
	10	2.6	2.1	2.8	2.7	1.6	0.8	0.6	1.0	0.9	0.4	0.6	0.4	0.7	0.6	0.2
	12	2.7	2.9	2.7	2.9	2.1	1.0	0.9	1.2	1.0	0.9	0.6	0.7	1.0	0.6	0.8
LSD	7	2.5	2.8	3.7	3.3	2.1	0.5	0.6	0.6	0.8	0.4	NA	0.4	0.2	0.5	0.2
	9	12.0	13.8	14.9	12.0	9.5	3.0	3.0	3.3	2.6	1.5	1.1	1.4	1.1	0.9	0.2
	10	14.5	15.7	14.8	16.1	13.9	4.3	3.0	3.4	3.6	3.3	1.4	0.5	1.0	1.0	0.9
	12	13.7	13.4	16.2	16.1	13.5	3.5	3.5	3.2	4.4	3.5	1.2	1.0	1.1	1.3	1.5
Marijuana	7	13.2	15.0	18.0	16.8	15.6	4.6	4.2	5.6	5.0	4.5	NA	2.3	2.3	2.4	2.2
	9	39.0	47.0	47.8	44.4	46.1	23.0	22.6	29.3	25.2	24.5	12.5	12.8	17.4	13.7	13.5
	10	49.3	51.9	54.6	51.9	54.4	32.2	32.9	35.6	33.6	34.6	19.1	18.8	22.0	18.9	19.2
	12	53.0	57.2	58.2	55.5	56.0	35.5	37.8	38.8	37.2	36.0	20.4	20.4	22.8	20.9	21.3
Tobacco	7	37.5	46.2	49.0	46.4	43.6	16.4	18.7	19.5	16.9	13.9	NA	9.6	10.0	8.3	6.7
	9	57.7	63.5	64.8	63.8	63.6	34.5	38.0	41.2	39.4	38.7	24.7	27.0	29.6	27.3	27.1
	10	58.3	61.2	61.1	61.6	64.4	39.3	37.7	39.0	39.6	43.5	30.4	27.9	29.8	30.1	33.0
	12	55.1	56.9	58.2	57.1	59.4	39.1	39.2	40.7	39.6	40.8	31.9	32.0	33.4	31.3	33.1

*From a report prepared by Mrs. Lillian Blackford, San Mateo County, California, Department of Public Health: Alcohol-Amphetamines-Barbiturates-Heroin-LSD-Marijuana-Tobacco: Student Drug Use Surveys, 1968-1976.

Expert Committee on Drug Dependence reported that nonmedical drug use is "self-limiting" and is often discontinued after experimental use or a short period of casual use.[27] The probability of discontinuance varies with the drug used. DuPont stated it is no longer accurate to conclude that the experimental use of drugs inevitably leads to addiction.[28] Marin and Cohen also indicate that illegal drug use generally starts at the high school level but that in some places it may occur as early as the fifth or sixth grade, at ages 10 and 11. They claim that most young persons merely try drugs out by tasting or testing them. They believe that if adolescents are tuned into the world, are energetic, and are minimally adjusted, the use of drugs should not create serious problems. However, knowledge of the types of student users and of the extent to which they are using, misusing, and abusing drugs is necessary not only to further understand the nature of prevention but, more importantly, to design school programs.

Classification of users and abusers

David E. Smith, founder and medical director of the Haight-Ashbury Free Medical Clinic, has categorized student drug users as nonusers, experimenters, periodic users, compulsive users, and relapse users.

Nonusers use no drugs. Frequently this categorization of students refers only to those not using the illegal drugs, but occasionally it includes alcohol and tobacco. Actually if all legal drugs were included, it is conceivable that there are no nonusers of drugs.

Experimenters try drugs for short periods of time and then abandon their use. This is the largest group of users. Their numbers as well as the extent of their experimentation will vary with the drug used.

Periodic users use drugs regularly at social-recreational and religious-ritual affairs, but not necessarily every weekend. They may use prescription or over-the-counter drugs for medical reasons. They may use drugs in a group setting. The usage tends not to be habitual, although regular, and may fit only one segment of their life-style. This is the largest group of users of drugs who do so regularly, for example, at periodic cocktail parties or occasional marijuana parties. In numbers they may not be large, except possibly for the prescription and over-the-counter drug users. These individuals generally can stop using drugs if they so desire.

Compulsive users are habituated or addicted to the use of one or more drugs. They may be called "potheads," "acidheads," "speed freaks," or alcoholics, depending on the drug used. They use and seek drugs regularly. They are heavy users and drugs are part of their life-style. They constitute a very small percentage of the population.

Relapse users have ceased to be compulsive users and are fighting the craving for drugs. They also form a small but increasing percentage of the population, including alcoholics in Alcoholics Anonymous and ex-addicts in rehabilitation centers.

Numbers of drug users and abusers

Data clearly identifying the numbers and percentages of junior and senior high school students using various kinds of drugs are not available. However, there have been a number of scattered studies that have been carefully researched and provide helpful information. Generalizations made from these studies provide substantive indicative data. The best estimates, however, are probably "guestimates," for so many variables are involved in the collection of such data. Social, economic, racial, ethnic, and religious factors differ so widely in communities, as do the types of drugs used, that conclusions made in the discussion that follows should be reviewed in the light of these variables.

One of the more extensive and complete surveys on drug usage was compiled for grades 7 to 12 over a 9-year period (1968-1976) in San Mateo County, California.[4] Tables 1-3 and 1-4 report some of the data for the years 1972-1976 for grades 7, 9, 10, and 12. In addition, Table 1-5 provides interesting summary material from several recent studies. Table 1-6 introduces findings from a recent study of adolescent alcoholic drinking behaviors. These data, together with the in-

TABLE 1-5. Compiled data of high school student drug use

| | Percentages[*] | | | | | | | | | | | | | | | |
| | Never used | | | | | | | | Ever used | | | | | | | |
Drugs	Jacksonville, Fla.[2]	National study[52]	Illinois study[21]	White paper[62]	N.Y. state[26]	Six suburban groups[8]	Toronto H.S.[59]	AVERAGE	Jacksonville, Fla.[2]	National study[52]	Illinois study[21]	White paper[62]	N.Y. state[26]	Six suburban groups[8]	Toronto H.S.[59]	AVERAGE
Alcohol—all types	—	20	—	42	—	15	12	**22**	—	80	—	58	—	85	88	**78**
Beer	34	—	30	—	18	—	—	**27**	66	—	70	—	82	—	—	**73**
Wine	45	—	22	—	18	—	—	**28**	55	—	78	—	82	—	—	**72**
Hard liquor	59	—	36	—	35	—	—	**43**	41	—	64	—	65	—	—	**57**
Amphetamines	89	—	81	68	90	81	92	**84**	11	—	19	32	10	19	8	**16**
Barbiturates	93	—	85	81	88	77	80	**84**	7	—	15	19	12	23	20	**16**
Cocaine	94	—	—	95	96	93	—	**95**	6	—	—	5	4	7	—	**5**
Heroin—morphine	99	—	97	98	97	95	97	**97**	1	—	3	2	3	5	3	**3**
LSD—psychedelics	96	—	84	91	92	88	95	**91**	4	—	16	9	8	12	5	**9**
Marijuana	59	71	65	79	71	63	66	**67**	41	29	35	21	29	47	34	**33**
Solvents	97	—	91	93	92	—	98	**94**	3	—	9	7	8	—	2	**6**
Tobacco	62	—	70	42	18	62	63	**53**	38	—	30	58	72	38	37	**47**
Tranquilizers	93	—	91	92	93	—	90	**92**	7	—	9	8	7	—	10	**8**

[*]Data for each location and study derived from sources cited in references.

TABLE 1-6. Percentages of adolescent alcohol drinking levels by demographic characteristics[*]

| Characteristics | Drinking levels | | | | | |
	Abstinence	Infrequent	Light	Moderate	Moderate/heavy	Heavy
Sex						
Boys	23.2	13.7	15.6	16.4	16.0	15.1
Girls	31.1	18.8	17.6	14.6	11.5	6.3
Age						
13 and under	37.6	23.6	14.4	12.7	7.3	4.3
14	27.8	18.8	16.6	15.4	11.7	9.7
15	24.7	14.1	17.4	16.2	16.0	11.5
16	22.6	11.2	17.1	17.3	17.4	14.5
17	17.2	11.4	20.3	17.5	19.0	14.6
18 and over	20.5	6.9	15.1	16.5	20.2	20.2
Race/ethnicity						
Spanish-American	31.6	14.7	18.1	13.0	11.8	10.9
White	24.8	16.6	17.0	16.4	14.6	10.7
Black	40.7	17.6	14.8	11.4	9.5	5.7
American Oriental	27.1	15.2	14.0	15.6	11.6	16.5
Oriental	34.5	9.3	21.5	16.4	4.8	13.5

[*]Extrapolated from Rachel, J. V. and others: A national study of adolescent drinking behavior, attitudes and correlates, final report, North Carolina: Center for the Study of Social Behavior, April, 1975; prepared for the National Institute on Alcohol Abuse and Alcoholism.

formation found in Table 1-2, serve as the basis for the following generalizations regarding the extent of drug use among junior and senior high school students:

1. The percentage of compulsive and relapse users is relatively small and the numbers and percentages of these users are probably the lowest of all categories. In some ghetto areas the percentage of heroin users may be 6% or higher, while in other communities it may be 1 to 3% or less. The percentages of use of LSD, amphetamines, and barbiturates may be a little higher; marijuana, which has been increasing in usage, may possibly have been used by as many as 10 to 15% or more of the population in some communities. Alcohol abuse is growing in incidence, with 3 out of 10 adolescents in grades 7 to 12 having problems, according to one national study.[52]

2. The numbers and percentages of periodic users is probably somewhat higher than that of the compulsive and relapse users, but the data are not sufficient to clearly indicate how much higher.

3. The experimenters probably form the largest group of users. The percentages according to the drug used are as follows: alcohol, 60% to 90%; tobacco, 30% to 72%; marijuana, 14% to 64%; LSD, 3% to 21%; amphetamines and barbiturates, 2% to 20%; heroin, probably 2% to 6%; and cocaine, 1% to 4%. Nyswander and Millman[46] claim that it has been reported that 60% of students enrolled at several New York City high schools have used heroin. The use of alcoholic beverages has increased, and adolescent consumption is becoming a serious societal problem. Smart states some reports reveal that there are as many as 450,000 teenage alcoholics and a larger number of problem drinkers.[58] Girls drink less than boys but more of them are involved, drinking becomes more frequent with increasing age, and young people are starting to drink at earlier ages. Blum reports that second graders were using alcohol and tobacco.[6]

4. The percentage of nonusers differs with the types of drugs used. Table 1-5 shows the average percentage of nonusers to be as follows: alcohol, 22%; amphetamines and barbiturates, 84%; heroin, 97%; LSD-psychedelics, 91%; marijuana, 67%; and tobacco, 53%.

Polydrug abuse

Multiple drug use, as revealed in Table 1-7, is not uncommon among adolescents. Many teenagers who drink also use other drugs, especially marijuana, and the reverse is also true. Smith and Wesson define polydrug abuse as "the use of one or more psychoactive drugs including heroin and alcohol to the point where the individual's health or economic functioning is seriously compromised.[59] Single and colleagues have said:

There is a high probability that an adolescent who has used illicit drugs has also used one or more other illegal drugs as well. However, it is even more likely that the illicit drug user has also used legal drugs, such as alcohol and tobacco. The overwhelming majority of illicit drug users has used beer or wine (94%), hard liquor (90%), or tobacco (89%).[57]

• • •

Knowledge of the extensiveness of drug use and abuse as well as of the types of drug users among youth identifies the need for the development of varieties of preventive procedures and of differing educational programs. However, the meaning of drug education is widely misunderstood and is in need of clarification. Responsible individuals attempting to develop programs have been confused. This has caused difficulties in determining the differing roles of the school and of the community and has led to problems in communication and coordination of school and community efforts.

The meaning of drug education

Drug education is often identified synonymously as drug information or drug knowledge. Frequently phrases such as "give them the facts" and "scare the hell out of them" are used. Former President Nixon identified drug education in this manner, "There is no priority higher in this administration than to see that children and the public learn the facts about drugs in the right way and for the right purposes."[44] Others believe

TABLE 1-7. Patterns of multiple drug use*: product moment correlations† among adolescent use of 15 legal and illegal drugs (total N.Y. State weighted sample—wave 1, fall, 1971)

	1	2	3	4	5	6	7	8	9	10	11	12	13	14	15
1. Beer or wine		299	464	214	180	106	115	090	128	122	097	074	046	101	116
2. Cigarettes			400	433	378	283	232	239	328	334	212	182	148	267	259
3. Hard liquor				368	300	185	180	160	235	215	157	119	094	171	169
4. Marihuana					776	471	435	382	536	534	293	300	252	397	336
5. Hashish						560	528	446	570	598	327	356	273	444	329
6. LSD							674	624	550	584	354	467	391	526	374
7. Other psychedelics								588	528	535	370	469	327	513	349
8. Methedrine									509	541	361	509	373	536	380
9. Other amphetamines										696	408	390	295	484	397
10. Barbiturates											432	427	361	509	417
11. Tranquilizers												277	220	419	318
12. Cocaine													476	450	285
13. Heroin														370	248
14. Other narcotics															248
15. Inhalants															
Total N ≥	7517	7534	7658	7581	7517	7671	7663	7647	7661	7676	7667	7671	7654	7606	7630

*From Single, E., Kandel, D., and Faust, R.: Patterns of multiple drug use in high school, J. Health Soc. Behav. **15**:347, December, 1974.
†All significant at .001 level; decimal points omitted.

drug education to be learning that goes on in a classroom in which there are 30 to 40 students and a teacher who didactically warns them of the evils and hazards of using drugs. Some people think drug education is a talk by a noted speaker, physician, pharmacologist, psychiatrist, or other authority describing the effects of drugs on the human body to an assembly with 500 to 1000 students in attendance. The showing of a film and the distribution of a pamphlet are other references that some individuals believe to be education. There are many other points of view regarding the meaning of drug education, but perhaps these illustrate some of the varieties of understandings that exist.

Actually all of the activities described have educational possibilities. However, what learning takes place under these circumstances may be solely factual, or informational. It may be accurate as well as inaccurate in its content. It may be a series of biased, prejudiced, and false exhortations. The evidence is overwhelmingly supportive of the fact that without the concern for the personal attitudes, without individuals being actively engaged in the learning process, factual information by itself is meaningless, is useless, and will have little effect on the way persons behave toward drugs. In fact, data indicate that such "facts" may create "pro" attitudes toward drugs by removing the uncertainty of the hazards and thereby increasing the experimental use of drugs.

Unfortunately much of the so-called "drug education" that has occurred in the schools has been of the informational kind. This may be one of the main reasons for the ineffectiveness of many of the drug education programs. However, in recent years there have been numerous approaches away from this emphasis. The introduction of values clarification, peer counseling, self-concept, decision-making, and alternatives to drug use are a few of the new procedures.

Learning about drugs can be considered an overly simplified definition of drug education. It must also include learning about one's self and give attention to a whole array of problems affecting young people. Such learning may take place inside or outside the school. It may occur in a formal or an informal manner for children, youth, parents, teachers, counselors, administrators, and the general public. It may be provided for nonusers, experimenters, periodic users, compulsive users, and relapse users of drugs as part of primary, secondary, and tertiary prevention programs. It must focus on behavior change in students.

Formal education

Formal drug education generally refers to organized or planned learning that usually takes place in a classroom and may involve a teacher, a curriculum, a textbook, and such audiovisual aids as films, filmstrips, and tape recordings. Drug education as such usually is not considered to be a separate subject area in the curriculum for kindergarten through grade 12, but probably is taught as part of another subject such as health education, science, social studies, or as a separate unit of work in these same courses. It may be a specific course or series of presentations for teachers, counselors, nurses, parents, or community representatives in a college or in a university. It involves the use of a variety of teaching techniques, including speakers. Such education may also occur outside the school without the involvement of school personnel: a city health department may hold a series of meetings concerning drugs for parents, industrial leaders, and educators; a medical center may conduct formal sessions for the community at large or for physicians and paramedical personnel.

Formal drug education is more easily presented in schools or in the community when its purpose is to provide only pharmacological information. It becomes more complex and more difficult to conduct when the objectives include social, psychological, and possibly spiritual emphases—when the focus is on changing behavior or attitude. Thus expediency and the need for a simple, direct attack may be reasons for the factual emphasis in many formal drug education programs.

Informal education

Informal education refers to the learning that takes place without structure and without much, if any, planning. It may occur in the classroom, in the school, outside the school, in the home watching television, reading a newspaper or magazine, talking to a parent, or in the community talking to a friend, neighbor, or anyone else. It may take place in discussion on a one-to-one basis or in small groups. It is an activity in which a person usually participates voluntarily.

Behavioral approach

Drug education today must be centered on behavioral changes that include not only a knowledge or understanding of drugs but also attitudes toward drugs and drug practices. In the current vernacular of educators the appropriate goals must be stated in terms of their cognitive, affective, and action emphases. Education must cover more than merely the pharmacological and physiological effects of drugs on body systems. It must give consideration to student feelings, values, interests, and actions about and with drugs. It must include the why of drug use and abuse as well as the social effects of drugs on individuals and the community. It must provide students with alternatives to drug use. It should permit students to make their own decisions about the use of drugs after all the favorable and unfavorable aspects of such usage are presented. It should encourage the development of values. It should enable students to better understand themselves. This approach is referred to as the behavioral approach in drug education.

The available evidence clearly indicates that facts by themselves, information by itself, and knowledge alone are not sufficient to change or affect human behavior. Facts are singularly ineffective in changing the opinions of persons who are emotionally committed to their own way of looking at an issue. This is especially true of those users and abusers of drugs who may feel they are more sophisticated about drugs than the teacher or the speaker who may be presenting drug information. However, factual data

are prerequisite to intelligent action if such information is accurate, if it is acquired within a context that provides proper motivation, and if the student understands the facts to be meaningful, applicable, and useful in the environment in which he lives. Thus in drug education a teaching approach of much wider scope than merely the presentation of facts becomes mandatory.

Schools have encountered difficulties with, have not been aware of, or have not frequently used the behavioral approach. The result has been that drug education programs have been primarily information oriented and ineffectual in their impact on the drug problem. This may be the most significant justification for the criticism that has been made about the ineffectiveness of drug education programs. One of the purposes of this book is to help schools develop behaviorally centered curricula with behaviorally stated objectives so that the desired impact on students can be achieved.

Both formal and informal drug education must take place in the schools as part of programs of primary and secondary prevention in order to provide differential learnings for the different types of student drug users found in schools (Chapter 7).

Generally it may be concluded that formal education should be the main educational focus for nonusers and for experimental drug users, provided there are numerous opportunities for informal education as well. Informal education, which should also be a part of the services phase (Chapter 8) of the drug program, should be used to try to reach the periodic, compulsive, and relapse drug users.

The dilemma of the schools can be resolved by giving attention to the total school drug program introduced in this book. Such a program must provide differential phases to accommodate the variety of drug users and abusers as well as the nonusers in the local school community. It should focus on the primary and secondary prevention aspects of the problem. It must include both formal and informal education, services to identify and assist drug users and abusers, consid-

eration for improvement of the school atmosphere, and coordination of the total drug
program within the school and with the community.

REFERENCES

1. Arnold, M.: The trouble in drug education, Natl. Observer **10:**16, 1971.
2. Barr, C., and others: Student drug and alcohol opinionnaire and usage survey, grades 6-12, Jacksonville, Fla., Jan., 1976, Duval County School Board.
3. Barrins, P. C.: Drug abuse: the newest, most dangerous challenge to school boards, Am. School Board J. **157:**15-18, 1969.
4. Blackford, L.: Alcohol-amphetamines-barbiturates-heroin-LSD-marijuana-tobacco: student drug use surveys, 1968-1975, San Mateo, Calif., 1976, Department of Public Health.
5. Bland, H. B.: Problems related to teaching about drugs. In Hafen, B. Q., editor: Readings on drug use and abuse, Provo, Utah, 1970, Brigham Young University Press.
6. Blum, R. H., and others: Drug education: results and recommendations, Lexington, Mass., 1976, Lexington Books.
7. Bureau of Narcotics and Dangerous Drugs, U.S. Department of Justice: Guidelines for drug abuse prevention education, Washington D.C., 1970, U.S. Government Printing Office.
8. Calhoun, J. F.: An examination of patterns of drug use in six suburban groups, Int. J. Addictions **10:**521-538, 1975.
9. Cornacchia, H. J.: Teaching in difficult areas of health, J. School Health **41:**193-196, 1970.
10. Drive to curb hard drugs gets no. 1 priority, U.S. News and World Report **72:**37, April 3, 1972.
11. Drug abuse education; a failure so far, Los Angeles *Times*, January 25, 1974.
12. Drug education handbook, Denver, 1970, Alcohol and Drug Dependence Division, Colorado State Department of Public Health.
13. Drug education in Maine, Augusta, 1970, Maine State Department of Education.
14. Drug trade news, Oradell, N.J., Oct. 7, 1971, Topics Publishing Co.
15. Drugs and the educational antidote, Nat. Sch. **85:**49-52, 1970.
16. Drug use has leveled off, San Francisco *Chronicle*, Nov. 26, 1976.
17. Education USA, Washington, D.C., Sept. 27, 1971, National School Public Relations Association.
18. Edwards, C. C.: Drug Educ. Rep. **1:**4, 1971.
19. Eisner, V.: Adolescent drug abuse, Calif. Sch. Health **4:**1-9, 1969.
20. Finlator, J.: The drug scene: the scope and the problem faced by schools. In Teaching about drugs: a curriculum guide, Kent, Ohio, 1970, American School Health Association.
21. Galli, N.: Patterns of student drug use, J. Drug Ed. **4:**237-247, Summer, 1974.
22. Gallup, G. H.: Seventh annual Gallup poll of public attitudes toward education, Phi Delta Kappan **57:**227-241, December, 1975.
23. Globetti, G.: The use of beverage alcohol by youth in an abstinence setting, J. Sch. Health **39:**179-183, 1969.
24. Greenberg, J. S.: Drug abuse and the schools, J. Drug Ed. **1:**171-175, 1971.
25. Halleck, S.: The great drug education hoax, The Progressive **34:**30, 1970.
26. Kandell, D., and others: The epidemiology of drug use among New York state high school students, Am. J. Public Health **66:**43-53, January, 1976.
27. The Journal, 3:5, December 1, 1974, Addiction Research Foundation of Ontario, Canada.
28. The Journal, 5:2, December 1, 1976, Addiction Research Foundation of Ontario, Canada.
29. Laun, W. L.: Priority topics for inclusion in health instruction programs, Ill. J. Ed. **60:**12-18, 1969.
30. Lawler, J. T.: Peer group approach to drug education, J. Drug Ed. **1:**63-76, 1971.
31. Lennard, H. L., and others: Mystification and drug misuse, San Francisco, 1971, Jossey-Bass, Inc., Publishers.
32. Lipscomb, W. R.: An epidemiology of drug use-abuse, J. Public Health **61:**1794-1800, 1971.
33. Louria, D.: Nightmare drugs, New York, 1966, Pocket Books.
34. Marden, P., and Kolodner, K.: National Drug Reporter **6:**3, November, 1976.
35. Marin, P., and Cohen, A. Y.: Understanding drug use: an adult's guide to drugs and the young, New York, 1971, Harper & Row, Publishers.
36. Matchett, W. F.: Who uses drugs? A study in a suburban public high school, J. Sch. Health **41:**90-93, 1971.
37. McGrath, J. H., and Scarpitti, F. R.: Youth and drugs: perspective on a social problem, Glenview, Ill., 1970, Scott, Foresman, & Co.
38. Meeds, L.: Education: key to the drug problem, Soc. Ed. **33:**664-666, 1969.
39. Miller, T. J.: Drug abuse: schools find some answers, Sch. Management **14:**22-28, 1970.
40. Mullin, L.: Alcohol education: the school's responsibility, J. Sch. Health **38:**518-522, 1968.
41. National Commission on Marijuana and Drug Abuse: Drug use in America: problem in perspective, Fourth Report of the National Commission on Marijuana and Drug Abuse, Washington, D.C., 1974, U.S. Government Printing Office.
42. National Drug Reporter **5:**3, November, 1975.
43. National Drug Reporter **6:**3, November, 1976.
43a. National Institute on Drug Abuse: Marihuana and health: in perspective, Summary and Comments on the Fifth Annual Report to the U.S. Congress from the Secretary of Health, Education and Welfare, Washington, D.C., 1975, U.S. Government Printing Office.

44. Nixon, R. M., Quoted in Tune in: drug abuse news, Washington, D.C., 1971, National Institute for Mental Health, National Clearinghouse for Drug Abuse Information.
45. Nowlis, H. H.: Strategies for prevention, Contemporary Drug Problems 55:20, Spring, 1975.
46. Nowlis, H.: The student and his culture. In McGrath, J. H., and Scarpitti, F., editors: Youth and drugs: perspective on a social problem, Glenview, Ill., 1970, Scott, Foresman, & Co.
47. Nyswander, M. E., and Millman, R. B.: Slow detoxification of adolescent heroin addicts in New York City. In Proceedings of the Third National Conference on Methadone Treatment, Washington, D.C., 1970, National Institute of Mental Health.
48. Peterson, R. C.: Suggestions for educators. In Resource book for drug abuse education, Washington, D.C., 1969, National Institute of Mental Health, National Clearinghouse for Mental Health Information.
49. Petrillo, R. F.: Comprehensive action model to combat drug abuse in high school, J. Sch. Psychol. 8:226-231, 1970.
50. Plesent, E.: A community and its schools' efforts to understand and deal with drug abuse, J. Drug Ed. 1:85-91, 1971.
51. Prettyman, R. L., and others: Drug abuse and the school scene, Sci. Teacher 37:45-47, 1970.
52. Rachel, J., and others: A national study of adolescent drinking behavior attitudes and correlates, final report, North Carolina: Center for the Study of Social Behavior, April, 1975, National Institute on Alcohol Abuse and Alcoholism.
53. Randall, H.: Patterns of drug use in school-age children, J. Sch. Health 40:296-301, 1970.
54. Resource book for drug abuse information, Washington, D.C., 1969, National Institute of Mental Health, National Clearinghouse for Drug Abuse Information.
55. Ryan, J., editor: What the public spent for drugs, cosmetics, toiletries in 1975, Product Management 5:25-31, August, 1976.
56. Sandusk, J. F.: Size and extent of the problem, J.A.M.A. 196:707-709, 1966.
57. Single, E., Kandel, D., and Faust, R.: Patterns of multiple drug use in high school, J. Health Soc. Behav. 15:344-357, December, 1974.
58. Smart, R. G., The new drinkers, Toronto, Canada, 1976, Addiction Research Foundation of Ontario, Canada.
59. Smart, R. G., and others: Trends in drug use among metropolitan Toronto high school students: 1968-1974, Ontario, Canada, 1974, Addiction Research Foundation of Ontario, Canada.
60. Smith, D. E., and Wesson, R. R.: Editor's note, J. Psychedelic Drugs 7:111-114, April-June, 1976.
61. A teacher resource guide for drug use and abuse for Michigan schools, Lansing, 1970, Michigan State Department of Education.
62. U.S. Dept. of Health, Education and Welfare, National Institute on Drug Abuse, Domestic Council on Drug Abuse Task Force: White paper on drug abuse, September, 1975, Washington, D.C., 1975, U.S. Government Printing Office.
63. U.S. Senate, Hearings before Subcommittee on Alcoholism and Narcotics of the Committee on Labor and Public Welfare, Drug Abuse Prevention and Treatment Legislation, 1975, Washington, D.C., 1975, U.S. Government Printing Office.
64. Warner, R., Jr.: Reported in Arnold, M. R.: The trouble in drug education, Natl. Observer 10:16, 1971.
65. Yolles, S. F.: Prescription for drug abuse education, J. Drug Ed. 1:101-103, 1971.
66. Yolles, S. F.: Statement on control of drug abuse before the Subcommittee to Investigate Juvenile Delinquency of the Committee on the Judiciary, United States Senate, Sept. 17, 1969.

PART TWO

THE DRUG SCENE

2
Society and drugs

The exploding problem of drug abuse in the United States is of paramount public concern. Drug experimentation and drug dependency have spread with frightening speed among all age, social, racial, and economic groups; drug use and abuse by our young people threatens the physical and mental fiber of the next generation of citizenry. Former President Nixon warned, "Any nation that moves down the road to addiction . . . that nation has had something taken out of its character."[18] Pointing out that, although the United States produces no heroin, it uses more heroin than any other country in the world, Mr. Nixon in March of 1972 declared the control of narcotics traffic to be "the number one priority" for law enforcement in his administration. In 1976, national data indicated that there were approximately 9 million alcohol abusers, 2 million polydrug or nonnarcotic drug abusers, and 500,000 heroin addicts in the United States.*

Drug abuse, including alcohol abuse, is currently so extensive that all youths are exposed to it even though they are not actually involved.

Here is an enormous challenge to education. To ignore this challenge or to pretend that it does not exist or that it is not so widespread and serious, is irresponsible. To fail to deal adequately with this problem is to fail one of the most pressing educational needs of our time. Our schools—administrators and teachers as well as students—must provide viable programs that will positively direct the young away from drug abuse. One of the keys to productive educational programs is the involvement of youth. Many programs have failed because the young were left out of the planning or given only token responsibility. School personnel must try to understand the values, life-style, and world of the drug user and want to help find realistic answers to his problems, answers that offer *alternatives* to drug abuse. However, they must realize that not all drug use is destructive or a sign of deviance or personality disturbance. Schools must help students, both as individuals and as a group, to become involved in making wise choices about drugs. Efforts must extend beyond the school grounds to the fostering of better communication between young people and adults. The school must become a catalyst in changing and modifying community attitudes. Adults need information and education about drugs as much as if not more than youths.

Drug use and abuse patterns have shifted so significantly that much of the information once used as a basis for education and prevention programs has lost credibility and now must be supplemented and reinterpreted in the light of more sophisticated thinking.

*White Paper on Drug Abuse. A Report to the President from the Domestic Council Drug Abuse Task Force, Washington, D.C., September, 1975, U.S. Government Printing Office.

WHAT IS THE DRUG PROBLEM?

The problem of drug abuse is the complex interaction of pharmacological, psychological, and sociological variables and affects all strata of society, not just youth. Ours is a drug culture but, unfortunately, many of our reactions to the problem are based on emotional responses rather than on factual information placed in perspective. The lack of information and perspective has acutely compromised the effectiveness of many, if not most, of our educational and training efforts. Historically, the moralistic attack on drug-abusing addicts and youth seems to have lacked insight or logic, and has even added more confusion to an already complex medical, social, and legal problem. As drug abuse educator Helen Nowlis[19] has pointed out, most people believe that drugs are good or bad, safe or dangerous, legal or illegal, and that individuals are either drug users or nonusers and either good citizens or criminals.

Most persons in our society have fallen into the simple dichotomy of either-or and have been largely unwilling or unable to make the subtle distinctions necessary for understanding and intelligent action. Any useful or meaningful action or program relating to what we carelessly label "drug abuse," for want of a better title, must be based on careful discrimination not only among drugs and types of drug use and overuse but also among the different types of people who use drugs, including how and why they use them. We must be concerned with what specific drug is being abused and more concerned with what it is that the person thinks the drug is doing for him.

CONFLICTS OF REALITY: DIFFERENT WAYS WE THINK ABOUT DRUGS

What is really meant by drug use, drug abuse, and drug misuse? It should be fairly obvious that the words are used in so many different contexts that many of the great debates about the drug issue are largely semantic. The terms have lost their meaning, if they ever had much, and have caused endless confusion, misunderstanding, and hysteria.

The issue, as stated somewhat more aca-demically by sociologists, is whether or not those drugs that are defined as addicting, habituating, or indicative of psychological dependence and criminality have been so defined *not* because of the drug's inherent chemical nature but because of the *cultural framework* within which these drugs presently exist. Sociologists suggest that many of the so-called dangers of drugs are in large part defined by the social circumstances of their use.[4] It is certainly true that we approve of some drug use and that we do not approve of others regardless of health factors.

We believe that to fully understand the problems and complex issues of drug abuse education one must first become aware of hidden determinants in our cultural patterns that are crucial in forming our attitudes about just what the drug problem is and what should be done about it. Each of us has a mental set, a belief system, that affects the way we see social issues and the way we formulate solutions to problems. One of the false positions that each of us adopts in this age of technical and scientific expertise is assuming that our "expertness" is more than simply our opinion when it is nothing more than that. So let us look at some common opinions about drugs and drug abuse and consider their validity.

Conceptual views of drug abuse

Popularly held opinions about drugs have been divided into three general models or belief systems. They are as follows: (1) legal-morality model, (2) medical-psychiatric model, and (3) sociological-psychological model. The basic ideology of these models can be found in the "conventional" wisdom about drug abuse of the uninformed, average person and in the technical and popular literature.

Legal-morality model

The legal-morality model is a rigid perspective through which some people perceive, identify, and label the behavior and life-style of others. Such perceptions have actually fostered much of the present crisis surrounding certain drug use in this country.

According to this view, which is held by many of the "solid citizens" of our society, anyone who overuses drugs or indulges in drugs that are presently in disfavor with the dominant majority of society is a sinner and a criminal who should be punished and sent to jail. This community stereotype of the drug user, which has evolved within the last 50 years, represents a fusion of several strands within the American experience, including an essentially biblical interpretation of "man's weakness and fall from Grace." The drug user is viewed as essentially a sinner[9] or a disciple of the devil.

The foremost aim of the legal-moralists is to provide more severe criminal penalties in order to deal with the increasing use and sales of illegal drugs such as marijuana. This group maintains, in the face of scientific evidence to the contrary, that marijuana is a serious threat to our society and strongly resists the findings of the President's Commission on Marijuana. If such a position seems overly dramatic, remember that just a few decades ago we had newspaper headlines about "mad dog drug fiends" who, "crazed" on marijuana, rampaged about town in an orgy of raping, looting, and killing. Harry Anslinger, the former director of the then Federal Bureau of Narcotics, called the "dope fiend" America's "Public Enemy Number One."[14]

Increasingly, however, thoughtful persons were able to see through the shallow, vindictive stereotypes that falsely label without really explaining. An excellent analysis of the formative period in our nation's "drug history," including the creation of the drug fiend stereotype, is provided by Lindesmith in his book *The Addict and the Law.*[14] We shall not take time here to explore historical developments, but we will consider the implications of the legal-morality view for the many communities that discover "our kids take drugs!" One of the results of these implications is that youthful drug abusers have been segregated into a community of deviants and punished.

The emphasis of the official legal-morality view has been primarily functional and ex-pedient: how can the user or trafficker in illicit drugs be identified, apprehended, and punished? The most preferred form of punishment is that which permanently removes this social pariah from the larger community. He, like Adam and Eve, is literally to be cast out of concerned humanity because of his transgression. An extreme example of this was the sentencing of a young man in the state of Texas to a thousand years in prison for the possession of a small amount of marijuana.

Spokesmen for the legal-morality model have never appreciated the term "clinic," nor do they feel that any medical definition should be applied to what they see as essentially a problem for criminal justice. Indeed, some critics have gone so far as to suggest that the development of free clinics for drug-involved youth in this country raises a grave moral issue and that such clinics aid and abet persons who should receive whatever help, if any, in a government penal institution such as the original Federal Narcotic Rehabilitation Program at Lexington, Kentucky. The legal-moralists believe that local medical assistance provides drug addiction and illegal drug use with a convenient source of "official respectability" and acts as an excuse to maintain individuals in a perpetual state of disease.

Much of the present controversy over the effectiveness of treatment with the drug methadone (Chapter 4) is confused by the issue of whether a person with drug problems ought to be *treated* at all or if he ought to be simply *forced* to conform to the law. Methadone, it has been stated over and over again, maintains individuals in a perpetual state of disease and hence is immoral.[23]

The legal-morality view is best observed in the speeches and writings of those who feel it is their duty to enforce the community's prohibitions against particular types of drug misuse. In fact, the view of legal-moralists has been incorporated into much of the legal code surrounding the use and sale of drugs in this country. The legal-morality assumptions, explicitly stated or not, underlie almost all of our present national and state legislation, except that expressly concerned with providing treatment. Maximum sentences of 40 years and life imprisonment are found in many state laws, and in some states there are provisions for the death penalty on conviction for the sale of narcotics or of any of a number of specified dangerous drugs to a minor. Only recently has there been a thrust in legislation to reduce the penalties for first-time possession of marijuana for personal use.

Meanwhile, the pharmaceutical drug industry in America makes compulsive users and abusers out of millions of us. Physicians admit they overprescribe. Massive advertising and miseducation have convinced people that pills can improve almost every aspect of life—curing a cold, getting rid of a headache, putting one to sleep or waking one up, and making us all feel happy even if we are not. But to persons who adhere strictly to the legal-morality belief system, a certain special type of person, a "drug user," invariably falls into the classification of a deviant and a law breaker. Even though many persons who at one time subscribed to this punitive, rigid attitude have recently become more tolerant, the view of the drug user as a criminal still pervades most of our attitudes in teaching about drugs. We should be aware of this and rationally decide whether this is a reasonable state of affairs.

Most of the drugs used by the young have been outlawed for them by their elders, a fact that not only polarizes the existing ideological conflict between generations, but that technically makes criminals of the young. Smith sees this fact alone as creating a pivotal issue for adolescent rebellion. This is one of the sorry results of our national policy. Yet in no other form of deviance is the distinction between what constitutes criminal behavior and what is not criminal behavior so blurred as it is with drug use.

Too often the community's response to adolescent drug activity (Chapter 5) is not guided by an informed articulation of its causes. Instead a vaguely conceived panacea of "education" is proposed without any real understanding of what education is supposed to do, or even what it means. Too often "educating the community about youth and drugs" involves the assumption that drug use or nonuse is a matter of personal decision making and principally of individual wrongdoing. Such an attitude obscures rather than grapples with the complex social and group dimensions of drug use. Focus on the individual drug abuser alone denies that his drug use has important causal links with peers and with the peer-group social system. Drug use is largely a group experience. Yet the orientation of the legal-moralists is to support what has been called the "rotten apple" view of mankind. The sociologist Skolnick says, "Under this doctrine, crime and disorder are attributable mainly to the intentions of evil individuals; human behavior transcends past experience, culture, society, and other external forces and should be understood in terms of wrong choices, deliberately made."[22] Educators must become more aware of the social surroundings in which drug taking occurs and of the social as well as the personal meaning of its use. Education must be *about* drug taking as well as *against* drug taking.

Medical-psychiatric model

We shall return to some of the issues passed by, dealing with them in more detail in later chapters, but let us look at a second model, the medical-psychiatric. Although more benign and humanitarian than the legal-morality view, which stresses detection, isolation, and punishment, the medical-psychiatric view nevertheless still defines the problem in essentially individual and personal terms. The pathology still resides in the individual. Use of and addiction to heroin can be viewed as a disease in the following analogy: Almost nobody "catches" the disease (starts using dope) except from someone else who has it (uses). Therefore it is presumed that if somehow addicts or users can be kept separated from nonusers, the chances of the disease spreading are minimized.

When drug abuse is viewed as a disease, within the medical-psychiatric framework, it becomes an affliction that requires hospitalization and treatment. Doctors, psychiatrists, and other health professionals strongly urge a transfer of social control from the justice department to the medical profession. We are in basic accord with this view but maintain certain reservations that will be described later.

Today there is a crying need for inexpensive (to the patient), nonjudgmental, and humanitarian medical care for drug-dependent persons, particularly addicts.[25] But most physicians do not understand drug abuse treatment and do not want to get involved. Also the medical establishment in this country has long been disenfranchised by criminal justice in the drug abuse area. Passage of the Harrison Narcotic Act and the activities of the then Federal Bureau of Narcotics forced the medical profession, through dire threats, to abdicate completely its role and responsibilities in establishing and maintaining standards by which physicians could treat drug addiction and adverse drug reactions. Even today, over half a century after the passage of the Harrison Act, physicians are being threatened with the most extreme sanctions and brought to trial for attempting to treat drug abusers in normal medical settings.*

There has been in the last 15 years a slow shift from emphasizing the criminal nature of addiction toward the "new humanism"— a concern for the well-being of the individual and not just of the state. The increasing acceptance of this approach may in part be due to the fact that it offers advantages to law enforcement and to the bureaucracy as well as to the health care professions. Behind the new rhetoric are many old, punitive practices. Even so, more institutions are demonstrating genuine care and concern for the plight of the addict. The way has opened for massive assistance programs from the federal health institutes, and financial support has been developed for many communities previously unable to undertake remedial projects.

A second half of the medical approach, the psychiatric, still views the problem as residing within the disturbed psyche and flawed personality of the user, particularly in the case of the narcotic addict. A focus on unstable personality as a critical factor in drug usage has resulted in a whole range of treatment strategies devised originally for those identified as mentally ill. Again we must point out that trying to tinker with the body or the mind of the user bears little relevance to the underlying social causes. Nevertheless the medical perspective on drug use is a major advance when the user is classified as sick rather than as criminal.

Sociological-psychological model

A third major concept is the sociological-psychological model. This is essentially a behavioral approach that views drug use as a social activity arising out of group and individual needs. Although such use can lead to a serious pathological condition on the part of the user, perhaps warranting medical and psychiatric intervention, the usage itself is seen as a normal response to the environment and to peer pressure. Whereas the legal-moralistic view stresses free will, free choice, and individual volition, the sociological-psychological model considers the taking or not taking of various drugs to be largely the consequence of environmental circumstances in which the individual plays a limited role. The normal, healthy, curious child will naturally experiment with drugs in our contemporary permissive atmosphere. He will take drugs because of "peer-group pressure" and the aura of mystery and forbiddenness surrounding drugs. At a time when drug use is epidemic, the possibility is strong that he will become a statistic in the total epidemiology of disease. Rather than focusing on the user himself, the sociological-psychological approach examines the individual and social characteristics of the user population. Drug abuse or illegal drug use is often a central ritual in the lives of those attempting to develop a unique or counter-culture style of life.

---

*The Koning and Frazier trial is an example discussed in Smith, D. E., and Bentel, D. J.: Drug Abuse Information Project, the fifth annual report to the legislature, San Francisco, 1972, University of California, San Francisco Medical Center.

Factors affecting drug use and abuse

An attempt will be made to briefly examine and assess the role of different drugs in American life among adults as well as among the young.

Abuse of medicines and drugs

Many legitimate medicines and drugs are widely abused by adults and youth (Chapter 1). Among these drugs are stimulants such as amphetamines, diet pills, and "stay-awake pills" and depressants such as barbiturates, sleeping pills, and tranquilizers. These preparations are often used for reasons other than to alleviate specific diseases and can be dangerous. The number of drug-induced injuries runs into the thousands each year, and there are an estimated 1 million cases of drug poisoning annually. Half of these cases involve small children who get their hands on poisonous drugs, but the remainder is largely the result of adults attempting to treat or overtreat themselves.

The increasing, almost universal use of chemicals to alter the physical and emotional state has become accepted practice in the United States. The American people are subjected to massive amounts of advertising propounding the self-prescribing of drugs and medicines for various conditions ranging from the common cold and arthritis to tension headaches, irritability, depression, and even to "staying regular." Innumerable types of drugs, both prescription and nonprescription, are readily available.

The home medicine cabinet contains an average of 22 different drugs. For many Americans the medicine chest has become the one place to find comfort, energy, and sleep. One out of six Americans reaches for the pill bottle at the first sign of nervousness or anxiety. By taking more than the amount prescribed by a doctor, frequently refilling prescriptions, and repeatedly turning to the medicine cabinet when they are upset, millions of people flagrantly misuse drugs yet would never consider themselves in the same category as a "junkie" or other deviant.

Children become accustomed to seeing their parents freely use or misuse these different substances, and for many different reasons. Most parents give medicines to children, including a variety of vitamins, pain killlers, sedatives, and "children's aspirin" for mild childhood upsets. These medicines are selected for children from a variety of pleasant forms—candies, gums, and syrups—and condition children to seek drugs as a "first line" solution to many physical and mental problems. The home medicine cabinet nearly always contains one or more analgesics (aspirin) and sedatives, which can be dangerous and even fatal if not adequately guarded from children.

Illegal use of drugs

The legality of drug use is a factor that cuts through this complex issue of drugs without clarifying any crucial points or distinguishing between drugs on the basis of abuse potential. It is simply a fact of legislation that some drugs are outlawed and some are not. Legally, some nonnarcotic drugs are classified with narcotics and carry the same harsh penalties for possession or use. But making the use of a drug a crime solves neither the problem of use nor that of control.

As early as 1957, for example, government officials recommended that marijuana not be classified as an opiate, additionally suggesting pointed inquiry into the wisdom of punishment for the mere possession of marijuana. The findings of the recent President's Commission on Marijuana, 15 years later, support these earlier recommendations.[17] Meanwhile, millions of Americans have smoked marijuana, many regularly, with apparently minimal harm. Yet sale, use, or possession of marijuana is still a felony in most states and may result in a prison term on conviction.

The "legal pushing" of socially acceptable and widely distributed drugs is big business and involves the liquor and pharmaceutical industries. Alcohol use has resulted in chronic alcoholism for approximately 9 million persons and has contributed to 15,000 deaths and 200,000 traffic injuries yearly. Ten billion barbiturate and amphetamine tablets are produced annually to be prescribed by doctors for health care; yet these, too, are frequently misused. Thus millions of people legally use and abuse purchased or prescribed drugs (alcohol and pharmaceuticals) and millions more illegally use and abuse them.

Clearly, when so many people live in violation of the law, and when abusable substances can be found in almost every home, the law is either not enforced—which is mostly the case—or is enforced selectively. Faced with an impossible task, law enforcement can exercise only token control, taking action only in areas where criminal activity is visible, where drug distribution and use patterns lie outside legitimate big business, or where persons with little influence, prominence, or prestige can be apprehended.

In general we believe that it is futile to seek regulation solely through police efforts. Law enforcement, although given great fiscal support, has been temporary and limited. Perhaps through better education we can seek more effective alternatives for social change.

Basic definitions of drugs and drug abuse
Drugs and medicine

A *drug* may be defined as any chemical agent other than foodstuffs that significantly affects the structure or function of a living organism. All drugs are chemicals or contain chemicals that interact with the complex biochemical system of the human body. Such compounds are also referred to as medicine. *Medicine* is any substance or preparation used in treating disease, whereas a drug is usually defined as any chemical substance that alters bodily functions or structures. In current terminology, medicine usually refers to chemicals used to treat specific ailments, whereas the term *"psychoactive"* drug generally refers to chemicals used to relieve pain or that affect the mind or are mood modifiers. Many thousands of psychoactive drugs are now available and thousands of new ones are on the horizon.

A medicine (drug) then is any substance used to treat illness, protect against disease, or promote better health, whereas a psychotropic or psychoactive drug mainly affects mental processes by producing alterations in states of consciousness. The term "psychotropic," like "psychoactive," refers to drugs with predominent effects on the mind rather than on the body.[7] Such effects are produced by stimulants, depressants, psychotomimetics, and so on. Although we will use psychoactive in this text, use of the term "psychotropic" might be preferred because it has the advantage of being widely employed, has a carefully defined scientific definition, and there is more general agreement as to its meaning.[7]

Functionally, drugs may be grouped into two major overlapping categories: (1) those drugs used for medical purposes (prescribed by a physician for a specific therapeutic effect, such as Seconal or secobarbital for sleep induction) and (2) those that are used for purely social purposes (no specific therapeutic use, such as caffeine in coffee, nicotine in cigarettes, and ethyl alcohol in beer, wine, and hard liquor). The social uses of drugs may be further divided into the categories legal and illegal, since it is clear that people also use drugs for social or nonmedical purposes that are prohibited by the law.

Drugs are chemicals that effect changes in the perceptions, feelings, and behavior of the organism. The kind and extent of these changes depend on the nature of the ingested substance, the amount present in the body at any one time, the route and speed of administration, the physiological characteristics and current physiological state of the individual, the physical and social setting when the substance is ingested, the reason(s) it is taken, and what changes the substance is expected to make in the feelings of the individual (Chapter 4).

Drugs, then, may be viewed as powerful catalysts that induce changes of an exceedingly complex social, psychological, and biochemical nature. Before we describe the role that drugs play in these complex events, all drug-related terms that are in everyday usage must be defined. Either through ignorance or intent, official and unofficial information about psychoactive drugs is often inaccurate, slanted, or hysterical rather than factual. Even the scientific terms used to describe drugs have been given such highly emotional connotations that they are used essentially as accusations. A straightforward, culture-free definition of the words "drug use," "drug misuse," and "drug abuse" is needed.

Drug use, drug misuse, and drug abuse

The term "drug use" means no more than the consumption of a drug. A "drug user" then is just about everybody.

The term "drug misuse" refers to the periodic or occasional improper or inappropriate use of either a social or a prescription drug. Misuse means the *improper* use. For example, society might condone the behavior of a star player of a football team who gets "smashed" (drunk) after losing a game. Yet from a medical point of view, this would still be inappropriate behavior and would be drug (alcohol) misuse, even if society might define such behavior as appropriate under the circumstances. In addition, if this person were underage, his use of alcohol would be illegal drug-taking.

The term "drug abuse" is an epithet as well as a social concept. The user of the term typically writes in whatever meaning it has for him. For many, it simply means the use of some drugs (illegal or illicit) that are more favored by a minority (typically youth) and disfavored by the majority (the older "establishment"). Drug abuse refers to the use of drugs that society has outlawed, in contrast to the use of other abusable drugs that are socially acceptable. For some, drug abuse means the ill effects or unacceptable behavior accompanying certain drug use, as reported by the popular press. For still others, it has strong political overtones and becomes a partisan rallying cry, a call for action to prevent the destruction of the conventional American value system and way of life. Thus the concept of drug abuse has consisted of part myth and part hysteria, obscuring any real understanding of a serious social and medical problem.

Although the term "drug abuse" is used to describe just about any relationship between man and chemical of which someone disapproves, we must take a position that distinguishes certain man-drug relationships as abuse from others that are not abuse. Smith's definition of drug abuse will be used in this book to mean the *use of any drug to the point where it interferes with an individual's health or with his economic or social adjustment.*[24] Notice that this term does not touch on whether or not the use of the drug is legal. By our health-oriented definition, marijuana smoking is not *necessarily* drug abuse, for although an outlawed drug such as heroin does possess a high degree of inherent abuse potential, so do cigarettes and alcohol, which are legal. Our concern is whether drugs are harmful, not whether they are socially acceptable. First we ask, does a substance harm the body? If so, in what ways and to what degree? Does the substance have the capacity to cause either physical or psychological dependency?

Drug addiction, drug dependence, and habituation

Before defining drug dependency, let us first consider the word "addiction." The term has acquired many shades and degrees of meaning; we even speak of being addicted to golf. Clearly the flexibility of modern usage has influenced the preciseness and utility of the word. Dr. Harris Isbell[12] of the Addiction Research Center in Lexington, Kentucky, says that national laws and international treaties imposing special controls on drugs have lumped together substances of such diverse natures that it becomes difficult and confusing to try to discuss these varying forms of drug abuse under a single term. For these reasons, the Expert Committee on Addiction-Producing Drugs of the World Health Organization has recommended that the terms "addiction" and "habituation" be dropped and replaced by the term "*drug dependence.*"

Drug dependence, Dr. Isbell adds, "is defined as a state of psychic and physical dependence, or both, which arises in a person following chronic administration of that drug either periodically or continuously."[12] Since the characteristics of drug dependence will vary with the particular agent involved, and since the damage to the individual and to society will also vary with particular drugs, it is always necessary to specify the particular type of drug dependence in each case. For example, one must speak of drug dependence of the "morphine type" or of the "barbiturate type."

At this point we should distinguish *physical dependence* from *psychological dependence*. In physical dependence, the user experiences acute physical symptoms such as nausea, vomiting, anxiety, watery eyes and nose, withdrawal and abstinence syndrome, and an overwhelming compulsive desire to seek the drug if deprived of it for any period of time. To maintain normal body functioning without discomfort, the drug is needed at regular intervals.

In psychological dependence, or what we still like to term "habituation" (despite the WHO definition), the individual demonstrates a strong emotional motivation to continue the use of a drug either because of the pleasure that it gives, or because it relieves real or imagined discomfort. If the drug is withheld, the user may experience anxiety, but will suffer no acute or otherwise serious physical discomfort. Escape from tension, the dulling of unpleasant reality, and euphoria (being "high") are some of the other reasons drugs come to be used habitually. (To this end they may even prove to exert significant therapeutic properties.)

Unfortunately such drugs often contribute their own dependence, the inner need for repeated use. Nicotine in cigarettes, alcohol, caffeine, marijuana, and amphetamines, each of which possesses no inherent addictive properties, are all often involved in psychological drug dependence and often result in injury to body tissue as well.

Psychological dependence on a drug is not necessarily abuse, although it might become so. Psychological dependence is what we are referring to when we say that a person has a bad "habit." Nail biting and cigarette smoking (particularly chain smoking) are compulsive habits suggesting psychological dependence. That regular, first cup of coffee to start the morning is a type of dependence. Yet there is nothing inherently addicting in the drugs in coffee. The body and the mind, however, may be habituated to the ritual of drinking as well as to the lift that caffeine produces. Navy chiefs and Scandinavians have in common a reputation for the use of coffee bordering on the excess. Coffee drinking becomes a compelling social ritual. But the drinking of coffee is also associated with allergies and kidney malfunction, making its habitual use a health problem for some people, and thus, drug abuse.

When cigarette smoking is associated with spells of coughing, poor health, emphysema, and even cancer, then its sustained use also constitutes drug abuse. Millions of Americans, in increasing numbers, are abusing cigarettes despite substantial medical evidence documenting their danger (Chapter 4). Since such a wide variety of substances consumed by humans on a daily basis are capable of inducing this same psychological dependence, we believe that, as a conceptual aid, the term "habituation" is useful, since it strongly suggests a habit!

In closing our discussion of drug dependence, we hope it is understood that there is not simply one unified phenomenon that can be labeled drug dependence. A variety of different types of drug dependence exists, each having its own typical syndrome of use or abuse. Each of the drugs that we will discuss has specific characteristics, particular problems associated with it, and often a particular style of use and social setting, or lifestyle. Therefore the common or general term "drug abuse" has extremely limited relevance or utility.

SUMMARY OF DRUG TERMS

The World Health Organization Expert Committee on Addiction-Producing Drugs created the following definitions that are used worldwide*:

addiction A state of periodic or chronic intoxication produced by the repeated consumption of a

---

*Drug dependence, its significance and characteristics, W.H.O. Bull. **32**:721-723, 1965.

drug and involving tolerance, psychological dependence, usually physical dependence, an overwhelming compulsion to continue using the drug, and detrimental effects on both the individual and society. Its characteristics include (1) an overpowering desire or need (compulsion to continue taking the drug and to obtain it by any means); (2) a tendency to increase the dose; (3) a psychic (psychological) and generally a physical dependence on the effects of the drug; and (4) detrimental effects on the individual and society.

dangerous drugs A legal term that applies specifically to barbiturates, amphetamines, and other drugs (except narcotics) which are officially determined to have a potential for abuse because of their depressant, stimulant, or hallucinogenic effect on man.

desire (for drugs) A persistent but not overpowering wish for a drug to an undeniable compulsion to take the drug and to obtain it by any means.

drug A medicine or a substance used in the making of medicine and when used within the context of the illegal use of drugs, has been interchanged freely with the term "narcotics."

drug abuse The illegal self-administration of drugs, narcotics, chemicals, and other substances to the possible detriment of the individual, of society, or of both.

drug dependence A state arising from repeated administration of a drug on a periodic or continuous basis.

habituation A condition, resulting from the repeated consumption of a drug, which involves little or no evidence of tolerance, some psychological dependence, no physical dependence, and a desire (but not a compulsion) to continue taking the drug for the feeling of well-being that it engenders. Its characteristics include (1) a desire (but not a compulsion) to continue taking the drug for the sense of improved well-being which it engenders; (2) little or no tendency to increase the dose; (3) some degree of psychic dependency on the effect of the drug, but absence of physical dependence and hence of an abstinence syndrome; and (4) detrimental effects, if any, primarily in the individual.

physical dependence A condition in which the body has adjusted to the presence of a drug and, when forced to function without the drug, reacts with a characteristic illness, called "abstinence syndrome," or "withdrawal illness."

psychic dependence The individual who receives satisfaction from his first use of a drug tends to make repeated use of the drug. Through continued repetition he may find it necessary to utilize the drug as an instrument in his adjustment to life, relying upon it for fulfillment which others achieve without the help of drugs.

tolerance A condition in which body cells protect themselves against toxic substances by developing resistance to them. Tolerance is manifested when repeated doses of the same amount of a drug become diminishingly effective and progressively larger doses are required to secure the desired effect.

COMMONLY ABUSED DRUGS

Although we will be dealing at much greater length in Chapter 5 with various categories of drugs and individual drug syndromes, the following will briefly introduce five important categories of widely abused drugs. They are the central nervous system stimulant group; the central nervous system (sedative-hypnotic) depressant group with its subgroup of inhalants, the volatile hydrocarbons; the psychedelic or hallucinogenic group; the narcotic drugs; and finally, the common over-the-counter or nonprescription drugs.

Central nervous system stimulant drugs

A serious drug abuse problem among middle-class youth is the use and abuse of the central nervous system stimulant drugs, our first category of abusable drugs. This group consists largely of the amphetamines, of which methamphetamine is the most commonly used. Cocaine, a central nervous system stimulant used in medicine as a local anesthetic, is another drug in this group that is growing in popularity. It has the same abuse potential as the amphetamines and can produce both a cocaine psychosis and a cocaine anxiety reaction. However, because of its high cost and low availability, cocaine is less widely abused than the amphetamines. Methamphetamine (Methedrine, Desoxyn), or "speed" and "crystal" as it is called on the street, stimulates all parts of the central nervous system. "Meth" excites the individual, suppresses his appetite, and prevents him from sleeping, particularly when injected rather than taken orally (oral use of amphetamines is much more common than intravenous use). Because of the massive stimulation of the nervous system by the amphetamines and perhaps indirectly because appetite and sleep patterns are disturbed, prolonged use of these compounds may cause a state of acute toxic psychosis.

Toxic psychosis, a major break with reality, may be characterized by hallucinations, tremendous panic or fear reactions, and paranoia to a point where the indivudal feels that various individuals are trying to harm him. One does not become physically dependent on the central nervous system stimulants in the classic sense of the word. However, when prolonged dosage is discontinued, the individual falls into a state of exhaustion, then eats ravenously, and then often lapses into a prolonged depressive reaction.[24]

Minor stimulants. The nicotine contained in cigarette tobacco places cigarettes in the category of minor stimulants. Although it is the nicotine that gives the physiological lift to the smoker, it is the high temperature of the gases inhaled by the smoker and the tar and particulates that cause most of the serious health problems. It is estimated that approximately 50 million people in the United States smoke tobacco cigarettes, and a large number of these individuals suffer heart and lung disease as a consequence of their smoking. As stated by DuPont, "Alcohol and nicotine are the two most widely used drugs in the United States today and the number one and number two drug problems in American society. Efforts should be encouraged to integrate broader health care programs for both treatment and prevention, focusing on the broader topic of substance abuse rather than narrowly focusing on just illegal drugs."*

Caffeine is another widely used minor stimulant consumed primarily in the form of coffee, although it is formed as the psycho-

active drug in such over-the-counter drugs as No-Doz and in soft drinks such as Coca-Cola. Caffeine used in excess can produce chronic anxiety and may aggravate heart disease.

Central nervous system depressant (sedative-hypnotic) drugs

The second major category is central nervous system depressants, or sedative-hypnotics. The most commonly abused sedative, which may lead to chronic physical dependence, is ethyl alcohol. Alcohol still represents the biggest drug problem in the United States. It, and not the psychedelics, is the major problem drug with school-age youngsters.

Alcohol. In the United States, ethyl alcohol is the most widely used social drug; it is legal and accepted by our culture. Used in large amounts, alcohol leads to a state of acute intoxication, in which the depression of various elements of the central nervous system seriously interferes with the individual's motor and mental functioning. As now recognized, the disease of alcoholism is one in which chronic, repeated intoxication with alcohol has seriously compromised the individual's ability to function normally or to be casual about his drinking. It is important to note that one can become physically dependent on alcohol. Physical dependence is present if the use of a drug reaches the point where the body's metabolism depends on that agent in order to function. If that particular chemical agent is withdrawn, a physical abstinence syndrome is seen, characterized by extreme anxiety, hyperactivity, and often hallucinations. The most severe withdrawal state seen in medicine today is that of withdrawal from alcohol, not heroin. Delirium tremens, a physical condition caused by abrupt withdrawal during physical dependence on alcohol, is responsible for a high death rate. Persons in the final stages of alcoholism often die of delirium tremens.

Millions of Americans are addicted to alcohol. In the United States it is the foremost addictive drug; yet because of public demand

---

*White Paper on Drug Abuse, A Report to the President from the Domestic Council Drug Abuse Task Force, September, 1975, Washington, D.C., U.S. Government Printing Office.

an age limit is the only restriction placed on its use.

Alcohol abuse produces more problems than all other drugs combined and is the leading drug abuse problem among young people. Unfortunately, it is also increasing among the youth population; the trend is more and more toward drug mixing, such as alcohol and other sedative-hypnotic combinations, or alcohol and marijuana. Alcohol can produce an overdose crisis and, when consumed in high dosages, can produce physical dependence. Crisis intervention may be necessary as well as detoxification from alcohol addiction. Aftercare treatment modalities are varied and range from the use of Antabuse to Alcoholics Anonymous. All of these techniques are described in greater detail in subsequent chapters. In addition, the reader is directed to an excellent book by Becker and co-workers, developed at San Francisco General Hospital, for more information on the alcohol problem and what to do about it.*

Barbiturates. Other commonly abused sedatives are the barbiturates. Prescribed by physicians for sleep or relaxation, these agents are commonly abused by adults. The use of the barbiturates can produce a state of disinhibition similar to that caused by excessive dosages of alcohol. The user may also consume the drug repeatedly, taking progressively larger doses to the point where he also becomes physically dependent. Withdrawal from barbiturates presents a severe medical situation and can result in convulsions and death. In fact, withdrawal from sedatives generally is more dangerous than withdrawal from heroin. Withdrawal from barbiturates, as from alcohol, may be a life-or-death matter.

Inhalants—the volatile hydrocarbons. Other types of sedatives include the volatile hydrocarbons, which are inhalants. For example, certain young people sniff glue and a variety of other substances such as gasoline, kerosene, and paint thinner. This is

*Becker, C. E., Roe, R. L., and Scott, R. A.: Alcohol as a drug: a curriculum on pharmacology, neurology and toxiocology, New York, 1974, Medcom Press.

actually inhalation of an anesthetic-like chemical, toluene, which in higher vapor concentrations depresses the central nervous system and causes many of the same abuse problems as alcohol. Such sedative abuse is a problem in certain school areas and in lower socioeconomic groups, although youth involved in the hippie subculture use few sedatives and, in general, reject alcohol as a primary intoxicant, along with the inhalants. Inhalants are typically abused by younger brothers and sisters who cannot obtain more sophisticated drugs.[13] Unfortunately, there is a growing trend among youth toward drug mixing or polydrug abuse. Increased adverse drug reactions are seen with this pattern, particularly when alcohol is mixed with other sedative-hypnotics.

Psychedelic (hallucinogenic) drugs

LSD (lysergic acid diethylamide) is the prototype of the psychedelic or hallucinogenic drugs, a new group of selective central nervous system stimulants. The use of this relatively new drug has spread widely among middle-class youth throughout the nation, and there are potentially hundreds of LSD-like chemicals that can be assembled from a variety of laboratory, plant, and animal sources. For example, LSD is made in the chemical laboratory and is a semisynthetic derivative of ergot, a mold of rye grain. Mescaline, which produces LSD-like mental effects, is derived from the peyote cactus. Bufotenine, another psychedelic substance, is derived from an animal source—the skin of a toad.

A dose of LSD as small as 250 micrograms (this amounts to only a speck that could rest on the head of a pin) generates startling perceptual alterations, synesthesia (the translation of one sensory phenomenon into another, such as feeling color or sound, or hearing light), and other major psychological changes that can last for up to 8 hours. For example, an individual under the influence of LSD may see colored vibrations coming from music produced by a record player. He may experience disorientation in time and place. Cognitive changes produce striking alterations in value judgments and severely disorient the user. Such disorientations may or may not be perceived as pleasurable.

Because of the action of LSD on the central nervous system, the individual, in fact, sees and perceives his environment in a way that he has never seen it before. Many individuals describe this as a valuable experience, but many others have what they consider a "bad trip." That is, the perceptual alterations produce panic to the point where the individual, under the influence of LSD, loses control of his mental processes and reacts in a manner often destructive to himself. Subjectively he might be described as "crazy." To predict which individuals will react positively to LSD and which individuals will react negatively is difficult because such an equation involves not only the drug itself, but also the personality of the individual as well as the setting in which he takes the drug. The drug trip may change from minute to minute. The use of LSD in unsupervised circumstances increases the likelihood of an adverse reaction.

Two patients illustrate the different types of reactions one sees with unsupervised LSD use. A 19-year-old girl from a middle-class background in her second year of college had used alcohol, occasionally smoked marijuana, but never used any other drug. She was vaguely unhappy with school, but described no other mental problems and had no history of psychiatric care. One day she was given some LSD by a friend. Although she knew nothing about the chemical, she took the drug and described the experience as beneficial, or a good trip. No long-term residual effects followed this drug experience.

In the second example a 19-year-old boy of a similar background was persuaded by a friend to take LSD in an equally casual fashion. After taking the drug, he became frightened. The perceptual alterations and distortions he observed in his environment (everyone looked like a meaningless body) made this reaction a bad trip. After recovery, he continued to feel that life was meaningless

and developed a severe depression, resulting in an attempt at suicide. Ten months after his experience with LSD, the boy was still significantly depressed and under psychiatric care.

Marijuana. Where does marijuana belong in this discussion of sedatives and narcotics? Marijuana is pharmacologically *not* a narcotic and *does not* produce physical dependence. Whether or not it is a psychedelic drug is a subject of argument even among experts and many authorities believe it is a sedative-hypnotic similiar to nitrous oxide.* Among middle-class youth the drug is used primarily because in limited doses it produces a mild euphoria and is a pleasant relaxant. Occasionally, as with alcohol, an individual may take large doses and achieve a classic state of intoxication with central nervous system depression.

Marijuana and its various preparations are known by different names all over the world. The weed marijuana *(Cannabis sativa)* grows just about everywhere. Known and used for its special properties over the centuries, marijuana is grown as a commercial crop (although it is classed as a weed) in Mexico, India, Nepal, Ceylon, and Afghanistan. It grows wild and is illegally cultivated in the United States as well. There is evidence of Chinese hemp cultivation as early as 3000 B.C., but whether or not is was raised for its psychoactive properties is unknown. Historically, its commercial uses have been as the fiber for hemp ropes and for the oil from its seeds.[5]

Until a decade or so ago, the use of the drug marijuana in the United States was limited to nonwhite minorities, primarily Mexican-Americans who brought the habit with them from Mexico, and to a few avantgardes and jazz musicians. Smoking marijuana was not prestigious and was considered the vice of the criminal and the degenerate. Violence and sadism were attributed to its

*Meyers, F. H.: Pharmacological effects of marijuana. In: Smith, David E., editor: The new social drug: legal, cultural and medical perspectives on marijuana, Englewood Cliffs, N.J., 1970, Prentice-Hall, Inc.

use as with heroin. Marijuana users were classified with the worst dope fiends, and legal penalties, until the present, have been severe.[3,21]

Pharmacology. From a health viewpoint, the abuse potential of marijuana is less than other social drugs such as alcohol. The use of marijuana among both middle-class youth and adults of today is similar to that of alcohol by the older generation. It is a social drug that is taken in group settings for its mild high, or intoxication. Prolonged or heavy dosage of marijuana can produce impairment of physical or mental functioning, although most of the marijuana available is of too low a concentration to cause such reactions. In contrast to alcohol, marijuana does not suppress appetite nor does one become physically dependent on the drug. From a health viewpoint, it is ironic that in many states the possession of one drug, marijuana, is a crime, and indeed a felony upon conviction of a second offense, yet possession of another drug, alcohol, which has many similar properties and even greater demonstrated abuse potential, is socially accepted. This suggests, perhaps, a need for more rational criteria in making judgments about drugs. In recent years, more states have moved to decriminalize personal possession of marijuana in order to reduce the negative consequences of criminalization on the individual and to allow society to concentrate its financial resources on more serious drug problems.

Narcotic drugs

The fourth major category of drug abuse includes drugs of the narcotic type, the most common of which is heroin. Narcotics include the opium derivatives such as morphine, semisynthetic opiates such as heroin, and the purely synthetic opioids such as Demerol, the chemical name of which is meperidine. Heroin, as with other morphine-like analgesics, is a narcotic derived from the sap of the opium poppy.

Opium. Long known to man, perhaps as long as 6000 or 7000 years, opium has probably been the most singularly important herbal medicine in history. It is almost a magic drug in the way in which it relieves pain, replacing suffering with a feeling of euphoric well-being. The juice of the opium poppy *(Papaver somniferum)* not only has solved many medical problems but also has served to maintain the credibility of early and rather unreliable medicine. Besides its other euphoric properties, opium induces sleep and corrects dysentery.[20]

Pharmacology. Prolonged or regular use of the opium drugs alters body chemistry so that the organism's metabolism becomes dependent on its continued use. If use of the addicting chemical is discontinued, a disruptive general physiological reaction called the abstinence syndrome occurs. The body hunger for the addicting drug may produce great mental and physical discomfort. In the case of heroin addiction, acute discomfort may occur over a period of several days unless relieved by the administration of the addictive drug or various other psychoactive drugs that help alleviate the withdrawal symptoms. These symptoms do pass after several days, but the psychological craving for this drug of choice and for the life-style surrounding it may persist for months or even years.

Heroin addiction used to be associated primarily with the youth of the economically and socially deprived areas, that is, the ghettos of the Negro and Mexican-American communities. It appears that young persons who become addicted to heroin utilize the drug as an escape from their poverty-striken surroundings. Today heroin use is found increasingly in many of our schools and is one of the most significant and serious drug problems among the middle-class youth of school age. One of the major problems of addiction, or of dependency, is that the user must have the drug on a regular basis or experience a physical and mental crisis. In some types of drug dependence, such as with some sedative-hypnotics, rapid withdrawal of the drug may precipitate a life-threatening emergency for the user. One addicted to barbiturates, or "downers," as they are called by youth (Seconal or Nembutal, the generic drugs secobarbital and pentobarbital, respectively), may lapse into coma and convulsions and, in extreme cases, may die.

With narcotics such as heroin, withdrawal (that is, deprivation of the drug) will cause moderate to severe discomfort, depending on how much pure drug the user is accustomed to ingesting. Moderate withdrawal typically causes aching muscles, nausea, cramps, and vomiting. This may be accompanied by the symptoms of flu—runny nose, runny eyes, muscle cramps, and general malaise. Rarely is such withdrawal of narcotics life threatening, but the process fosters a strong emotional and physical resistance to "getting off dope." Death may also result from an overdose of heroin, a situation causing respiratory depression and heart stoppage, but death is not usually precipitated by withdrawal.

Because of increased physical tolerance, the narcotic user may continue to maintain his drug habit long past the point where he no longer gets a thrill, or euphoric effect. He keeps using drugs, in large part, because such use helps him avoid the discomfort of withdrawal and because it has become a habit and a way of life.

Criminalizing the heroin addict has not proved to be an effective solution to the narcotics problem and has driven the cost of heroin so high that the average habit of an addict costs $50 per day. The narcotics addict often resorts to property theft or prostitution to support a habit, thus making a substantial contribution to crime in the United States. Currently there is discussion of decriminalizing heroin possession and setting up heroin maintenance programs to reduce the cost of addiction to society and better help the addict.*

Over-the-counter or nonprescription drugs

Our last major category is the over-the-counter drugs. When considering categories of drugs that are the source of considerable abuse, this category is almost always over-

*The Drug Abuse Council: Heroin maintenace: the issues. Community approaches to drug abuse treatment and rehabilitation, J. Psychedelic Drugs 6(2), April-June, 1974.

looked, or at best, given little consideration. Few books on drug abuse, in fact, even mention the over-the-counter drugs. The limited coverage of this area in this volume is not intended to minimize the extensiveness and importance of the use of these substances (see Chapter 1). They are readily available and abuse does occur with some degree of frequency. Further information about these medications may be found in the *Handbook of Non-Prescription Drugs.* [10]

Chemical comforters, as Nowlis[19] states, change the way a person feels about himself and the world, which says as much about the world in which the user lives as it does about the drug he chooses. The largest number of these chemical comforters, or mood-altering drugs, are the over-the-counter pain relievers, tranquilizers, antidepressants, antianxiety drugs, stimulants, and sedatives found in almost every medicine cabinet in the nation. An enormous variety of these nonprescription preparations is used by millions of Americans on a daily basis. The essential difference between prescription drugs and proprietary (over-the-counter or nonprescription) drugs is the provision in the latter case for self-diagnosis.

Providing drugs for self-medication is currently at least a $2.5 billion a year industry. [10] Over-the-counter (which we shall refer to from here on as OTC) preparations are chemicals considered to be safe for general unsupervised use by the public. These are drugs of a relatively mild nature used to treat minor "everyday" (the ads say) ailments. The directions for use provided in the package or on the label of each product are considered sufficient to protect the consumer and to direct proper usage.

One assumption now being challenged is that OTC drugs are weak enough that abuse potential in all cases is extremely limited. Recent investigations, however, disclose that these drugs, when used in high dosage, may be abused, are being abused, can be toxic, and can even be lethal. All OTC drugs have multiple effects, depending on the dose and the physical as well as the psychological and social setting of the user. All of these drugs have side effects that may be serious. At higher and higher dosage levels, all may be dangerous. Many of them should be taken rarely or not at all. Few healthy persons, for example, should have to regularly use laxatives or sleep inducers.[15]

Aspirin. One of the most widely used medicines in the world is aspirin. Americans consume nearly 30 million pounds annually—almost 7 pounds per person per year. More than 1000 medical products sold in the United States contain aspirin. Also, some 200 deaths annually in this country result from overdoses of aspirin, with children the most frequent victims. This drug, invaluable as it is, often is misused. Pathologically, aspirin causes minute hemorrhages in the viscera and affects the central nervous system. Excessive use has been linked to kidney damage, ulcers, and anemia. The symptoms of aspirin poisoning are headache, dizziness, ringing in the ears and loss of hearing, nausea, vomiting, gastric hemorrhage, mental confusion, and, in some instances, convulsions, delirium, and coma. Severe cases are difficult to treat and require highly specialized medical care and laboratory examinations.

Antihistamines. There are few cough syrups that do not contain antihistamines. Antihistamines dry the mucus of the respiratory tract and may be helpful in the early congestive stages of the common cold. They are mild sleep inducers and often act as minor tranquilizers (that is, they counteract tension without acting on the central nervous system). Antihistamines also relieve symptoms of hay fever and other allergies, motion sickness (Dramamine is an antihistamine), insomnia, and Parkinson's disease.

Habitual or excessive use of antihistamines may result in drowsiness, dizziness, ringing in the ears, lack of coordination, fatigue, blurred or double vision, euphoria, nervousness, insomnia, and tremors. There may also be a loss of appetite, nausea, vomiting, abdominal pain, constipation or diarrhea, dryness of the mouth, urinary frequency and burning, headache, tightness of the chest, heaviness, and weakness of the hands.

Cough medicine. Cough remedies are among the most common nonprescription drugs available. All are mixtures containing from two to five or more drugs, including antitussives, antihistamines, expectorants, and decongestants. Cough elixirs (not syrups) are sometimes used as "kick-inducers." Some mixtures may contain as much as 50% ethyl alcohol (the equivalent of 100-proof whiskey). Since many states still have no limitation on the purchase of these cough mixtures, many medical authorities believe they should be made prescription items because of their abuse potential.

Diet pills. Dieting has become an American way of life. In their compulsion to lose weight, people are often indiscriminate in their use of the many popular OTC diet pills. The major ingredients of these nonprescription preparations are stimulants that act on the body in various ways. For example, sugar substitutes such as saccharin are widely used, although they have been known to have a harmful effect on children, pregnant women, and persons with kidney failure.

Diuretics, used in diet preparations, purge the body of excess water, but they have a wide range of possible side effects, including rash, headache, constipation, dizziness, restlessness, fatigue, sweating, and a tingling feeling in the arms and legs. On rare occasions convulsions and blood and kidney diseases have developed. Diuretics can also frequently cause the user to lose too much natural salt. Although an individual may lose weight using a diuretic, this effect is temporary. The body will usually begin to retain water once again when its use is discontinued.

Caffeine. Long-haul truck drivers and students are the most flagrant, although hardly the sole, abusers of the popular OTC pep pill preparations such as No-Doz, Vivarin, and Comeback. These nonprescription drugs are concentrated caffeine preparations, although they contain less caffeine than the average cup of coffee.

Commercial or industrial caffeine is a white powder obtained from tea leaves. If taken orally, it stimulates the cortex of the brain, temporarily increasing alertness. The user thinks faster and performs mental functions more easily. In short, he is more awake. The sense of touch is intensified and drowsiness and fatigue disappear for a while. Caffeine, however, is habit forming. Moreover, large doses may cause rapid and irregular heart action, muscle twitching, agitation, and possibly even convulsions. Caffeine also stimulates the flow of gastric juices and should not be used by persons with peptic ulcers. Caffeine certainly is no substitute for rest.

Sleeping pills. There are countless sleep-inducing prescription drugs such as barbiturates, but numerous sleeping aids such as Sominex can be purchased over the counter. Such preparations usually contain an antihistamine (methapyrilene hydrochloride) to induce drowsiness and scopolamine, an anticholinergic drug that has a number of sedative properties. Sleeping pills, after prolonged use, generally disrupt healthy, normal sleeping habits. Possible side effects of sleeping pills include blurred vision, rapid pulse, dizziness, and drying of the mouth. Excessive doses of scopolamine and methapyrilene in the form of these nonprescription relaxants can produce delirium. Medical researchers have studied recent cases in which patients who took popular brand-name sleeping pills suffered toxic reactions that appeared to be the early stages of acute schizophrenia. There is no conclusive evidence to indicate that their disorders resulted from the drug, although it may have helped precipitate the psychotic reaction.

Influence of mass media

We have mentioned just a few of the OTC drugs, one category of abusable substances, and the dangers inherent in their use. The researchers Mannheim and Mellinger,[15] studying patterns of legal family drug use, found American medicine cabinets and bathroom shelves practically pharmaceutical houses, stocking every imaginable drug. From diet pills to headache powders, the average American home is a drugstore. Industry promotes such use. The mass media expend large sums of money selling drug

products to the public. They create a belief structure in which the normal, accepted way to achieve pleasure, health, happiness, relief from life's pains and anxieties, as well as to achieve sexual prowess is to smoke, drink, eat, or swallow a drug. Do the media have impact? Particularly, do the media have impact on youth?

During 1969, Dr. Donald Kanter, then professor of consumer psychology at the University of Southern California, served as a research consultant to the Coronado Unified School District in a study to clarify for educators the processes that occur when drug advertising (direct or indirect) impinges on students.[11] The results of this initial research with hundreds of students clearly indicated, "There is no doubt . . . that there is a relationship between drug use and certain kinds of advertising. . . . The nature of the relationship is complex."

1. Drug and cigarette advertising affects the very young (subteens) and encourages them to experiment with certain palliatives.
2. Experimenting takes the form of increasing dosage, to see what kind of a kick can be obtained.
3. Pleasure and relief are depicted in many advertisements, particularly drug and cigarette commercials. These depictions of relief and personal satisfaction acts as reinforcing agents to general teenage usage.
4. Teenage initial experimenting and drug advertising do not seem directly related; but early excessive usage of Bufferin, Midol, etc., widely advertised products, could be the seedbed for later experimentation. "To ignore advertising's reinforcing function in the general world of the teen-ager as well as the subteen seems also incorrect."

SUMMARY

It should now be apparent that drug abuse is a much broader issue than it is popularly understood to be. Most persons wish to see drug abuse as only the misbehaving of the young despite the fact that our entire society indulges in temperate drug use and also in drug abuse. Most people support the myth that they themselves would never succumb to what are assumed to be the temptations that drugs hold only for the evil or the degenerate. The doper, the junkie, and even the chronic alcoholic are seen as almost an untouchable caste, a population of deviants with some inherent character flaw that makes them deserve what they get because they are immoral, weak willed, or have criminal leanings.

Yet anyone, given the right set of circumstances, might become a junkie or a chronic drug user and many people have who do not even recognize the extent of their own involvement. Much of our current understanding about drugs and the young is hypocritical. One need only examine the statistics on the number of conventional housewives who are abusing amphetamines and barbiturates as well as alcohol. Society, for unexplained reasons, still seems reluctant to accept the responsibility for creating and sustaining conditions that both encourage addictive behavior and work aggressively against attempts at therapeutic modification. Addiction and dependence and habituation are primarily social and health issues, not criminal ones.

REFERENCES

1. Bauer, W. W.: Today's health guide: a manual of health information and guidance for the American family, Chicago, 1965, American Medical Association.
2. Becker, C. E., Roe, R. L., and Scott, R. A.: Alcohol as a drug: a curriculum on pharmacology, neurology and toxicology, New York, 1974, Medcom Press.
3. Blum, R. H.: Society and drugs, San Francisco, 1969, Jossey-Bass, Inc., Publishers.
4. Carey, J. T.: The college drug scene, Englewood-Cliffs, N.J., 1968, Prentice-Hall, Inc.
5. Chein, I., and others: The road to H; narcotics, delinquency, and social policy, New York, 1964, Basic Books, Inc., Publishers.
6. Cornacchia, H. J.: Consumer health. St. Louis, 1976, The C. V. Mosby Co.
7. DiPalma, J. R., editor: Drill's pharmacology in medicine, New York, 1971, McGraw-Hill Book Co.
8. The Drug Abuse Council: Heroin maintenance: the issues. Community approaches to drug abuse

treatment and rehabilitation, J. Psychedelic Drugs 6(2), April-June, 1974.
9. Goldfarb, J.: The medieval legacy of crime and delinquency, speech delivered at the School of Criminology, University of California at Berkeley, 1967.
10. Handbook of non-prescription drugs, Washington, D.C., 1976, American Pharmaceutical Association.
11. Kanter, D.: Innovative solution to teen- and sub-teen-age drug abuse, 1968-70, from material prepared under the Elementary and Secondary Education Act, Title III Project by Coronado Unified School District.
12. Isbell, H.: Paper presented at the International Physicians' Conference on Drug Abuse, University of Michigan, Ann Arbor, Nov., 1970.
13. Kitzinger, A.: Narcotics and dangerous drugs: a manual of basic information for teachers, Sacramento, 1964, California State Department of Education.
14. Lindesmith, A. R.: The addict and the law, Bloomington, 1965, Indiana University Press.
15. Mellinger, G. D.: Society's dilemma: pills, pills, pills, unpublished paper presented to the Contra Costa Mental Health Association, Diablo Valley College, May 25, 1967.
16. Meyers, F. H.: Pharmacological effects of marijuana. In Smith, D. E., editor: The new social drug: legal, cultural, and medical perspectives on marijuana, Englewood Cliffs, N.J., 1970, Prentice-Hall, Inc.
17. National Commission on Marijuana and Drug Abuse: Marijuana: a signal of misunderstanding, first report of the Commission, Washington, D.C., 1972, U.S. Government Printing Office.
18. Nixon, R. M.: Quoted in San Jose Mercury News, San Jose, Calif., Mar. 21, 1972.
19. Nowlis, H.: Perspectives on drug use, J. Soc. Issues 27:7, 1971.
20. Over the counter drugs—easy does it. In Attack, Spring 1971.
21. Ray, O. S.: Drugs, society, and human behavior, St. Louis, 1972, The C. V. Mosby Co.
22. Skolnick, J. H.: The politics of protest, New York, 1969, Ballantine Books.
23. Smith, D. E., and Bentel, D. J.: Drug Abuse Information Project, the third and fourth annual reports to the legislature, San Francisco, 1969-1970, University of California, San Francisco Medical Center.
24. Smith, D. E., and Luce, J.: Love needs care, Boston, 1971, Little, Brown & Co.
25. Smith, D. E., and others: The free clinic: a community approach to health care and drug abuse, Beloit, Mich., 1972, Stash Press.
26. White Paper on Drug Abuse. A Report to the President from the Domestic Council Drug Abuse Task Force, Washington, D.C., September, 1975, U.S. Government Printing Office.

3
Psychosocial factors and the adolescent

The misuse and abuse of drugs by young people involve a variety of psychological and sociological factors that need understanding in order to be familiar with the drug problem. No attempt herein will be made to completely segregate the psychological from the sociological aspects because both are frequently interrelated and such a separation would be impossible. Instead those essentials will be identified that should be known and utilized by school and community personnel in their drug programs.

PATTERNS OF DRUG ABUSE

The patterns of drug abuse, particularly among adolescents and disaffiliated youth, have changed dramatically in the last 10 years, as discussed in Chapter 1. Prior to the 1960s, whatever constituted drug abuse was relatively constant and predictable, with illegal drug use largely confined to racial, ethnic, and philosophical minorities submerged in urban ghettos. The white middle-class representative of the dominant culture usually restricted his use to alcohol, tobacco, and a few prescription psychoactive drugs.[5]

Contemporary drug-use patterns have become much more widespread and varied. The available evidence suggests that drug use has become a *majority* phenomenon among both youth and adults.[2] Cohen states dramatically, "Even excluding alcohol, coffee and cigarettes, it is now safe to estimate that more than 50% of the total American population over 13 years of age has at least tried some powerful mind-altering drug via prescription or on the illicit market."[6]

In May 1970 the National Institute of Mental Health estimated that there were 125,000 "active narcotic abusers" in the nation. The number of persons directly involved with other dangerous drugs was placed somewhere between one-quarter and one-half million. The number having experimented with marijuana was estimated to be 20 million persons and in 1976 was closer to 30 million. In addition, the Pentagon reported that about 50% of the American troops in Vietnam smoked marijuana. The soldiers themselves say that the percentage was even higher.

Large universities report marijuana use by more than 50% of their undergraduate student bodies. High school, junior high, and even elementary school students are using a variety of drugs and intoxicants at an increasing rate.

Tables 3-1 through 3-3 provide a comparison of marijuana, alcohol, and tobacco use by region and by age between 1971 and 1976, utilizing a study sponsored by the National Institute on Drug Abuse.

In addition to the usual drugs of abuse described in Chapter 2, young persons are continually experimenting with other preparations. Some have smoked catnip, nutmeg,

TABLE 3-1. Marijuana experience (percent)*

	Adults (18+)				Juveniles (12-17)			
	1971	1972	1974	1976	1971	1972	1974	1976
Ever used marijuana	15	16	19	21.3	14	14	23	22.4
Current user (within month)	5	8	7	8.0	6	7	12	12.3
Began smoking within last year†	†	†	2	2.8	†	†	9	8.2

*Response Analysis Corporation: Main findings, part I; Non-medical use of psychoactive substances, RAC 3698B, Sept., 1976, Trenton, N.J. Available through The National Institute on Drug Abuse, Public Information Office, Rockville, Md.
†Not included in 1971 and 1972 surveys.

or oregano or have injected deodorant, milk, or mayonnaise in their reckless search for a high. Not infrequently such experiments result in death.

On the school grounds today there is a readiness to use a wide variety of drugs. Although alcohol, especially wine, is the favored and most consumed intoxicant, almost anything, including heroin, is likely to be used: sniffing of glue, gasoline, and lighter fluid is fairly common. The use of barbiturates and amphetamines begins to develop. The smoking of marijuana enters into the repertoire. If no drugs are available, youngsters—at least some of them—seek out substitutes. We obtained reports of youths using nutmeg or crushed aspirin in cokes, sniffing the vapors of burned plastic combs, consuming the cotton inserts from Vicks and Valo inhalers, smoking tea, injecting wine intravenously, "dropping" amphetamines, barbiturates, and hypnotic compounds, and sniffing paint thinner and a variety of unclassified materials. Recently, there has been an increase in phencyclidine (P.C.P.) abuse among youth. P.C.P. is a dissociative anesthetic used in veterinary medicine which, when used in excess, can produce a toxic psychosis often associated with violent and self-destructive behavior.*

Adults are serious offenders, too. Tens of thousands of adults are being given prescriptions for amphetamines or barbiturates in situations where accepted medical practice

would indicate that the prescription should not have been issued. Many persons with prescriptions for such drugs take them more frequently and in greater doses than their doctors intended. The result is a substantial amount of harm to the individual involved, in many cases leading to irreversible personality damage or near addictive patterns or both, involving extreme dangers to the user and others.

One survey found that 25% of all American women over 30 years of age currently had prescriptions for amphetamines, barbiturates, or tranquilizers; the percentage was found to be as great as 40 to 50% for those of higher income families. Thus we reiterate a point made in other chapters— drug use of some sort has become a *social norm* in our drug-oriented culture. Before there can be real understanding of the drug problem, the concept of drug usage as a minority phenomenon must be discarded. Given the right conditions, almost anyone is susceptible. The popular notions that drug abusers are a distinct breed of people or a separate social group and that they are to be identified as deviants and as willful, aggressive troublemakers must be buried.*

Society's view of drug abuse must change as profoundly as the nature and extent of the drug problem has changed. No longer is it acceptable to label the psychoactive chemicals nicotine and alcohol as nondrugs, thus perpetuating their enormously harmful in-

*Burns, R. S., Lerner, S. E., Corrado, R.: Phencyclidine—states of acute intoxication and fatalities, West. J. Med. **123:**345-349, November 1975.

*White Paper on Drug Abuse. A Report to the President from the Domestic Council Drug Abuse Task Force. Washington, D.C., September, 1975, U.S. Government Printing Office.

TABLE 3-2. Marijuana experience among particular subgroups (percent)*

	Have ever used		Current users	
	1974	**1976**	**1974**	**1976**
Age (adults)				
18-25	53	53	25	25
26-34	29	36	8	11
35-49	7	6 (34+)	1	1 (34+)
50+	2	—	—	—
Age (youth)				
12-13	6	6	2	3
14-15	22	21	12	13
16-17	39	40	20	21
Sex (adults)				
Male	24	29	9	11
Female	14	14	5	5
Sex (youth)				
Male	24	26	12	14
Female	21	19	11	11
Region (adults)				
Northeast	22	24	7	9
North Central	17	19	7	7
South	13	17	4	6
West	29	28	11	11
Region (youth)				
Northeast	26	21	14	13
North Central	21	26	11	16
South	17	16	6	7
West	30	30	19	17
Population density (adult)				
Large metropolitan	25	26	9	9
Other metropolitan	19	23	8	9
Nonmetropolitan	11	13	3	4
Population density (youth)				
Large metropolitan	27	25	14	18
Other metropolitan	22	24	11	11
Nonmetropolitan	18	18	10	8
Education (adults)				
Below high school graduate	9	12	3	4
High school graduate	20	22	7	8
Currently in college	61	48	33	24
Some college completed	27	30	10	12
College graduate	23	30	6	10

*Response Analysis Corporation: Main findings, part I; Non-medical use of psychoactive substances, RAC 3698B, Sept., 1976, Trenton, N.J. Available through The National Institute on Drug Abuse, Public Information Office, Rockville, Md.

TABLE 3-3. Comparison of alcohol, tobacco, and marijuana use (percent)*

	1971	1972	1974	1976
Adults				
Alcohol	74	75	78	85.1
Tobacco	70	67	72	79.5
Marijuana	65	59	68	61.7
Youth				
Alcohol	69	71	78	83.3
Tobacco	58	58	62	61.8
Marijuana	48	50	54	54.3

*Response Analysis Corporation: Main findings, part I; Non-medical use of psychoactive substances, RAC 3698B, Sept., 1976, Trenton, N.J. Available through The National Institute on Drug Abuse, Public Information Office, Rockville, Md.

fluences under the comfortable disguise of respectability, and at the same time to point with alarm and indignation at drug abuse in the youth culture and to demand that offenders and malefactors be rooted out and punished.

This ill-formed, sometimes hypocritical attitude has not worked and will not work in remedying the causes of the current and ominous drug epidemic. Until there is a more realistic understanding of the drug problem there will be no solution.

THE WORLD OF THE ADOLESCENT

To understand the youthful drug abuser one must understand the world of the adolescent with its cultural group life so distinctly different from the adult. Most adults at least vaguely realize that a separate and different adolescent culture exists but the extent of their awareness creates more puzzles than solutions. They may not recognize the world of the adolescent for what it is—a compelling social force often more influential in the life of the youngster than parent, home, or the mores, rules, and practices of adult society.

This is not a condition that youth has deliberately sought. He has been pushed or, perhaps more accurately, sucked into this position to fill a vacuum in his life created by our twentieth century society. Society does not incorporate youth into full membership. Therefore if a young person is to have the group affiliation and status that he needs for his psychological security, he must create his own group with its own rules, standards, and conduct. As Henry has noted:

In many primitive cultures and in the great cultures of Asia, a person is born into a personal community, a group of intimates to which he is linked for life by tradition; but in America everyone must create his own personal community. Where one is born into an inalienable personal community, social appeal is relatively unimportant, but in American culture, where no traditional arrangement can guarantee an indissoluble personal community, every child must be a social engineer, able to use his appeal and his skill at social maneuvering to construct a personal community for himself.*

It is necessary, then, to see the adolescent social system as an ad hoc arrangement by the young for dealing with their own problems or with their peer group.

Two views of adolescence

Two major competing views attempt to define the relationship of the adolescent social system to adult institutions, the transitional or functional and the segregationist. One group holds that adolescence is merely a transitional period whereby youth are gradually socialized into the adult world. This "functional" view sees youth passing through a series of socializing institutions that prepare him for adult life. The other, or "segregationist," view sees the adolescent as segregated from the social institutions of adult life and subordinated to second-class citizenship.

As Smith has put it, "The primary function of youth culture is that of bringing the normal movement of youth from the parental family to the marital family."[22] According to this functional view, adolescence is a transitional period wherein young persons are weaned from the dependent situation of a child to the independent status of an adult. Adolescent deviance, including the abuse of outlawed drugs, is understood in terms of blocked access to adult status and adult com-

*From Henry, J.: Culture against man, New York, 1963, Random House, Inc.

modities. In fact, Bloch and Niederhoffer[1] have interpreted adolescent cliques in school and adolescent gang behavior as the functional equivalents of puberty rites in primitive societies. Whereas puberty rites function to prepare youth for adult responsibilities, the gang provides adolescents with the symbolic equivalent of adult behavior denied them in bars, cars, and travel. Because American society has not made adequate preparation for the induction of adolescents into adult status, juvenile delinquency is an attempt, symbolically, to become adult by imitating certain superficial symbols of adulthood. The functionalists, rather than seeing this deprived status as inimical and destructive, see in segregation and powerlessness the necessary preparation and training of young adulthood. Parsons illustrates this point in noting: "At the same time [youth] is frustrated by being deprived of power and influence in the current situation, though it recognizes that such a deprivation is in certain respects essential, if its segregation for purposes of training is to be effective."[16] This is the Protestant ethic of delayed gratification: sacrifice now for future rewards.

The other view of the adolescent is the segregationist one in which the young person is separated from the social institutions of adult life and subordinated to second-class status. One of the functions of the high school, Reuter[19] observed, is to exclude adolescents from meaningful participation (and also competition for the labor market) in society. The trade union movement has been particularly effective in limiting the job market. This segregationist view contends that the proliferation of extracurricular activities (athletics, band, etc.) has operated to contain and entertain adolescents who have no function in the modern economy. Friedenberg[11] draws an analogy with colonial exploitation.

Extensive literature on the historical development of the adolescent social system in our industrial society is available. Under preindustrial conditions, each person was a useful member of society from an early age. This is no longer true as a consequence of two

significant developments: (1) The shocking exploitation of children in eighteenth century industrial England created social pressures for reform, resulting in our contemporary child labor laws. Children are no longer allowed to work as they did in the past. (2) The transition from an agricultural to an industrial economy, with its accompanying shift from rural to urban life, also helped create a marginal, noncontributing adolescent group.

Youth has lost its economic importance as a producer, with an accompanying loss of social position, pride, and self-esteem. The adolescent is a total dependent, with all the internal and external implications inherent in total dependency.

The growth of technology is also significant because it has changed the character of the occupational structure. The need for technical training, requiring years of education, means that occupational knowledge and skills are no longer transmitted from father to son. Most youngsters do not even understand the work their parents do. So the vocational preparation of youth has also passed from the family to the school system.

The inevitable consequences of these various changes have been the removal of an enormous and growing group of young persons from the mainstream of life and the denial to them of meaningful participation in the general community. Youth's self-created alternative is the adolescent society, with its own set of standards and values. In the last decade some of the older youth have become so segregated from the adult world that, as Messer has noted, "The generation gap seems to have widened to the extent that it is now a cultural gap."[15] This cultural gap is most apparent in the proliferation of hippie communes, "long hair" communities such as Haight-Ashbury, and the rapid diffusion of these life-styles to younger adolescents. The parent who puzzles over the generation gap and decries adolescent rejection of his value system fails to grasp the reasons why the dichotomy he so resents has become established. Invariably he will assign the wrong reasons for the emergence of practices unacceptable to his world—including that of drug abuse.

A meeting ground for both functionalist and segregationist positions is found in a consensus among students of adolescence that youngsters are subjected to an overly long and prolonged period of dependency. On that, at least, everyone agrees.

Rationales for drug abuse

Young people may use drugs for one or more of the following general purposes: (1) to achieve detachment from personal problems and troubles and to produce a state of well-being, (2) to establish an involvement with the subculture that offers an identity and an identification in society, and (3) to express hostility toward respectable society and as a protest against the injustices and restrictions imposed by the establishment. These reasons may be and are affected by a variety of psychological and environmental or social influences, including (1) personal conflicts, (2) television, and (3) commercial exploitation.

Personal conflicts

Personal factors involved in drug abuse may center around overwhelming intrapsychic conflict, present especially during adolescence and centered around adult sexuality, hostility, dependency-independency issues, and identity diffusion. These conflicts are the results of demands for conformity placed on the individual by society.

Secondary factors, arising largely from the first group, may include the following:
1. Fear of competition and failure
2. Fear of homosexuality
3. Fear of threatening mental illness or mental disintegration
4. The need to rebel
5. The need to be caught and punished
6. The need to explore the limits of one's body and psyche and to challenge one's resources
7. The need for a hedonistic or orgiastic experience
8. The need to belong to a group or subculture
9. The need for instant relief or instant answers (Chemicals produce the most instant change.)

Television

A constant emphasis on drugs as the solution to every physical and mental problem has created an atmosphere leading to a normality of drug overconsumption that borders on the unreal. This atmosphere is an influencing factor in the drug abuse problem. Television has probably had a profound influence on our habits as drug consumers and has especially impressed the young. As a result of this influence, there is a total diffusion of the drug culture through every social and economic level.

Television is no longer just a machine but has become the national babysitter, the substitute parent, the teacher, the preacher, the indoctrinator, and almost an extension of our bodies. Children spend an enormous amount of time in front of television before they are old enough to select and judge. They are stuck in front of the television set, which then acts as a tranquilizer so that mother can get on with her housework or so that parents may entertain their friends without interruption. On Saturday mornings channels on television are directed at children. By the time a child has reached 6 years of age, he may have seen on television over 20,000 acts of violence. He learns that violence is all right and that death is reversible because, "if the guy gets killed today, he still comes back next Saturday."

The child's fantasies about his own omnipotence are maintained by the fact that he can, at will, change the channel or switch off the program he does not like. Children deprived of communication with their parents or with other children lack the ability to express themselves verbally; their own initiative, inquisitiveness, and exploratory behavior is stifled. They begin to speak in monosyllables and, by identifying with the television set, talk in terms of "turning on," "tuning out," "tuning in," "turning off," and "dropping out." This, of course, has also become the language of the new psychedelic generation.

Society is in endless search of escape; one of the quickest temporary means of escape is drugs. Television offers drugs as the solution to all disaffections of body and mind. Seductive pharmaceutical advertisements promise to make one feel more tranquil, happier, younger, sexier, and more attractive. The advertising industry has for many years employed some of the best psychologists. They know that one good way to persuade people to buy is to promise relief from suffering and from feelings of inadequacy. Sex, strength, youth, and virility are implied; we are gulled into a delusion that chemicals are safe, when many are not.[13]

Commercial exploitation

The continuing intensification of group consciousness among adolescents during the last 25 years has led to their economic exploitation and is another factor related to the drug problem. Business and industry have effectively used the teenage group pressure for conformity to create a multimillion dollar market. The word "teenager" itself seems to have had a commercial origin, recognizing an identifiable subgroup within society that might be exploited.[13]

In 1946 Eugene Gilbert invented a business that involved the sale of information concerning the tastes and behavior of teenagers to commercial organizations. In 1958 MacDonald reported that Gilbert was making between $500,000 and $1 million a year for his services. His clients included Borden's milk, *Seventeen*, Hollywood V-ette, Vassarette brassieres, Van Heusen shirts, and the U.S. Army. In 1944 the magazine for adolescents, *Seventeen*, bulging with advertisements directed at teenagers, published its first issue. In 1958, 17 million teenagers purchased $9.5 billion worth of commodities with their own funds.[14] It is estimated this figure is much higher today.

Advertisers exploit peer-group status and personal insecurities expertly in the promotion of their products. In most instances the appeal is made not to the individual, but to the group; the youngster is reminded again and again that a particular product will enable him to stand in good stead with his peers. He can prevent isolation and minimize that left-out feeling by buying or accepting the commodity being offered.

Advertising offers to solve many adolescent problems—loneliness, sex, intimacy, personal community, instability—through the purchase of commodities such as face creams, perfumes, pimple preparations, hair oils, after-shave lotions, deodorants, soaps, mouthwashes, and shampoos. These products are fetishized solutions to real adolescent problems.

The inevitable consequence of the commercial exploitation of adolescent group psychology has been to intensify the conformity urge. Group drug abuse and the teenage drug epidemic reflect the same kind of motivation that causes the typical teenage girl to own an average of seven bras, the first of which she bought at the age of 13 years.

Psychological motivations

Young people, in their efforts to achieve detachment from personal problems and troubles, identify a number of specific reasons for the use, misuse, and abuse of drugs, including curiosity, peer-group pressure, insecurity, escape, boredom, rebelliousness, and "kicks."

Curiosity. Curiosity about drugs is engendered by our adult drug culture, which includes the use of tobacco, alcohol, tranquilizers, sleeping pills, diet pills, and pep pills, all advertised openly and widely by the media. What other teen- and subteenagers say about the fun they have turning on also creates curiosity.

Peer-group pressure. It is almost becoming a puberty rite to have experimented with drugs by the time one is 13 years old. The real change in recent months has been the large numbers of elementary school children turned on by others in elementary school or by older brothers, sisters, and friends. The "I dare you to" has become simply "why don't you have fun like we do and you can belong to our 'in' group."

Insecurity. A timeless condition among

teenagers has been a sense of insecurity and the desire for affection and identity (recognition). Failing to find security at home, feeling a lack of affection and concern for who and what they are and to whom, teenagers have throughout history resorted to various types of behavior designed to satisfy these needs. In numbers increasing for almost a decade, thousands of insecure young persons have resorted to drugs to find a sense of security, to attain affection (from others in the drug culture), and to identify with peers who are also involved.

Escape. Drugs of all kinds, including marijuana, LSD, hashish, and other psychedelics, have the ability to provide an escape from reality; they can reduce and, for the moment at least, can wipe out the internal conflicts and the normal insecurities of young people (thus preventing these persons from coming to grips with their problems at the time, place, and age where they normally need to "face up" if they are to mature). These persons can escape in this way without losing consciousness, and, for the duration of their high, they can live in a new and marvelous world—one recreated again and again by getting "stoned."

Boredom. Boredom with school or routine living lacking the interest and stimulation to engage the youngster in meaningful experience drives some young persons to drug experimentation.

Rebelliousness. Youth sees drugs as a way to get parents or teachers "up tight," frightened, or anxious, resulting in overreaction by parents, society, school officials, and civic and law enforcement personnel. Instead of curing the situation, this leads to further "bugging" of the adult world by the youngsters, which results in new levels of overreaction (for example, demands for new and more stringent laws and sentences when the present ones are ineffectual and unenforceable).

Risk-taking behavior. Last and probably most important, both for the experimenting young group and for those who become dependent, is using drugs for kicks, substituting synthetic fun for the development of

meaningful relationships with other people. Some youth lose their shyness in this way; through such risk-taking behavior, some lose their drabness or plainness and become, for a time, beautiful and handsome.

Student needs justify behavior

According to some students, drugs aid in the formation of friendships and the development of a better understanding of people. Rap sessions and interpersonal communications are "easier when zonked out on pot." The drugs create an atmosphere of relaxation and pleasure (hedonism). The question is whether the pleasure-to-risk ratio always favors the user.

The enrichment of life that students claim they gain through the use of drugs includes an enhancement of creativity and an increased appreciation of beauty and nature. Drugs are said to have inspired some persons to write, paint, compose music, and perform. It is possible that sensitivity in these areas may be heightened, although this is not the norm.

The contemporary quest for a deeper insight into the self and the universe incorporates the use of drugs. Some students use drugs as a panacea for emotional troubles, as a method for improving one's personality, or to cure hangups. Although chemicals produce the instant results desired, any enlightenment gained is always artificial and does not last. The use of drugs in do-it-yourself psychology has been a two-way street with sometimes traumatic results.

Search for identity

Time and again one hears teenagers asking the questions, phrased according to their age and verbal skills, "Who am I?" and "What am I doing here?" Some social scientists have called this the search for identity or for meaning. More and more young people, freed from considerations of economic survival, find it hard to accept the basic value system that modern civilization has emphasized—materialism and the quest for affluence and material achievement. Less and less are young persons satisfied with a system that seems to push them toward a greater amount of education designed to help them attain more prestigious jobs, leading to higher income and social status. To many teenagers, it makes no sense, especially because it has not led to widespread personal satisfaction and happiness in the adults most visible to them. This rejection of the values associated with material acquisition has led to confusion, to a vacuum in meaningful goals, and to a search for something "inside." Often it is also associated with a low self-concept and an identity crisis, which contributes to drug taking behavior. A further discussion is included in Chapter 9.

Values

Offspring of the middle class are particularly sensitive in perceiving that the "old myths" are unrewarding and meaningless. Members of the psychedelic revolution have been conspicuously concerned with values, with, as they put it, "where we're at." This preoccupation reflects their search for new personal identities and new ideologies to guide their lives.

Since the establishment possesses virtues as well as shortcomings, and those virtues and shortcomings are relative, not absolute, perhaps a different kind of teaching about our national ideals, achievements, and failures would help to counteract the youthful disillusionment that leads to disaffiliation. An honest and forthright examination of our national qualities in social science textbooks and classrooms, in a constructive rather than either a flag-waving or a negative perspective, certainly would provide less basis for a counter-society of hostile, contemptuous youth. Meanwhile a close link exists between the social-cultural attitudes of young persons and their abuse of drugs. This is discussed further in Chapter 7.

Rejection of the culture

Among the young there is widespread disillusionment with American ideals and American values, which appear phony to them in the light of reality. They perceive that the basic American ideologies often clash conspicuously with ongoing practices, and, in the adolescent manner of making absolute judgments from limited or two-dimensional evidence, they cross off entirely the establishment's claims to righteousness.[19] When as conspicuous an example as the Vietnam war involves them personally and acutely, threatening their very existence and trampling on their ideals, rejection of the establishment and everything it stands for results. From this disaffirmation it is an easy, even natural, step to challenge the sanctions against drugs and then to create a rationale of complete justification for their use. In 1967 Blumer touched on this point when he described the collective beliefs of young drug users he had studied:

. . . they viewed with contempt the use of opiates and rejected with evidence the claim that use of harmful drugs led naturally to opiate use. They pointed out that the break-up of home life, with which many of them were very familiar, was due to other factors than the use of drugs; they were able to show that the limitations of their career opportunities came from other conditions than the use of drugs as such. They met the fear of arrest by developing greater skill and precautions against detection in the use of drugs. Added to these stances was a set of collective beliefs that justified their use of drugs, so that such use resulted in harmless pleasure, increased conviviality, did not lead to violence, could be regulated, did not lead to addiction, and was much less harmful than the use of alcohol, which is socially and openly sanctioned in our society.*

An example of how teenage rejection of the American culture has led to drug abuse is in the identification of white students with the "Negro revolt" and their sharing of the Negro and lower class culture. As the civil rights movement developed and the American culture crisis grew in scope, marijuana smoking acquired increasingly political and ideological significance for college students affiliated with the New Left. The transfer of drug habits to the recruit was an inevitable consequence of joining up with causes. The contagiousness of drug abuse amply justifies the term "epidemic" in referring to the lightning spread of its use among youth groups.

The alternate drug scene has an undeni-

---

*From Blumer, H.: The "Ad" Center Project report on drug abuse, Berkeley, 1968, University of California Press.

able attraction for youngsters hard pressed to cope with our enormously complex environment. It appears to offer the same kind of escape from the onerous demands of growing up that the circus offered to youth of a generation or so ago. So many young persons roll up their blankets and take off. On a Friday afternoon they spot the highways from San Francisco to Big Sur, dressed in costumes carefully chosen for their picturesqueness from Salvation Army and Goodwill Industries used clothing racks, thumbing rides to "where the action is." The action includes the use of drugs, and those who join such alternate cultures have been effective intermediaries in transmitting drug usage to the larger youth population.

The use of drugs is an apparent alternative. After all, our culture and communications media teach children that one solves almost all problems by turning on—drugs for headaches, constipation, sleeplessness, "nerves," and for whatever other maladies beset us. Taking drugs is the *common* palliative in our society, not a deviant one. Thus it is difficult to fashion public health approaches without realizing the cultural logic and appeal of mind-altering drugs, although their unlawfulness and uniqueness would seem to set them apart from the mainstream of drug use.

Affluence and permissiveness

Bored teenagers with a car, money, no responsibilities to a family or to the community, and no meaningful or rewarding work easily succumb to the thrill of drug experimentation. These youngsters have little directed play after school or on weekends, no chores, no music lessons, and no scouting tests to pass to strengthen the ego and to gain rewards; they turn to challenging, aberrant behavior, including a whole range of marginal or unacceptable behavior, part of which is the use of drugs. This behavior begins as early as the third grade. The absence of standards of behavior, dress, and speech go along with a lack of zest, challenge, and satisfaction to promote drug abuse. Open and unchallenged violation of laws, morals, and manners, as seen among many adults,

cause a child to question the whole set of social rules and to wonder whether crime does not pay very well indeed.

Since the Civil War there has been a continuing trend toward the elimination of corporal punishment in the rearing of children and an increasing rejection of the stern exercise of parental authority. The earlier puritanical conception of evil saw the child as "damned with all mankind in Adam's fall." This creature of original sin was full of disobedience and rebellion against God's laws. Corporal punishment was necessary to break his congenital will to do evil.

Even at the beginning of this century the baby was a dangerous bundle of impulses that had to be curbed. By the 1940s his aberrant manifestations were viewed more complacently as exploratory gestures by which he learned about the world. The trend since then has been consistently toward less authoritarian discipline and parental domination of children's lives. Increasingly children have been given independence and self-determination within the sphere of the family. "The child should learn to live his own life; his parents cannot live it for him."

Parents have had a traditional role in determining educational policies in the public schools; this has enabled parents to extend into the classroom an insistence on freedom of action for the child without meaningful punishment for transgressions. Whether as a consequence or merely concurrently, the 1950s saw sudden public concern over juvenile delinquency. It has been pointed out that the decline in parental authority could not be blamed for any sudden increase in delinquency because permissiveness had been a long-term, gradual development. Instead, it was suggested, the extension of public education to absorb all economic and racial classes might be the explanation. In 1900 only 11% of the nation's high school age population was in high school; in 1930, 51%; in 1960, over 90%. The majority of these children came from working-class and farm families; these adolescents were found by Coleman[8] to dominate the high school social system. Increasing exposure of middle-class children to this group, it was proposed, was resulting in the adoption of patterns of behavior unacceptable by prevailing white middle-class majority standards. Such behavior was alien, subversive, and consequently threatening. The negative reaction of adults to "rock 'n roll" in the 1950s was based on the alien quality of its sound and delivery, which was of Negro and southern back-country origin.

Whether or not permissiveness was a contributing factor to the youth drug epidemic, the youngster of the 1960s and 1970s who chose or was pressured into the drug scene by his peers had a high degree of autonomy in taking that route. Family pathology, particularly when one or more of the parents is alcoholic, is a major factor in the background of many young drug abusers and family therapy may be needed.

Summary of motives for drug use

There is no need to dwell on the motives leading to drug abuse. Curiosity, social pressure, rebellion against authority, and escape from social and emotional problems, the desire for kicks—all these are relevant in many cases but add little to our capacity to understand the recency and magnitude of contemporary drug abuse. Beyond these obvious aspects are cultural and psychological factors that come to the attention again and again, glibly articulated by college students and teenagers and subconsciously manifested by those in their preteens.

The theme of these factors is disenchantment and alienation, particularly in the area of values. Increasing numbers of young persons have been struck with a sense of futility regarding the basic institutions of society. They charge social and political hypocrisy and reject governmental and social policies that seem headed toward more war, hate, and injustice. Youth has begun to challenge the goals of the educational system that trains them for jobs incapable of guaranteeing personal satisfaction. They criticize parents, citing a basic lack of understanding and discrimination of what is really important. They are put off by organized religion—sym-

bolized by rite and dogma—because it seems to deny inherent human worth and to exist for hypocritical adults who attend church without seeming to be touched with love for God or for their fellow men.

The psychedelic scene is a middle and upper-middle socioeconomic class phenomenon that reflects youth's disillusionment. It operates from material oversufficiency, not economic deprivation. Pot and acid are not functional to the ghetto individual and the poverty-striken minority member. Their drugs of choice are alcohol, barbiturates, heroin, and other depressants or "consciousness-contractors." The use of psychedelics has not flourished among the economically underprivileged, perhaps because they need to forget what already is. Children from affluent families can suffer a different kind of pain—a need to find that which they do not have.

As emphasized by Pomazol and Brown,* drug use motivation is very complicated. For example, motivation to try or experiment with a drug may be more under the influence of social or peer pressure; however, with subsequent use a person may form and/or reject various beliefs about using a drug, which may in turn influence his own personal attitude about continuing the drug. Once that attitude develops toward continued use of the drug, the drug-taking behavior does not stop unless preventive efforts are aimed at attitudinal change. Such an attitude may be very resistant to a pure factual or informational approach, and must be broader based.

THE "COP-OUT" FROM SOCIETY

By now it should have become obvious that illegal drug use, drug-using subcultures, social protest movements, politically inspired violence, destructive encounters between generations, and increasing rejection of our society by the young are merely symptomatic of a profound upheaval in contemporary life. Today's youth is attempting to resolve an identity crisis perhaps unparal-

---

*Pomazol, R. J., and Brown, J. D.: Understanding drug use motivation: a new look at a current problem, J. Health Social Behavior June, 1977.

leled in history. His abuse of drugs is directly associated with a sense of despair and rejection, with a failure to achieve self-realization and self-fulfillment, to discover a meaningful place in our contemporary world. Certainly our society is falling far short of providing him with such an environment.

It must be recognized, then, that the drug crisis is in large measure the product of complex, interacting social and psychological variables. But whatever their setting, most are aspects of the struggle and failure of youngsters to relate to what is for them a disrelated, disoriented, dehumanized, but enormously complicated culture. Their use of illicit drugs is frequently both a social protest and an escape mechanism. It is a self-defeating problem-solving procedure—but an attractive one. In the initial stages, at least, drug usage is exciting and pleasurable. Many drugs are relatively cheap and easily available; the rationale for their use is seductive. Carey's study[4] of the college drug user identifies the frequently recreational use as one of the unique features of the contemporary drug scene. But the significant fact here is that such use has developed within the context of a life-style that offers an alternative to an unacceptable social world epitomized by the organization man.

One of the fallacies that appears in discussions of drug education is that drug use and abuse are somehow different from the conventional problems of youth and education. Drug use seems to bear little relationship to the larger context of adolescent peergroup relationships and the school environment. As a consequence, proposals emerging from such discussions may not penetrate the realities. They do not come to term with the social causations. Drug education must be made to relate to the actual, specific causes of drug abuse before it can achieve any significant influence.

Unfortunately, few persons either in teaching or in administration have the training and experience to equip them to deal effectively with youthful drug abuse. Moreover, much uncertainty exists regarding the proper role of the school. This is particularly true in dealing with the increasing drug traffic on the school grounds. Unfortunately the specifics of these difficult individual situations are likely to obscure the need for dealing with the problem in its larger social dimensions.

THE SCHOOL ENVIRONMENT*

The school is the staging ground for the adolescent social system. In the usually small neighborhood elementary school the youngster continues the association with his young friends from down the street or around the block. His social relationships are extended to the school grounds; parental and neighborhood influences still strongly affect his environment, which tends to be familiar and secure.

When the individual leaves the neighborhood school to enter the large, impersonal, and heterogeneous junior or senior high school, he is without a well-defined and continuous identity for the first time in his life. In this new and confusing setting he must both meet academic requirements and strive to establish identity and status with his peers. Here the adolescent may be chosen or rejected, he may not know whether he has been chosen or rejected, and those he numbers in his personal community one day may not be there the next. This situation makes for great uncertainty in interpersonal relations. It also makes for great sensitivity to group standards and practices and reinforces the compulsion to conform. The fact that the adolescent social system creates a world of superficial social contacts rather than a climate of loyalty and intimacy explains the tremendous pressure for conformity. It helps to explain the epidemic appeal of drugs once they are accepted or used by the prestige members of the peer group. The compulsion to "go along" is very strong.

The school can no longer effectively intervene in the affairs of students because (1) the power of the administration has been diffused by the size of the school and the fragmentation of classes and (2) because the authority

---

*See Chapter 9 for specific ways to modify the school atmosphere.

of the teacher over student conduct has been restricted. Consequently when the youngster enters this new and expanded student community where he must scramble for membership, the strongest influence in his life is apt to be the peer group that takes him in. If it is a drug-using group, then there is a strong possibility that he will soon be a drug user.

Rejection of the school culture

The diffusion of drug use among high school populations has grown apace with student rejection of traditional school culture. The old symbols of participation associated with that culture—athletics, the block letter, membership on committees, student government offices, rallies, and the "rah rah" emphasis long identified as "school spirit"— have been drained of meaning for many youngsters sharply aware of the racial crisis, the deteriorating environment, war, violence, and poverty. These issues have been imposed upon their consciousness by the mass media and by first-hand personal observation. For drug-prone youngsters the traditional school culture is empty, although great variation exists between urban and rural school situations. Its failure is not that it does not provide the opportunity to grow, achieve, and find emotional outlets, but that it provides the *wrong kind* of opportunity. This is also discussed in Chapter 9.

Results of the irrelevance of school to the lives of students have ranged from the undramatic withdrawal of students from school activities and even from school itself at one extreme, to the highly dramatic hippie movement and student political radicalism at the other. A thorough reexamination of the assumptions underlying the traditional high school culture has long been needed. The research for such analysis is not adequate, but nevertheless some information is available. One thing appears clear—the extracurricular activities to which the school attaches the greatest rewards (athletics, student government, etc.) are those that serve the school, not the student. Athletes perform a role that enhances the prestige of the school

and establishes solidarity with the local community. To the extent that their energies are channeled into such service rather than into their own growth, social prestige is gained at the expense of personal development.[12]

In contrast, activities that bear little relationship to enhancing the school's public image—art and science, for example—foster only individual growth; hence they carry little prestige. The system increasingly turns off students, so that now the star halfback passes among them unnoticed, and the student body president's denunciation of the lack of school spirit goes unheard. Instead the students seek identification with alienated groups: hippies, radicals, black militants, Chicanos, antiwar groups, youth for Jesus, and so on. And, of course, they also choose alternative groups (including some of the aforementioned and others not so easily identified by label) that embrace drug use.

The traditional school culture has fostered a climate of adolescent irresponsibility because most of the areas of student initiative have been usurped by the school.[20] Such a climate facilitates an adolescent ethos of kicks, fun, and impulse release with little regard for consequences. Under circumstances where adolescents are not expected to be responsible agents, it is unlikely that they will be.

The schools have been largely concerned with the "technology game"—teaching young persons the skills necessary to enter the commercial enterprise system. But fewer and fewer young people want to learn what the schools are teaching. The concepts of grades and pure achievement are no longer incentives for students, but lead to the rejection of the school culture.

Schools could get students so totally involved that grading would become largely irrelevant. In fact, Paula Gordon has stated:

In general then I see a change in grading as being a means to vastly increasing a young person's mobility out of a failure syndrome as well as a means of removing one of the underlying causes that may have landed him there in the first place. It is also important because a young person's desire to achieve would then no longer be based on a fear of failure as it may be seen to be at present. . . .

Such a change in grading systems would not do away with the notion of failure altogether. It would simply make a sense of failure dependent upon internally established criteria rather than externally imposed ones. In this way also, self-development and growth would be nurtured, rather than thwarted as they often are under present systems.*

Soskin,[23] a psychologist who developed an innovative drop-in center for school-age children states:

Schools—like shopping plazas, these educational super markets for the young—could only have been conceived by efficiency-minded adults who think in terms of persons as units to be processed through a system rather than children to be guided humanely and wisely to the full ripening to the human potential. Hundreds of thousands of tired and troubled teachers, as their classes grow more restless and querulous and as daily absence rates mount despite their most conscientious efforts, must be asking themselves about the adequacy and relevance of the educational experiences we provide our young. For, despite the architectural innovations and the electronics innovations and the "system" innovations, the stark fact is that our schools are in grievous trouble, and our young people are trying to tell us this, if we could only comprehend the meaning of their anger or alienation.†

Development of a school program responsive to human needs

Soskin,[23] among others, believes that schools, as their primary purpose, ought to teach young persons to understand themselves better. Experience in living and the complexities and subtleties of interpersonal relationships ought to be explored to help young persons develop more quality in their lives. Schools should begin to deal with essential human traits and values (Chapter 7). These include openness, honesty, dependence, and trust instead of fear, anger, and loneliness. Alternatives to the "speeding" of modern life as well as to the compulsion for achievement could be provided. Schools should do more than merely program young minds to unquestioningly absorb the dominant cultural values. Getting grades—pure achievement—should be secondary to fostering self-acceptance, enjoyment of life, self-expression, and creativity.

The most important thing that needs to be done to improve education is to make it more responsive to basic human needs. The educational experience must be both relevant and stimulating. When it fails to be meaningful, stimulating, and relevant to the problems and life experiences of the child, he becomes bored, dissatisfied, and may be seriously handicapped emotionally and spiritually. Charles Silberman's *Crisis in the Classroom* (1970) is only the one in a series of studies documenting the nonproductive and psychologically destructive nature of much of our educational system today.

Contemporary emphasis in education has tended to be on information and on a limited form of critical analysis. What has been missing is an emphasis on assimilating and using such information in daily living and on developing goals, values, and ideals that would give a basis for the enjoyment of a meaningful and happy life.

Young persons need direction and guidance. Answers to basic questions are being sought by them, but are not being found. These questions concern the meaning of life, the significance of actions, the reasons for being discriminating in what one does, the relevance of a moral life, the ways of finding inner peace and self-understanding, and the place of happiness, humor, and love. School should be a place where the student can deal with such realities.

There seems to be a tendency today for educators, parents, and adults in general to shy away from taking personal stands, from stating personal opinions, from arguing against what they know is wrong and false, and from defending what they have learned from their own experience to be true. Such evasive tendencies may be seen as related to an inner uncertainty as to what is right or true. The trend seems to be toward a "hands off" policy of giving youth the facts they presumably need, presenting them with a neutral view of alternatives, and turning them loose to make their own choices and mis-

---

*From Gordon, P., editor: Guide to ideas on drug abuse programs and policies, ed. 2, Berkeley, Calif., 1970, Committee for Psychedelic Drug Information.
†From Soskin, W. F.: Project community and the children of the good life, Unpublished monograph, Berkeley, Calif., 1970.

takes, but punishing them, of course, if they do not follow the majority and conform.

Persons, whether teachers, parents, or other adults, do not develop expertise overnight in giving moral guidance, especially when they may be uncertain as to what their own convictions are. Educational programs that do not have an ethical basis do youth a definite disservice. It would seem that education must renew its focus upon the understanding, inculcation, and awakening of ideals and goals. It is essential that the lives of exemplary individuals and exemplary societies and civilizations, both Eastern and Western, be studied with such objectives in mind. Young people are looking for direction and purpose, and the prescripts that they receive today appear to be having little or no positive impact upon their lives.

The techniques of critical analysis have made students more inclined to take apart and find fault rather than to approach problems and situations in constructive and creative ways. The educational process has failed if the young person leaves secondary school unable to cope constructively with the day-to-day problems he is certain to face. The educational process has failed if the young person is left without a sense of direction and some basic personal values by which he can guide his life.

Ideally, the educational process should play a key role in the child's spiritual, emotional, and characterological development. Ideally, the educational experience should help to inculcate a young person with an attitude of caring about what happens to himself and to others. At present the educational experience, as well as the home experience, too often fails to stir these natural feelings. Human needs and aspirations seem to be bypassed. If children are to be rendered "drug abuse proof," higher goals and values must be internalized for them.

Educators can play a key role in helping young persons to develop goals and values, a sense of direction, a capacity for meeting problems, solving them, and finding a sense of inner satisfaction in life. The more humor, love, care, and simple respect for their students that teachers bring to their classrooms,

the more human the educational process will become. Real interest is contagious; so are happiness, hopefulness, trust, humor, love, and an attitude of caring. If these attributes become a manifest part of the teacher's life, the child will begin to naturally acquire some of the same attitudes and attributes.

The drug problem is but one symptom of a deeply rooted discontentment. When life itself is not valued, then health itself will very likely also be disregarded. Health education can stress the merits of *not hurting;* it can help to inculcate persons with deeper regard for health. It can also help by instructing them to exercise safeguards and to discriminate as far as what they do to their minds and bodies. But it would seem most unlikely that health education alone can provide the motive force needed for the young to find themselves and to begin to build values and to discover meaning in living.[20]

ALTERNATIVES TO DRUGS*

"Youngsters use drugs because they want to, and they would stop doing it if there were something better." This hypothesis may appear weak in that it ignores the complex psychosocial aspects that we have discussed at length, but if we say the same thing in a little different way it will sound more credible. Let us say that if there were satisfying alternatives for youth, such alternatives would serve to interrupt a drug-using lifestyle. Alternatives could be used to help develop legitimate personal aspirations, which are more effective than drugs. Cohen[7] has provided a table of alternatives that matches motives with relevant concerns. Opposite from each level-motive category in Table 3-4 are examples of types of alternatives that might replace, ameliorate, or prevent drug abuse. Dohner[9] includes other alternatives such as self-reliance development, vocational skill training, and meditation through the achievement of a state of heightened consciousness by focusing attention, daydreaming, and "mind-tripping." The National Institute on Drug Abuse has iden-

---

*See Chapters 7 and 9 for other specific activities; see also References at end of this chapter.

TABLE 3-4. Alternatives to drugs*

Level of experience	Corresponding motives (examples)	Possible alternatives (examples)
Physical	Desire for physical satisfaction; physical relaxation; relief from sickness; desire for more energy; maintenance of physical dependency	Athletics; dance; exercise; hiking; diet; health training; carpentry or outdoor work
Sensory	Desire to stimulate sight, sound, touch, taste; need for sensual-sexual stimulation; desire to magnify sensorium	Sensory awareness training; sky diving; experiencing sensory beauty of nature
Emotional	Relief from psychological pain; attempt to solve personal perplexities; relief from bad mood; escape from anxiety; desire for emotional insight; liberation of feeling; emotional relaxation	Competent individual counseling; well-run group therapy; instruction in psychology of personal development
Interpersonal	To gain peer acceptance; to break through interpersonal barriers; to "communicate," especially non-verbally; defiance of authority figures; cement two-person relationships; relaxation of interpersonal inhibition; solve interpersonal hangups	Expertly managed sensitivity and encounter groups; well-run group therapy; instruction in social customs; confidence training; social-interpersonal counseling; emphasis on assisting others in distress via education; marriage
Social (including sociocultural and environmental)	To promote social change; to find identifiable subculture; to tune out intolerable environmental conditions, e.g., poverty; changing awareness of the "masses"	Social service; community action in positive social change; helping the poor, aged infirm, young, tutoring handicapped; ecology action
Political	To promote political change; to identify with antiestablishment subgroup; to change drug legislation; out of desperation with the social-political order; to gain wealth or affluence or power	Political service; political action; non-partisan projects such as ecological lobbying; field work with politicians and public officials
Intellectual	To escape mental boredom; out of intellectual curiosity; to solve cognitive problems; to gain new understanding in the world of ideas; to study better; to research one's own awareness; for science	Intellectual excitement through reading, through discussion; creative games and puzzles; self-hypnosis; training in concentration; synectics—training in intellectual breakthroughs; memory training
Creative-esthetic	To improve creativity in the arts; to enhance enjoyment of art already produced, e.g., music; to enjoy imaginative mental productions	Nongraded instruction in producing and/or appreciating art, music, drama, crafts, handiwork, cooking, sewing, gardening, writing, singing, etc.
Philosophical	To discover meaningful values; to grasp the nature of the universe; to find meaning in life; to help establish personal identity; to organize a belief structure	Discussions, seminars, courses in the meaning of life; study of ethics, morality, the nature of reality; relevant philosophical literature; guided exploration of value systems

*From Cohen, A. Y.: J. Psychedelic Drugs **3**:16-21, 1971.

TABLE 3-4. Alternatives to drugs—cont'd

Level of experience	Corresponding motives (examples)	Possible alternatives (examples)
Spiritual-mystical	To transcend orthodox religion; to develop spiritual insights; to reach higher levels of consciousness; to have divine visions; to communicate with God; to augment yogic practices; to get a spiritual shortcut; to attain enlightenment; to attain spiritual powers	Exposure to nonchemical methods of spiritual development; study of world religions; introduction to applied mysticism, meditation; yogic techniques
Miscellaneous	Adventure, risk drama, "kicks," unexpressed motives; pro-drug general attitudes, etc.	"Outward Bound" survival training; combinations of alternatives above; pronaturalness attitudes; brainwave training; meaningful employment, etc.

tified a variety of individual and community alternatives.*

There is, however, as Cohen points out, another major alternative not specified here, and that is stopping drug use. Even junkies stop using drugs when the use itself or the life-style of using becomes simply unbearable. They are faced with too many "rip offs" (exploitation), too many hassles (interpersonal confrontations), and often too many "bummers" (unpleasant drug experiences). Exposing this side of drug use could act as a deterrent to new users.

Our emphasis here is not to demonstrate the supposed evils of drug abuse but to show the benefits of nonuse. The concept of viable alternatives may be effectively applied in the field of drug education. The idea that making children afraid of drugs will stop them from using drugs has completely lost credibility. The real possibilities lie in educational alternatives, what people can do with and about their own lives. That is what drug abuse prevention should stress.

The present national policy that singles out particular drugs and makes their unauthorized possession or use a crime should be changed. We believe that the individual and social harm accomplished by imposing

criminal sanctions on drug users far outstrips the benefits of this approach. Handling drug users as criminals has created widespread disrespect for the drug laws, has resulted in selective enforcement, has possibly done more to encourage than to discourage illegal drug use, has undercut bona fide educational efforts to explain the important differences between the physical and mental damage caused by the different types of drugs, and has deterred drug abusers from seeking necessary help. There is a strong need for decriminalization of the drug laws.

Most of those who advocate a public health approach disapprove strongly of the unsupervised use of dangerous drugs, especially by young persons. Our conclusion is based rather upon a recognition that the present penal methods of handling the drug abuser are at best ineffective, and at worst counterproductive, and that other approaches must be tried.

As a first step in bringing the problem back into perspective, criminal penalties for the possession of illegal drugs for personal use only should be abandoned, just as criminal penalties for public intoxication are now being abandoned in many jurisdictions. This is in conformity with the 1975 federal government policy toward drug decriminalization and drug abuse.

If the confrontation over the role of criminal law in enforcing private moral judgments

*National Institute on Drug Abuse: Alternatives, Washington, D.C., 1976, U.S. Government Printing Office.

or choices of drugs were eliminated, the country might then be able to unite behind an intensified approach to research, prevention, treatment, and law enforcement; this last should be directed against the upper echelons of the illegal drug traffic: the importer, the pusher, and the dealer. Restrictions on scientific research inquiries into particular drugs might then be lifted and substantial public and private funds more easily directed toward the understanding of how drugs work on the mind and body and what effects, both short- and long-term, they produce. The education of young people against the reckless use of powerful substances that affect the mind could proceed in a free and open climate more calculated to affect behavior.

In the meantime, however, the present realities make it necessary to deal with the facts of illegal usage and with the stipulated penalties. The law makes the unauthorized consumption of a large number of drugs criminal. Those who use them are thus defined as criminals, irrespective of how leniently specific laws are enforced. Teachers should know the law, legal and government policy, and how the laws apply. This is discussed further in Chapter 5.

REFERENCES

 1. Bloch, H., and Niederhoffer, A.: The gang: a study adolescent behavior, New York, 1958, Philosophical Library, Inc.
 2. Blum, R. H., and others: Students and drugs, San Francisco, 1969, Jossey-Bass, Inc., Publishers.
 3. Burns, R. S., Lerner, S. E., and Corrado, R.: Phencyclidine—states of acute intoxication and fatalities, West. J. Med. 123:345-349, 1975.
 4. Carey, J. T.: The college drug scene, Englewood Cliffs, N.J., 1968, Prentice-Hall, Inc.
 5. Chein, I., and others: The road to H; narcotics, delinquency, and social policy, New York, 1964, Basic Books, Inc., Publishers.
 6. Cohen, A. Y.: Inside what's happening: sociological, psychological, and spiritual perspectives on the contemporary drug scene, Am. J. Public Health 59:2092, 1969.
 7. Cohen, A. Y.: The journey beyond trips: alternatives to drugs, J. Psyched. Drugs 3:16-21, 1971.
 8. Coleman, J. S.: The adolescent society, Glencoe, N.Y., 1961, The Free Press.
 9. Dohner, V. A.: Alternatives to drugs: a new approach to drug education, J. Drug Ed. 2:3-22, 1972.
10. Finlator, J.: Speech at the National Training Center

in Drug Education, San Francisco State College, July, 1970.
11. Friedenberg, E.: Coming of age in America, New York, 1963, Random House, Inc.
12. Gordon, W. C.: The social system of high school, Glencoe, N.Y., 1957, The Free Press.
13. Gottlieb, D., and Ramsey, C.: The American adolescent, Homewood, Ill., 1964, Dorsey Press.
14. MacDonald, D.: Profiles: a caste, a culture, a market, The New Yorker 34:57-94, 1958.
15. Messer, M.: Epilogues: running out of era; some non-pharmacological notes on the psychedelic revolution, J. Psyched. Drugs 2:157-165, 1968.
16. Parsons, T.: Youth in the context of American society, Daedalus 91:97-123, 1962.
17. Pomazol, R. J., and Brown, J. D.: Understanding drug use motivation: a new look at a current problem, J. Health Social Behavior, June, 1977.
18. Poveda, A. G.: Drug use among the major social types in high school, unpublished doctoral dissertation, University of California, 1970.
19. Reuter, E.: The education of the adolescent, J. Ed. Sociol. 14:67-68, 1940.
20. Smith, D. E., and Bentel, D. J.: Drug Abuse Information Project, the third, fourth and fifth annual reports to the legislature, San Francisco, 1969-1972, University of California San Francisco Medical Center.
21. Smith, D. E., and Wesson, D. R.: Diagnosis and treatment of adverse reactions to sedative-hypnotics, Rockville, Md., 1974, National Clearinghouse for Drug Abuse Information.
22. Smith, E. A.: American youth culture, Glencoe, N.Y., 1962, The Free Press.
23. Soskin, W. F.: Project community and the children of the good life, unpublished monograph, Berkeley, Calif., 1970.
24. Turner, R.: The social context of ambition, San Francisco, 1964, Chandler Publishing Co.
25. White Paper on Drug Abuse. A Report to the President from the Domestic Council Drug Abuse Task Force, Washington, D.C., September 1975, U.S. Government Printing Office.

DRUG ALTERNATIVE REFERENCES

Cohen, A. Y.: Alternative to drug abuse: steps toward prevention, Rockville, Md., 1975, National Clearinghouse for Drug Abuse Information.
DARTE (Drug Abuse Reduction Through Education): Alternatives from A to Z, National Search Headquarters, Morristown, N.J.
Jackson, L. S.: Alternative pursuits: implications for drug prevention. In Senay, E., and others, editors: Developments in the field of drug abuse: Proceedings 1974 of the National Association for the Prevention of Drug Abuse, Cambridge, Mass., 1975, Schenkman Publishing Co.
National Institute on Drug Abuse: Alternative pursuits for America's third century: a resource book on alternatives to drugs, Washington, D.C., 1974, U.S. Government Printing Office.

4
Pharmacological aspects of drug abuse

Drugs possess the potential for unlocking a variety of mental and physical experiences. They are also catalysts that energize complex body processes. Although we shall discuss the actions of just a few dozen psychoactive (mood-altering) drugs, the number of psychoactive (psychotropic) substances available runs in the thousands, and their effects are many. Under certain conditions, which vary with the individual, psychotogenic drugs can precipitate a pleasant, even a euphoric, experience. Under other conditions, those same drugs may conjure up a veritable nightmare of horror and misery. The obscure passages leading to an understanding of these effects are only partly explored. What is known, however, demands public awareness if our society is to deal effectively with the problems of drug abuse.

PHYSIOLOGICAL ACTION OF DRUGS
The nervous system[8,20]

To maintain a physiological and biochemical balance in the body, man is equipped with a complex, self-adjusting, and self-regulating biological system. All functions are thus kept within certain tolerance limits. For example, when physical exertion generates excessive heat, the body signals peripheral blood vessels (those close to the surface of the skin) through the nervous system to dilate and allow more blood to circulate and cool the body. When exposed to cold the body conserves heat in the central cavity by re-stricting peripheral blood flow through constriction of blood vessels.

These self-adjusting characteristics are called homeostasis. The mechanisms that exercise this complex control include the brain, the nervous system, and the endocrine system. Messages about the condition of the body must be transmitted to the brain, processed, and fed back to body centers through the nervous system to adjust conditions that are in imbalance. Such electrical messages are sped along the complex network of the nervous system. Chemical messages are communicated through the bloodstream by the endocrine system; the time of travel and duration of effect may vary from a few seconds to several weeks.

The nervous system may be conceptualized as a fine network of electrical wires (neurons) running throughout the body, along which millions of signals, or messages, pass each second. But where a wire is continuous, nerves are not. Nerve fibers consist of billions of cells, end to end, that almost but do not quite touch each other. There is a gap called the synapse. Nerve cells are long and thin—many hundreds of times longer than their own width. A message, or signal, travels from one end of a nerve cell to the other as an electrical pulse. To move that pulse across the gap to the next nerve, chemicals must be produced to fill the gap and to generate a corresponding electrical pulse in the adjacent nerve. It is these billions of signals across and along nerves that not only regulate our body chemistry but also create for us our whole world of perception and feeling. All of our experiences, thoughts, and emotions are nothing more than electrical activity that occurs in some part of the brain.

Normal nerve functioning depends on the regular manufacture by the body of the nerve chemicals, called nerve transmitters, their release to create an electrical impulse, and their breakdown after achieving the desired effect. The internerve cell gaps where the chemistry of nervous transmission occurs is also the point of chemical action for many psychoactive drugs. Some psychotomimetic drugs have characteristics similar to the nerve transmitters so they can occupy the spaces between the nerves and activate the nerves. Others block the transmitter effect because they occupy but do not activate the receptor site.

The messages that are transmitted through the nervous system must be sorted out and carried to the body organs for action. This is accomplished by the two divisions of the entire nerve structure—the central nervous system (CNS) and the autonomic nervous system (ANS). The CNS is voluntary and comprises the brain, which includes the forebrain, midbrain, hindbrain, and the spinal cord, which is an extension of the brain. The ANS is involuntary and comprises the sympathetic and parasympathetic segments that control visceral functions—heart, blood vessels, glands, abdominal organs, and others.

Encapsulated in the skull and continuing down the back as the spinal cord is the central nervous system. The CNS gathers the myriad items of information coming from stimuli inside and outside the body (all that is heard, seen, and felt), integrates it with information from internal sources, and then sends out messages to all the muscles and glands for action. The CNS "computerizes" what is happening to us and how we react.

A second integrating system is the ANS, which forms a network of nerves along each side of the vertebral column, the spine. The CNS and the ANS work together to perform certain chores; the ANS operates mostly to regulate organ functions and to maintain a stable internal environment. This might be called the "unconscious" nervous system, which maintains our body functions. When we run, without conscious thought, our heart beats faster. When we are cold, we get "goosebumps" where the hair shafts have been raised to preserve heat. These reactions are controlled by the ANS.

The ANS may be divided into two units—the sympathetic and parasympathetic systems. The first functions principally to mobilize the body for action; the second generally operates to maintain ongoing production of necessary materials via the digestive system.

Mobilizing the body for action is part of a process of stimulation. Forces or pressures both outside and inside the body activate the organs and parts through the nervous and endocrine systems. Body machinery is speeded up and mental alertness is increased. We breathe faster, our heart rate speeds up, and blood flow increases. We may grow flushed, as when angry or excited. Our blood pressure rises and our pupils dilate. Our appetite and other food and waste processing functions are suppressed for the moment. Some of the drugs that we call stimulants, such as cocaine and the amphetamines, produce just these effects on the CNS.

Sometimes, however, we say we are depressed. This is both a state of mind and a physical condition. Drugs called sedative-hypnotics, which are known as central nervous system depressants, act in just this way. Barbiturates and alcohol slow us down. Depressants may lower our body temperature, slow breathing, and decrease blood flow so that we look pale and anemic.

Additional drugs cause a variety of other body reactions through the nervous and endocrine systems. These drugs will be identified later.

Drug effects

The effects of drugs on people are dependent on four factors: individual dose response, biological variability, potency of the drug, and tolerance.

Dose response

A fundamental concept in understanding drug actions is the "dose response curve." This term refers to the fact that, as the amount of a drug in use is changed, there may be a change in the reaction of an individual, which may be shown as a curve on a graph. Generally speaking, the greater the dose, the greater the response. Ranging from a dose that is too weak to achieve any effect on an organism to a lethal dosage, the dose response may be plotted along two axes of a graph, or chart; one axis illustrates the low to high dosage and the other shows the small to great effect. The resulting figure is called the dose response curve. Different dose response curves are influenced by biological variability of individuals, the type and dosage of drug used, and other factors.

Since drug effects result from the collective action of many molecular interactions, the more molecules at the site of a drug's action, the more interactions will take place and the greater will be the effect of the drug. For each type of drug, however, there must be a minimum number of molecules to produce the smallest response; this amount is referred to as the threshold dose. Some drugs may necessitate a large amount of the substance for reaction. Threshold dose refers to the minimum amount of a drug needed to stimulate a bodily reaction. The threshold dose of LSD is 10 to 50 micrograms.

Other dose responses include therapeutic, toxic, or lethal: therapeutic refers to the amount of a drug that will aid in the solution of a medical problem; toxic means that the prescribed dose will have adverse effects on the body; and a lethal dose will result in death.

In contrast, at a certain point the organism may become drug saturated and increasing the dosage or the amount of the drug does not increase the response. The affected system shows maximal response, and additions of the drug have no further effect on it. But as the dosage level is increased beyond saturation for one particular response, new response systems may suddenly be affected. Some biological systems have higher thresholds than do others or are less accessible to the drug. Therefore to fix an exact dosage for a set response may prove to be both complex and uncertain.

Biological variability

In all living organisms there is substantial variability in biochemical response. This is particularly true with ingested drugs. Dose response curves vary widely between persons. Some individuals are generally more sensitive to drugs than others. Some persons will show the desired effect at lower dosage levels and others, equally drug sensitive, will have more bad side effects at the set levels.

Some persons have a much higher drug threshold, which additionally may mean that there is a longer delay before drugs become effective and start to work. Thus a person may continue to increase the dose for a time without feeling any effects, then—rather suddenly—succumb to overdose. Street people call this "OD-ing." Other individuals may "get off" on much smaller dosages and be able to maintain a high with no additional dose reinforcement.

With some drugs, like alcohol, the range between a subthreshold dose (not causing any result) and a lethal dose is very large. With cocaine, an example of the opposite extreme, the dosage range is small. It takes little to cause an effect and very little more to kill.

The *effective dose* is the amount of drug needed to cause a particular reaction or desired response in a certain percentage of persons. The lethal dosage is measured by the percentage of animals that die within a specified period of time. The safety margin is the dose range between an acceptable level of effectiveness and a dose that results in a 1% lethality level among animals.

The wide variability of response in these dosage ranges is not completely understood, but some of the most apparent considerations are the rate of absorption of the drug from the digestive tract and the activity of the drug-metabolizing enzymes in the liver. Dose-response is a complex relationship.

Potency

The potency of a drug is determined by the amount that must be given to obtain a particular response; the smaller the amount needed to achieve that result, the more potent the drug. Intrinsic chemical strength, efficiency, and maximum effect are not measures of potency. If the dosage of a drug is increased past the point of maximum therapeutic effect, the drug effect may be prolonged, but the primary result is an added number and degree of undesirable side effects. It may become toxic to the individual. An excessive dose of aspirin, for example, does not stop a headache more efficiently, but rather produces gastric irritation and bleeding if usage is prolonged.

Cumulative effects result from the addition of a second dose before the body has assimilated the first dose. An example of this is alcohol. With this drug, the effects continue to increase as the dosage is increased.

Additive effects of drugs are similar to cumulative effects in that they represent an increase in response corresponding to an increase in dosage. But additive effects result from a combination of drugs acting on the same system. Although small doses of each of several drugs may be taken without adverse effects, together the effect may be the same as a larger dose of a single drug. Alcohol and the barbiturates are drugs that show additive effects; they may be lethal. The depressant effects of both together are more than the latent effect of either drug alone. Unfortunately the result of this little understood phenomenon is that many people unwittingly kill themselves.

Tolerance

Tolerance refers to a condition in which repeated administration of a drug results in a gradually diminishing effect. That is, the second dose does not produce as much effect as the first; the third dose is less effective than the second, and so on. To achieve the same result as previously, the dose must be increased. But increasing the dose also increases the unwanted side effects. With some drugs, like LSD, tolerance builds very rapidly; with others, such as morphine and barbiturates, it builds more slowly; with alcohol, tolerance is minimal. We learn how to handle higher and higher alcohol dosage levels, but we still get just as drunk. Marijuana, in quite the opposite way, seems to lead to sensitization rather than to tolerance. The more one smokes, the less one needs in order to get high.

Tolerance can occur with both stimulants and depressants, but physical dependence occurs only with depressants.

CATEGORIZING DRUGS

A drug is any substance other than food that, by its chemical or physical nature, alters structure or function in the living organism. Drugs can be classified in many ways, ranging from their chemical structure to their effects on biochemical, physiological, or behavioral systems, as well as according to their social uses. Physicians, pharmacologists, chemists, lawyers, psychologists, and users all have drug classification schemes that serve their special purposes. As Ray has explained:

> A compound such as an amphetamine might be categorized as an anti-appetite agent by many physicians since it reduces food intake for a period of time. It might be classed as a phenylethylamine by a pharmacologist since its basic structure is a phenyl ring with an ethyl group and an amine attached. The chemist wastes no time and says flat-out that amphetamine is 2-amino-1-phenyl propane. To the lawyer amphetamine may only be a drug of abuse falling in Schedule II of the 1970 federal drug law, while the psychologist may simply say that it is a stimulant.*

Drugs may be called by (1) their trade name—the manufacturer's own brand name, (2) their generic name—the pharmaceutical name of the compound, (3) their chemical name, (4) their pharmacological category, and (5) their common or street name. Thus we have Benzedrine (made by Smith, Kline & French Laboratories), generically *dl*-am-

*From Ray, O.: Drugs, society, and human behavior, St. Louis, 1972, The C. V. Mosby Co.

phetamine, chemically 1-phenyl-2-aminopropane, which is catalogued as a CNS stimulant and is called a stimulant or an "upper."

The molecular structure of a compound is described by its chemical name. This description is based on the rules of organic chemistry for naming compounds. Because of the complexity of chemical names, their use is usually confined to the laboratory.

The American Medical Association, the American Pharmaceutical Association, the U.S. Pharmacopeial Convention, Inc., and the Food and Drug Administration have standardized the legal names of drugs. These are official generic (or nonproprietary) names and, because of their simplicity, are much more commonly used than chemical names. A generic name is assigned to a specific chemical structure and may be freely used by anyone (is in the public domain) and is not protected by a trademark.

The brand name is the registered title of a drug and identifies a particular manufacturer and formulation of a generic product. Companies try to make brand names as simple and meaningful in terms of use as possible. These names are protected by trademarks.

Drugs that are available only on prescription are called legend drugs. Each prescribed drug must be marked with the legend "CAUTION: Federal law prohibits dispensing without prescription."

We have developed a classification that we hope will be useful to educators and still maintain pharmacological accuracy. Drugs are grouped into socially meaningful clusters of compounds. (See pp. 97-98.)

The first category is the central nervous system *stimulants;* they increase functional activity. These stimulants include the amphetamines (Table 4-2), amphetamine-like drugs, or equivalents, as well as the so-called minor stimulants, the social drugs nicotine (Table 4-4) and caffeine (Table 4-5). Cocaine (Table 4-3), used as a local anesthetic, is included in this group. Although cocaine is also an analgesic (pain killer), its primary activity is one of stimulation.

Caffeine in coffee, tea, and cola drinks and nicotine in tobacco are natural or "organic" stimulants; the amphetamines are synthetic stimulants. Stimulants are identified by their primary effect of excitation of the central nervous system, resulting in behavioral arousal and activation.

The second category is the nervous system *depressants* (Tables 4-6 and 4-7), sometimes known as *sedatives* or sedative-hypnotics. These hypnotic anesthetics induce the opposite physical effects of those produced by stimulants; they have a calming effect. Alcohol, popularly considered a stimulant, is a depressant, as are barbiturates.

There is confusion regarding the classification of marijuana. It is considered by law to be a narcotic; at high doses it has psychedelic properties and therefore people use it for this reason; but pharmacologically it has properties that enable it to be called a sedative-hypnotic. Therefore marijuana has been included at this point but is descriptively discussed later in the chapter. Table 4-8 has been prepared to identify some of its unique characteristics. The main physiological effects of marijuana are disinhibition, euphoria, which is interpreted by the user as a "high," and mild sedation, much the same as alcohol. The case of marijuana illustrates how so often drugs are classified on moral, ethical, political, or legal grounds.

Also included among the depressants are a variety of substances that emit intoxicating vapors—the *inhalants.* Most of these products contain volatile (evaporate into the air) hydrocarbons. Model airplane cement is the most common inhalant.

We have called the third category *psychedelics* (Table 4-9) instead of the more frequent term "hallucinogens." Many of the so-called hallucinogens do not technically cause hallucinations. An hallucination, according to *Dorland's Illustrated Medical Dictionary,* is "a sense perception not founded upon objective reality," such as the hearing of unreal sounds and the seeing of things that are not there. This would be true for some LSD trips, but most experiences with the mind-altering drugs are *distortions* of reality rather than *illusions.*

In the fourth category we place the better known *narcotics* (morphine; heroin) (Table 4-10), all produced from the juice of the opium poppy. The *opiates* are noted for their remarkable properties of sedating, suppressing pain, and unfortunately addicting the repeated user.

The fifth category, *tranquilizers* (Table 4-11), antidepressants, and diverse psychoactive agents, represent a more diverse and mixed collection of substances. They are lumped together rather than distributed through other categories because they possess certain common characteristics, although they are only cousins rather than brothers or sisters.

The tranquilizers and their cousins are all psychotherapeutic agents used in psychiatric medicine. One of the revolutions in pharmacology was the introduction in the early 1950s of the antipsychotic phenothiazine tranquilizers for treatment of the mentally ill. These drugs affected the mind but not the body. They virtually revolutionized the treatment of schizophrenia and made thousands of totally institutionalized mental patients ambulatory and minimally functional in society.

Although it will not be discussed here, our sixth and final major category deals with OTC (over-the-counter) drugs, some of which have already been listed in other categories (Chapter 2). The sixth category includes the mild analgesics, or pain relievers, the sleep aids and sedatives, the mild stimulants (caffeine and nicotine, also mentioned earlier), and the cough suppressants and cold remedies, such as antihistamines. These drugs will be discussed with the categories in which they fall pharmacologically.

The White House Paper (1975)* has recommended that federal efforts in both supply and demand reduction be directed toward those drugs which inherently pose a greater risk to the individual and society. Table 4-1 identifies the priority rankings as determined by the Domestic Council Drug Abuse Task Force.

---

*White House Paper on Drug Abuse. A Report to the President from The Domestic Council Drug Abuse Task Force, Washington, D.C., September, 1975, U.S. Government Printing Office.

TABLE 4-1. Summary of drug priorities *

	Dependance liability	Severity of consequences		Size of core problem
		Personal	Social	
Heroin	Hi	Hi	Hi	Hi 400,000
Amphetamines				
Needle	Hi	Hi	Hi	Hi
Oral	Low	Med	Med	500,000
Barbiturates				
Mixed	Hi	Hi	Hi	Med
Alone	Med	Hi	Med	300,000
Cocaine	Low	Low	Med	Low
Marihuana	Low	Low	Low	Low
Hallucinogens	Med	Med	Med	Low
Inhalants	Med	Hi	Med	Low

*White House Paper on Drug Abuse. A Report to the President from The Domestic Council Drug Abuse Task Force, Washington, D.C., 1975, U.S. Government Printing Office.

Though the data are flawed and the rankings therefore imprecise, a clear pattern emerges:
1. heroin ranks high in all four categories;
2. amphetamines, particularly those injected intravenously, also rank high in all four categories;
3. mixed barbiturates rank high three out of four categories;
4. cocaine, hallucinogens, and inhalants rank somewhat lower; and
5. marihuana is the least serious.

CENTRAL NERVOUS SYSTEM STIMULANT DRUGS
Amphetamines[4]

The amphetamines are known to most people as diet or pep pills. Like all psychoactive agents, they exert certain effects on both the peripheral and the central nervous systems. The peripheral actions of the compounds include an increase in blood pressure, dilation of the pupils, constriction of the blood vessels on such mucosal surfaces as the lips and the lining of the nose, relaxation and dilation of the bronchial muscles of the respiratory tract, relaxation or a spasmodic contraction of the gastrointestinal tract, and a secretion of sparse, thick saliva. The drugs' dilating action on the bronchial passages explains their former use in treating hay fever and asthma.

Although these peripheral actions are both marked and potentially therapeutic, amphetamines are generally employed today only for their more profound stimulative effects on the CNS. Of these, the three most pronounced actions are the suppression of appetite, the elevation of mood, and the forestallment of fatigue. The first property is used medically in the control of weight; the second is employed in the treatment of some forms of psychological depression.

TABLE 4-2. Amphetamines

Brand name	Generic name	Slang name	Usual single adult dose	Duration of action
Benzedrine	Amphetamine sulfate	Bennies, beans, whites, cross tops, truck drivers, cart wheels	2.5-5.0 mg up to 15 mg	4-6 hr
Dexedrine	Dextroamphetamine sulfate	Dex, dexies, oranges, hearts	2.5-5.0 mg up to 15 mg	4-6 hr
Dexamyl	Dexedrine, amobarbital	Christmas trees (spansule form)	2.5-5.0 mg	4-6 hr
Biphetamine-T	d- and dl-Amphetamine	Black beauties	2.5-5.0 mg	4-6 hr
Methedrine, also Desoxyn	Methamphetamine hydrochloride	Meth, crystal, crank, speed	2.5-5.0 mg	4-6 hr
Preludin	Phenmetrazine	Diet pills	2.5-5.0 mg	4-6 hr
Didrex	Benzphetamine		2.5-5.0 mg	4-6 hr
Tenuate	Diethylpropion		2.5-5.0 mg	4-6 hr

Method of administration—Swallowing pills or capsules and intramuscular (I.M.) or intravenous (I.V.) injection

Legitimate medical uses (present and projected)—Treatment of obesity, narcolepsy, fatigue, and depression

Potential for psychological dependence—High

Potential for tolerance leading to increased dosage—Yes

Potential physical dependence—???

Overall potential for abuse—High

Usual short-term effects—CNS stimulants; increased alertness; reduction of fatigue; insomnia; often euphoria

Usual long-term effects—Restlessness; irritability; weight loss; toxic psychosis (mainly paranoid); diversion of energy and money; habituation

Form of legal regulation and control—Available in large amounts by ordinary medical prescription that can be repeatedly refilled or obtained from more than one physician; widely advertised and "detailed" to doctors and pharmacists; other manufacture, sale, or posession prohibited under federal drug abuse and similar state dangerous drug laws; moderate penalties; widespread illicit traffic

Although amphetamines are now classified as dangerous drugs under state and federal law, they are readily obtainable through doctors' prescriptions. The American pharmaceutical industry advertises the drugs as panaceas for fatigue, boredom, depression, and many other human emotional problems. Some physicians continue to indiscriminately dispense them to their patients despite recent production controls. As a result, and despite their high abuse potential, millions of people today ingest amphetamines to induce euphoria. Even low-dosage amphetamine consumption can cause tremulousness, anxiety, drying of the mouth, alteration of sleep habits, and other unpleasant effects.

No fatalities have been recorded as a direct result of high-dose consumption, but these drugs commonly produce restlessness, hypertension, extreme anxiety, impaired judgment, hyperventilation (a state of excessively rapid breathing), hallucinations, and possibly psychosis. Sedatives may be profitably employed in treating acute toxicity, but patients may require isolation and reassurance that they are not suffering heart attacks or losing their sanity.

More serious and increasingly common in this country is *chronic amphetamine toxicity.* The chemicals are not addictive in small doses, but persons who take larger amounts do experience extreme psychological dependence and may even suffer mild physical withdrawal symptoms when deprived of the drugs. Such dependence is complicated by the fact that, as the body develops a tolerance to amphetamines, increasingly larger doses are required to maintain the drug effect. Prolonged high-dose amphetamine consumption often results in physical deterioration and in a toxic psychosis characterized by perceptual alterations, visual and auditory hallucinations, severe depression, and a state that resembles paranoid schizophrenia. It may also lead to organic brain damage and personality change, as studies of amphetamine abusers in Japan seem to reveal.[13]

Street use of amphetamines

Speed is a street name for amphetamines and any number of substances that provide the same CNS stimulation. Although the words "speed" and "Methedrine" were once used synonymously in the San Francisco Bay Area underground, young persons in Haight-Ashbury and elsewhere apply the term "speed" to any stimulant that will bring them up, just as they use the word "downer" to describe alcohol, opiates, barbiturates, and all other depressants. Speed is also referred to on Haight Street as "splash," "uppers," "rhythm," "crank," "meth," and "crystal"; the last three terms apply particularly to a powdered form of methamphetamine.

The "speed binge" can be divided into an action phase and a reaction phase. During the action phase the user may inject methamphetamine intravenously from one to ten times a day. With each injection he experiences a "flash," which he describes as a "full body orgasm." Between injections the user is euphoric, hyperactive, and hyperexcitable. This action phase may last for several days, during which time the individual does not sleep and rarely eats. It is terminated for a number of reasons. The user may stop voluntarily because of fatigue; he may become confused, paranoid, or panic striken and stop "shooting"; or he may simply run out of drugs.

Whatever the reason for termination, the action phase is followed by the reaction phase in which the user goes rapidly from a hyperexcitable state to one of extreme exhaustion. The "speed freak" may sleep for 24 to 48 hours and upon awakening eat ravenously. When his food and sleep needs are satisfied, he often enters a prolonged phase of extreme psychological depression. This depression is often so intolerable that he starts another speed binge. The cycle is repeated, leading to even deeper depression as well as the paranoid-schizophrenic psychoses characteristic of chronic amphetamine toxicity. He may suffer terrifying hallucinations, mistake friends for police officers, and lash out with murderous rage at any real or imagined intrusion. Some users start new runs at this point to escape their depressions; some people inject barbiturates to induce sleep. Other speed freaks should be hospitalized and restrained before they can do physical harm, especially if they were "going up" or "coming down" in crowded places. Reactions, of course, differ with the individual.

Cocaine: new uses of an old drug[26]

Cocaine, called the "champagne" of drugs because of its scarcity, cost, and great euphoric properties is the new "in" drug. Except for several highly publicized groups such as musicians, it traditionally was abused only in the inner-city ghetto. Seizures and undercover purchases have increased steadily in the last 5 years. Recently its widespread usage has developed among minority groups, middle-class white youth, and the very affluent.

Most of the cocaine that comes into the United States is derived from the leaves of the *Erythroxylon coca* tree, which grows mostly in Colombia and the Peruvian Andes. The drug moves northward, through Mexico, is smuggled over the border, and—increasing in value all the time—finally ends up in major cities all around the country.

Although used in medicine as a local anesthetic, cocaine has been described by "coke heads" (users) as having euphoric effects almost indistinguishable from amphetamines. In the Controlled Substances Act it is classified as a Schedule II substance—a drug having a high abuse potential with severe psychic or physical dependence liability. Although the subjective effects of cocaine are generally considered to be more intense and the abuse potential more significant than with the amphetamines,[8] there has been no definite evidence to support this position. An equivalency with amphetamines in terms of effect may be assumed. Stereotyped, repetitious, and compulsive behavior is common with both speed (amphetamines and methamphetamines) and coke (cocaine). Both cocaine and amphetamine users attempt to cope with the tense, "wired" effect of these CNS stimulants by using sedatives and narcotics, including heroin. The mixture of opiates and either cocaine or an amphetamine is known as a "speedball."

Cocaine produces a strong state of psychological excitation involving feelings of euphoria more pronounced than those seen with practically any other psychoactive agent, including heroin. Psychological depression, however, follows this state in a rather short time (30 minutes). This depression is in such marked contrast to the previous pleasurable sensations induced by sniffing and intravenous use of cocaine that users may be motivated to repeat the dose immediately in order to recapture the original state. A cycle may then develop, with the user injecting the drug at short intervals (as little as 10 minutes) in an attempt to maintain a constant euphoric state.

The repeated administration of cocaine tends to increase the severity of excitatory symptoms. Users may become so psycho-

TABLE 4-3. Cocaine

Generic name	Slang name	Usual single adult dose	Method of administration	Duration of action
Cocaine	"C," candy, coke, flake, snow, dust, Bernice, Charlie	Variable	Swallowing pills, I.M. or I.V. injection, sniffing	4 hr

Legitimate medical uses (present and projected)—Anesthesia of the eyes and throat
Potential for psychological dependence—High
Potential for tolerance leading to increased dosage—Yes
Potential for physical dependence—No
Usual short-term effects—CNS stimulant; increased alertness; reduction of fatigue; loss of appetite; insomnia; often euphoria
Usual long-term effects—Extreme irritability; toxic psychosis
Form of legal regulation and control—Same as narcotics

logically excited and agitated that they develop an intense anxiety state with gross paranoid features. In this state, hallucinations are not uncommon, and abnormal sensations induced by cocaine in the peripheral nerves may convince the hyperexcited that animals are burrowing under his skin.

Behavioral aspects of cocaine use

The technique for using cocaine consists of raising the powder to one nostril, closing the other, and sniffing deeply. What follows are 15 to 20 minutes of very pleasurable exhilaration and then several hours of nervousness and depression similar to the aftereffects of amphetamine abuse. Other aftereffects of high-dose cocaine use can include extreme irritability, loss of the sense of heat and cold, tightening of muscles, jerking or convulsions, and finally respiratory arrest and cardiovascular collapse. The last two symptoms, of course, are those of a fatal overdose. Although this has been relatively rare up to now, it becomes increasingly likely because of the various adulterants contained in most of the cocaine presently available.

Cocaine addicts have been reported to use up to 10 grams in a single day, a potentially lethal dose. Yet after a long period of abstinence (which is not accompanied by notable severe symptoms) the user may be able to tolerate the same dosage levels that have been reached gradually during an earlier period of chronic use.

Pharmacological investigations have failed to uncover any characteristic withdrawal syndrome after the cessation of chronic cocaine use. In a strict sense, then, the drug cannot be termed addictive. However, a pattern of psychological dependence on cocaine can develop with a number of adverse consequences for the user.

Cigarettes and tobacco[32,34]

Until the twentieth century cigarettes were neither a major article of consumption nor an important threat to public health. Individuals used tobacco mainly in the form of cigars, chewing tobacco, pipe tobacco, and snuff. In 1900 only about 4 billion cigarettes were manufactured; more than 580 billion are now being manufactured annually.

As a major article of consumption, then, cigarettes are relatively new. Their sudden enormous increase in popularity came about because they provide the user with many gratifications that other forms of tobacco do not. They are convenient, relatively clean, can be smoked quickly, and are mild enough so that they can be inhaled. Smoking cigarettes, however, can rather quickly become addictive for many persons—addictive in the sense of building up a psychological dependence and perhaps, for some individuals, a physiological dependence as well.

Characterization of the tobacco habit (nicotine)

Of the known chemical substances present in tobacco and tobacco smoke, only nicotine has been given serious pharmacological consideration in relationship to the tobacco habit. Lewin stated, "The decisive factor in the effects of tobacco, desired or undesired, is nicotine . . . and it matters little whether it passes directly into the organism or is smoked."[14]

Nicotine is present in tobacco in significant amounts, is absorbed readily using all routes of administration, and exerts detectable pharmacological effects on many organs and structures, including the nervous system. The physical and psychological effects of smoking vary. Wilder summarized the literature by noting ". . . observations that cigarette smoking obviously serves a dual purpose: it will mostly pick us up when we are tired or depressed and will relax and sedate us when we are tense and excited."[37]

Smokers and users of tobacco in other forms usually develop some degree of dependence on the practice. At the extreme point significant emotional disturbances occur if the smoker is deprived of its use. The evidence indicates this dependence to be psychogenic in origin. In medical and scientific terminology the practice should be labeled habituation to distinguish it clearly from addiction, since the biological effects of tobacco, coffee and other caffeine-containing beverages, betel nut chewing, and such, are not comparable to those produced by morphine, alcohol, barbiturates, and many other potent, addicting drugs.

Psychogenic dependence is the common denominator of all drug habits and the primary drive that leads to initiation of and relapse to chronic drug use or abuse. Although a pharmacological drive is necessary, it does not need to be a strong one or to produce profound subjective effects for habituation to the use of the crude material to become a pattern of life. Besides tobacco, the use of caffeine in coffee, tea, and cocoa is the best example of psychogenic dependence in the American culture.

Scientists became suspicious of cigarettes as a cause of illness and death as early as the 1930s. One of the reasons they were concerned was an increase in the incidence of lung cancer. In 1930 fewer than 3000 Americans were listed as dying from this disease; by the 1950s, this number had grown to 18,000 annually. In 1965 the number was approximately 50,000. In 1962 a damning indictment of smoking was issued by Great Britain's Royal College of Physicians of London and in 1964 this was followed by the report of the U.S. Surgeon General's Advisory Committee on Smoking and Health. Its conclusions were summed up in the sentence: "Cigarette smoking is a health hazard of sufficient importance in the United States to warrant appropriate remedial action."[33]

In the years since publication of that report an unprecedented amount of pertinent research has been completed, continued, or initiated in this country and abroad under the sponsorship of governments, universities, industrial groups, and other agencies. No evidence has been revealed that questions the conclusions of the 1964 report. The health consequences of smoking can, in the judgment of the Public Health Service, be summarized as follows[34]:

1. Cigarette smokers have substantially higher rates of death and disability than their nonsmoking counterparts in the population. This means that cigarette smokers tend to die at earlier ages and experience more days of disability than comparable nonsmokers.
2. A substantial portion of earlier deaths and excess disability would not have occurred if those affected had never smoked.
3. If it were not for cigarette smoking, practically none of the earlier deaths

TABLE 4-4. Nicotine

Source	Slang name	Usual single adult dose	Method of administration	Duration of action
Cigarettes	Fags, smokes, coffin nails	1-2	Smoking and/or inhalation	1-2 hr
Cigars		1		
Pipe tobacco		1 pipe		
Chewing tobacco		1 "chaw"	Chewing plug or loose tobacco	1-2 hr
Snuff		1 pinch	Sniffing or chewing	1-2 hr

Legitimate medical uses (present and projected)—None (used as insecticide)
Potential for psychological dependence—High
Potential for tolerance leading to increased dosage—Yes
Potential for physical dependence—No
Overall potential for abuse—Moderate; potential for compulsive use high
Usual short-term effects—CNS stimulant; relaxation or distraction in the process of smoking
Usual long-term effects—Lung and other cancer; heart and blood vessel disease; cough; habituation; diversion of energy and money; air pollution; fire
Form of legal regulation and control—Available but advertising banned on TV; minimal regulation by age, content, and labeling of packages

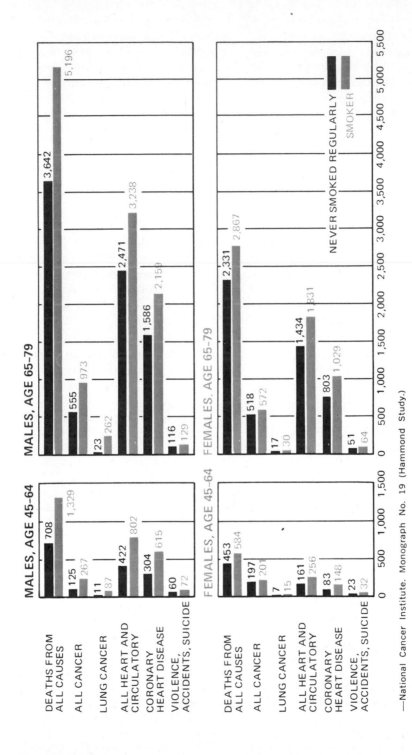

FIG. 2. Death rates of smokers versus those of nonsmokers. (From U.S. Department of Health, Education and Welfare: Chart book on smoking, tobacco, and health, Washington, D.C., 1969, Government Printing Office.)

—National Cancer Institute. Monograph No. 19 (Hammond Study.)

from lung cancer would have occurred; this is also true for a substantial portion of the earlier deaths from chronic bronchopulmonary diseases (commonly diagnosed as chronic bronchitis, or pulmonary emphysema, or both) and a portion of the earlier deaths of cardiovascular origin. Excess disability from chronic pulmonary and cardiovascular diseases would also be decreased.

4. The cessation or appreciable reduction of cigarette smoking could delay or avert a substantial portion of the deaths that occur from lung cancer, a substantial portion of the earlier deaths, and a substantial portion of the excess disability of cardiovascular origin.

Smoking-related diseases, produced primarily by the hydrocarbon tars contained in the inhaled smoke, have been defined by the Public Health Service as cancer of the lung, larynx, lip, oral cavity, esophagus, bladder, and other urinary organs; chronic bronchitis and emphysema; arteriosclerotic heart disease, including coronary artery disease; specified noncoronary cardiovascular disease; cirrhosis of the liver; and ulcer of the stomach. These are the diseases, for whatever cause or reason, that occur significantly more often among cigarette smokers than among nonsmokers.

Figs. 2 to 6 are adapted from studies by the American Cancer Society, based on 3,764,571 person-years of experience and 43,221 deaths occurring in 1,003,229 persons.[21]

As may be seen, death rates within each age group and for every cause of death listed are greater for smokers than for those who never smoked regularly. The differences are striking for the 65 to 79 year age group, and for those diseases most clearly associated with cigarettes, such as lung cancer and coronary heart disease. A study reported at the 1967 World Conference on Smoking and Health by E. C. Hammond[7] of the American Cancer Society shows that important differences exist between the life expectancies of smokers and nonsmokers, and also between the life expectancies of heavy smokers and light smokers.

The 25-year-old man who never smoked regularly can expect to live 48.6 more years, which is 4.6 years longer than the man who smokes 1 to 9 cigarettes a day; 5.5 years longer than the 10 to 19 cigarette-a-day smoker; 6.2 years longer than the 20 to 39 cigarette-a-day smoker; and 8.3 years longer

Age	Never Smoked Regularly	Cigarette Smokers By Daily Amount			
		1-9	10-19	20-39	40+
25	48.6	44.0	43.1	42.4	40.3
30	43.9	39.3	38.4	37.8	35.8
35	39.2	34.7	33.8	33.2	31.3
40	34.5	30.2	29.3	28.7	26.9
45	30.0	25.9	25.0	24.4	23.0
50	25.6	21.8	21.0	20.5	19.3
55	21.4	17.9	17.4	17.0	16.0
60	17.6	14.5	14.1	13.7	13.2
65	14.1	11.3	11.2	11.0	10.7

FIG. 3. Estimated life expectancy of males age 25 to age 65 years in the United States. (Data from the American Cancer Society's epidemiology study of over 1 million men and women; reprinted from Proceedings, world conference on smoking and health, New York, 1967, National Interagency Council on Smoking and Health.)

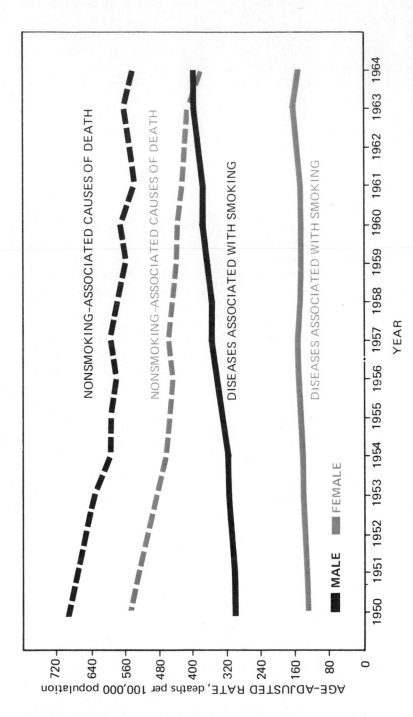

FIG. 4. Smoking-related diseases versus other causes of death, 1950 to 1964. (From U.S. Department of Health, Education and Welfare: Chart book on smoking, tobacco, and health, Washington, D.C., 1969, Government Printing Office.)

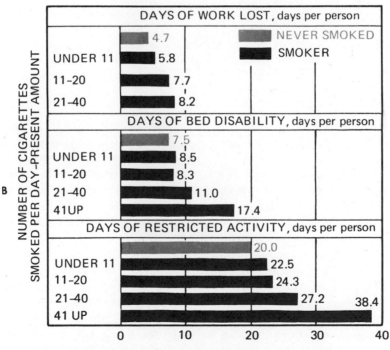

—National Center for Health Statistics.
Chart shows age-adjusted number of days per person per year, 1965.

FIG. 5. Smoking and disability. **A,** Males. **B,** Females. (From U.S. Department of Health, Education and Welfare: Chart book on smoking, tobacco, and health, Washington, D.C., 1969, Government Printing Office.)

AGED 55–64

SMOKED 20 OR MORE CIGARETTES PER DAY			
UNDER 1	2,962
1–4	2,613
5–9	1,880
10 UP	1,563
	1,187 NEVER SMOKED REGULARLY

FORMER SMOKER ■

SMOKED 19 OR LESS CIGARETTES PER DAY			
UNDER 1	2,017
1–4	1,854
5–9	1,669
10 UP	1,020
	1,187

AGED 65–74

SMOKED 20 OR MORE CIGARETTES PER DAY			
UNDER 1	6,339
1–4	5,488
5–9	4,260
10 UP	4,399
	3,118

SMOKED 19 OR LESS CIGARETTES PER DAY			
UNDER 1	4,607
1–4	4,796
5–9	3,682
10 UP	3,681
	3,118

YEARS SINCE LAST SMOKED

0   1,000   2,000   3,000   4,000   5,000   6,000

—National Cancer Institute. (Hammond Study.) Rates per 100,000 person-years.

FIG. 6. Death rates of males who were formerly smokers. (From U.S. Department of Health, Education and Welfare: Chart book on smoking, tobacco, and health, Washington, D.C., 1969, Government Printing Office.)

than the heavy smoker who uses two packs a day or more. Similar differences exist at other ages.

A high correlation exists between death rates and exposure to cigarettes, whether the exposure is expressed as the number smoked, the degree of inhalation, or the time elapsed since smoking began. Increased consumption of cigarettes is accompanied by higher death rates for both men and women. Among men 45 to 54 years of age, the death rate for those smoking 10 to 19 cigarettes per day is more than double that of non-smokers. In all age groups from 45 to 74, a greater number of cigarettes smoked per day is consistently associated with a higher death rate.

A pronounced increase in both male and female mortality from lung cancer and coronary heart disease corresponds with an in-crease in the number of cigarettes smoked. The death rates associated with cigarettes smoked per day provide one of the most striking examples of the dangers of smoking for women. Although those who smoke 1 to 9 cigarettes per day have death rates comparable to those who do not smoke at all, those who smoke more than this show consistently higher death rates. In the case of women in the 45 to 54 age group, the death rate for two-pack-plus smokers is almost double that of those who do not smoke.

There is also a consistent upward trend in the death rate in relation to the depth of inhalation. Those who inhale deeply have death rates more than double the rates of those who do not smoke.

The longer a person smokes, the greater the risk of early death. Men who began smoking before they were 15 years old have

TABLE 4-5. Caffeine

Source	Slang name	Usual single adult dose	Method of administration	Duration of action
Coffee	Java	1-2 cups	Swallowing liquid	2-4 hr
Tea		1-2 cups		
Colas		16 oz		
No-Doz and similar products		5 mg	Swallowing pill	2-4 hr

Legitimate medical uses (present and projected)—Mild stimulant; treatment of some forms of coma
Potential for psychological dependence—Moderate
Potential for tolerance leading to increased dosage—Yes
Potential for physical dependence—No
Overall potential for abuse—None
Usual short-term effects—CNS stimulant; increased alertness; reduction of fatigue
Usual long-term effects—Sometimes insomnia or restlessness; habituation
Form of legal regulation and control—Available and advertised without limit; no regulation for children or adults

death rates about double those of men who started in their thirties.

In 1967 the Public Health Service issued a report based on interviews with members of 42,000 households.[19] The findings show that a man who smokes more than two packs of cigarettes a day is away from work half again as many days as the nonsmoker, spends more than half again as many days ill in bed, and suffers nearly twice as many days of restricted activity. Comparisons between women smokers and nonsmokers yeild similar, or worse, statistics.

Chronic conditions are those illnesses that last for a long time—months, even years. In the Health Interview Survey, any illness that began more than 2 months before the time of the interview was considered a chronic condition. Both men and women cigarette smokers reported more cases of chronic illness than those who never smoked. More chronic illness existed among the heavy smokers than among those who smoked fewer cigarettes or had never smoked at all. Smokers also reported more chronic conditions per person.

When data from the Public Health Service's report are interpreted to reflect the entire population, some indication may be gained of the magnitude of the total economic burden associated with cigarette smoking. For the nation as a whole, in the year the survey was made, there were 399 million workdays lost because of illness. A total of 77 million of these days, or 19%, were excess in the sense that they would not have been lost if persons who smoked cigarettes had the same rate of illness as those who have never smoked. Using this same method of analysis, there were 88 million excess sick days related to smoking, or 10% of the national total, and 306 million excess days of restricted activity, or 13% of the national total.

The loss of human life, of productive time, and of wages, and the costs of hospitalization and medical care that are a consequence of smoking are appalling. It seems indeed ironic that the current great popular concern over drug abuse should be focused to such a small extent on the use of tobacco and its almost incalculable injury to our society. Unfortunately, studies conducted in 1976 show that smoking in the United States, particularly among young people, continues to increase.

Caffeine

Caffeine (Table 4-5) is a substance found in popular beverages, including coffee, tea, chocolate, and cola drinks. It is also an ingredient used in several over-the-counter drug products. It is commonly used and readily available for purchase.

CENTRAL NERVOUS SYSTEM DEPRESSANT (SEDATIVE-HYPNOTIC) DRUGS[28]
Barbiturates

Barbiturates are nonselective CNS depressants because they can dull all excitable areas of the nervous system. They should be considered sedative-hypnotic–general anesthetics because graded doses of the compounds produce the same four stages of depression as seen with alcohol. True barbiturates are derivatives of barbituric acid, a condensation of malonic acid and urea that was prepared by a German chemist in 1864. Over 2500 barbiturates were subsequently synthesized, 50 of which are in wide use today. Many barbiturate preparations are available commercially and approximately 300 tons of barbiturates are consumed in the United States each year.

Barbiturate intoxication is similar to that obtained with ethyl alcohol and involves motor impairment, dizziness, difficulty in thinking, slowness of comprehension and speech, emotional instability, and exaggeration of basic personality traits. Barbiturate use may lead to serious accidents because these drugs can impair coordination and performance while deluding users, as amphetamines do, into thinking their abilities are increased.

Many users become dependent on sedatives and sleeping pills and develop a tolerance that forces them to increase their dosages, resulting in severe physical symptoms when the drugs are withdrawn. As with amphetamines, the distinction between therapeutic use and the abuse of these chemicals is frequently blurred. The oral ingestion of a 100-milligram dose of short-acting barbiturates usually causes sleep if the drugs are used in an appropriate setting with that purpose in mind. But if sleep is neither achieved nor intended, individuals may show signs of euphoria and confusion, resembling alcohol intoxication. Many individuals take sleeping pills to induce this intoxication. The disinhibition characteristic of acute toxicity usually leads to sluggishness, slurring of speech, increased emotional lability, and

nystagmus, an involuntary oscillation of the eyeballs. Excessive irritability and moroseness are also common, as are hostility and paranoia.

In large doses these drugs produce a state of deep anesthesia that is followed by respiratory and circulatory depression. Such overdosage is particularly frequent in those whose toxic confusion leads them to forget the extent of the drugs' effects and in those who use the chemicals singly and in combination to commit suicide. Acute barbiturate toxicity and overdosage have become major problems in most urban centers. Twenty percent of these attempted suicides succeed. Barbiturates and their equivalents in combination with alcohol figured in the deaths of Marilyn Monroe, Judy Garland, Alan Ladd, and a host of other celebrities.

An equally grave problem is chronic barbiturate toxicity, which resembles alcoholism. Its symptoms consist of extensive neurological damage, greatly impaired coordination and emotional lability, skin rashes, and malnutrition.

Repeated intoxication with the barbiturates produces true physical dependence, and abrupt withdrawal of the drug from a dependent individual can produce severe and dangerous symptoms. The abstinence syndrome varies considerably, depending on the duration and magnitude of barbiturate use. Some patients experience only weakness and anxiety; others exhibit hallucinations, delirium, and convulsions. Some patients who have seizures may then show improvement, but more than half of those reported proceed to a psychotic reaction that mimics the delirium tremens of withdrawal from alcohol or the paranoid-schizophrenic reaction associated with amphetamines. Anxiety mounts during this period, and frightening dreams may be followed by insomnia. Visual hallucinations, disorientation of time and space, and agitation may then lead to exhaustion, cardiovascular collapse, and death. An individual addicted to the short-acting barbiturates can be safely withdrawn by substituting a long-acting barbiturate, phenobarbital, and slowly with-

TABLE 4-6. Barbiturates and barbiturate-like drugs

Brand name	Generic name	Slang name	Usual single adult dose	Duration of action
Amytal*	Amobarbital		15-100 mg tablets	4 hr
Amytal sodium*	Amobarbital sodium	Blues, blue dolls, blue bullets, blue devils, blue heavens	65 mg and 0.2 Gm capsules	4 hr
Alurate*	Aprobarbital		500 mg, 2.5 Gm, and 5.0 Gm ampules	4 hr
Brevital*	Methohexital sodium		500 mg, 2.5 Gm, and 5.0 Gm ampules	1 hr
Butisol sodium*	Butabarbital sodium		¼-½ gr tablets and capsules	5 hr
Sombucaps*	Hexobarbital		250 mg tablets	1 hr
Gemonil*	Metharbital		100 mg tablets	5 hr
Nembutal*	Pentobarbital sodium	Nembies, yellows, yellow jackets, yellow bullets, yellow dolls	30-100 mg capsules	3 hr
Mebaral*	Mephobarbital		30-500 mg capsules	5 hr
Pentothal sodium*	Thiopental sodium		Ampules in various doses	1 hr
Tuinal*	50% Amytal sodium and 50% Seconal sodium	Double trouble, rainbows, blues and reds	¾, 1½ and 3 gr capsules	4 hr
Seconal*	Secobarbital	Reds, red dolls, red devils, red bullets, red birds, pinks, seggy, seccy	½-1½ gr capsules	3 hr
Luminal*	Phenobarbital	Phennies	30-100 mg	6-8 hr
Doriden	Glutethimide	Goofers	500 mg tablets and capsules	5 hr
Equanil	Meprobamate		400 mg tablets	4 hr
Miltown	Meprobamate		400 mg tablets	4 hr
Librium	Chlordiazepoxide		5-10 mg capsules	5 hr
Somnos, Noctec, Lorinal	Chloral hydrate	Coral	500 mg capsules	5 hr

Method of administration—Swallowing capsules or tablets and I.V. injection

Legitimate medical uses (present and projected)—Treatment of insomnia and tension; induction of anesthesia

Potential for psychological dependence—High

Potential for tolerance leading to increased dosage—Yes

Potential for physical dependence—Yes

Overall potential for abuse—High

Usual short term effects—CNS depressants; sleep induction; relaxation and sedation; sometimes euphoria; drowsiness; impaired judgment, reaction time, coordination, and emotional control; relief of anxiety-tension; muscle relaxation

Usual long-term effects—irritability; weight loss; addiction with severe withdrawal illness (like D.T.'s); diversion of energy and money; habituation and addiction

Form of legal regulation and control—Available in large amounts by ordinary medical prescription that can be repeatedly refilled or obtained from more than one physician; widely advertised and "detailed" to doctors and pharmacists; other manufacture, sale and/or possession prohibited under federal drug abuse and similar state dangerous drug laws; moderate penalties; widespread illicit traffic.

*True barbiturate.

drawing the medication over a 7- to 21-day period (method of Smith and Wesson).*

Acute and chronic barbiturate toxicity has increased dramatically at all levels of our society. Many of the barbiturate compounds are classified as dangerous drugs, the illicit manufacture, sale, or possession of which is prohibited by state and federal law. Yet they are widely available by ordinary medical prescriptions, which can be refilled repeatedly or obtained from more than one physician.

Alcohol[4]

The favorite drug of abuse in American society and the most toxic chemical is ethyl alcohol. This drug, which results from the fermentation by yeast of a sugar, was known to Paleolithic man and has been employed as an intoxicant by almost every culture in human history. It is classified pharmacologically as a nonselective CNS depressant be-

---

*Smith, D. E., and Wesson, D. R.: Diagnosis and treatment of adverse reactions to sedative-hypnotics, Rockville, Md., 1974, National Clearinghouse for Drug Abuse Information.

cause it can depress all excitable areas of the nervous system. Several experts have noted that alcohol should be considered a sedative-hypnotic–general anesthetic because graded doses of the compound produce the four discernible stages of CNS depression. These include sedation and the relief of anxiety; disinhibition, possible excitation, and hypnosis; general anesthesia; and complete respiratory and vasomotor depression.

Small amounts of alcohol also increase the respiratory rate. This effect has led many to assume that the chemical has stimulative properties. More pronounced are alcohol's central effects, which are initially experienced as a lessening of inhibitions and a characteristic feeling of euphoria and self-confidence. These reactions are followed by increased sedation and an impairment of physical coordination. At a blood concentration of 0.2%, alcohol makes most drinkers comatose. If the drug's concentration increases further, drinkers may die of acute alcohol toxicity as their respiratory and cardiovascular functions are arrested.

TABLE 4-7. Alcohol

Alcohol source	Generic name	Slang name	Usual single adult dose	Duration of action
Beer, ale, malt liquor	Ethyl alcohol	Suds, brew	12 oz	2-4 hr
Wine, champagne, wine drinks	Ethyl alcohol	Grapes	12 oz	2-4 hr
Whiskey, gin, "hard liquors," liqueurs	Ethyl alcohol	Booze, hard stuff, juice, hooch	1-1½ oz	2-4 hr
Wood or grain alcohol	Ethyl alcohol	Rotgut		

Method of administration—Swallowing liquid
Legitimate medical uses (present and projected)—Rare; sometimes used as a sedative for tension
Potential for psychological dependence—High
Potential for tolerance leading to increased dosage—Yes
Potential for physical dependence—Yes
Usual short-term effects—CNS depressant; relaxation (sedation); sometimes euphoria; impaired judgment, reaction time, coordination, and emotional control; frequent aggressive behavior; driving accidents
Usual long-term effects—Diversion of energy and money from creative and productive pursuits; habituation; possible obesity with chronic excessive use; irreversible damage to brain and liver; addiction with severe withdrawal illness (D.T.s)
Form of legal regulation and control—Available and advertised without limitation in many forms; only minimal regulation by age (18 or 21 years), hours of sale, location, taxation, driving laws, and ban on bootlegging; minimal penalties

Acute alcohol toxicity is quite common in our society and most urban communities must deal with dozens if not hundreds of cases daily. Even more common is chronic alcohol toxicity, or alcoholism, which ranks as one of America's most serious health problems. Alcohol is both psychologically habituating and physically addicting in high doses and can cause organic brain damage and personality change. It also has one of the highest abuse potentials known to man. Of the over 90 million people in the United States who use alcohol, at least 9 million are estimated to be alcoholics.

One of the most damaging and least known aspects of alcohol abuse is that when a pregnant woman uses alcohol to excess, it produces impairment in fetal development. This abnormality has been described as the fetal-alcohol syndrome, as it has been determined that alcohol abuse has produced a number of birth deformities characterized by mental retardation, lowered birth weight, and delayed growth and development.* It should also be noted that excessive cigarette smoking during pregnancy produces lowered birth weight. The observation is that legal drugs such as alcohol and tobacco produce far more damage to the unborn fetus than the more widely publicized drugs such as marijuana and LSD. Unfortunately this information is not widely known in American society, particularly among younger people of child-bearing age.

Alcoholism has no easy cure. Chronic alcohol toxicity is rightfully regarded as a behavioral disorder in our society and has been explained by a number of theories emphasizing that alcoholics, like other drug abusers, are dependent people who have difficulty forming interpersonal relationships and handling stress. Studies made of alcoholics reveal that most of them have parents who themselves abuse alcohol. But no one has found a completely effective way to help alcoholics.

Johns Hopkins University has developed a twenty-question self-assessment inventory which provides a warning to the individual to determine if he/she is a problem drinker. The twenty questions found on p. 84 can be important in both the areas of prevention and early treatment for the alcoholic.

In addition, the National Council on Alcoholism believes that alcoholism should be diagnosed as any other disease, although there is no general agreement as to definition. The problem is difficult to assess for medical purposes; however, the California Medical Association has identified guidelines for use by medical audit committees in hospitals. Some of the conditions indicating the existence of alcoholism follow:

1. Physiological—includes high tolerance to alcohol (a fifth of whiskey, 2 quarts of fortified wine, 3 quarts of table wine, or twenty-three 12-ounce bottles of beer regularly ingested in one day for a person weighing 180 pounds) with a withdrawal syndrome (hallucinations, DTs)
2. Clinical—includes organ damage such as fatty liver, chronic gastritis, and cerebellar degeneration, among others
3. Behavioral—includes blackouts, uncontrolled drinking, and acute psychotic reactions; poor job performance, frequent arrests, repeated accidents, and marital problems*

Psychotherapy is one method of help, but few alcoholics have the motivation necessary to undergo complete treatment. Alcoholics Anonymous, which bases its appeal on group confession and catharsis and attempts to replace the alcoholic's dependence on drink with a dependence on the organization, is only moderately successful with confirmed drinkers. Drugs are also employed to treat alcoholism, especially in Europe. Some doctors have administered hallucinogenic agents to alcoholics, hoping to give them intense spiritual experiences. Others have used

---

*Becker, C. E.: The fetal-alcohol syndrome, California Society for the Treatment of Alcoholism and Other Drug Dependencies Newsletter 3(1), January 1976.

*Adapted from Practical Criteria for the Diagnosis of Alcoholism in Hospital Practice, California Medical Association: West. J. Med. **120:**348-349, May, 1974.

THE TWENTY QUESTIONS "ARE YOU AN ALCOHOLIC?"

These questions must be answered as honestly as you will allow yourself to answer them; a "sometimes" usually constitutes a "yes."

1. Do you lose time from work due to drinking?
2. Is drinking making your home life unhappy?
3. Do you drink because you are shy with other people?
4. Is drinking affecting your reputation?
5. Have you ever felt remorse after drinking?
6. Have you ever gotten into financial difficulties as a result of your drinking?
7. Do you turn to lower companions and an inferior environment when drinking?
8. Does your drinking make you careless of your family's welfare?
9. Has your ambition decreased since drinking?
10. Do you crave a drink at a definite time daily?
11. Do you want a drink the next morning?
12. Does drinking cause you to have difficulty in sleeping all night?
13. Has your efficiency decreased since drinking?
14. Is drinking jeopardizing your job or business?
15. Do you drink to escape from worries or troubles?
16. Do you drink alone?
17. Have you ever had a complete loss of memory as a result of your drinking? (e.g., no recollection of driving home)
18. Has a physician ever treated you for drinking, or warned you to quit?
19. Do you drink to build up your self-confidence?
20. Have you ever been to a hospital or institution due to drinking?

If you have answered YES to any *one* of the questions, it is a definite warning that you may be a problem drinker.

If you have answered YES to *two,* your chances are excellent that you are on your way to contracting alcoholism.

If you have answered *YES* to *three* or *more,* you are definitely a *serious* problem drinker and probably an alcoholic.

Antabuse, which inhibits the complete metabolism of alcohol and thereby floods the body with its toxic by-product, acetaldehyde, producing illness when alcohol is consumed. As described by Becker and co-workers, depressed alcoholics should not be given Antabuse, as they may commit suicide while using this medication.* This agent is likely to deter people from drinking when it is taken with alcohol, but its use is generally restricted to highly motivated spree drinkers who are willing to risk suffering the sickening effects of Antabuse if they try some alcoholic beverage. Unmotivated alcoholics rarely request drug or nondrug treatment. In fact, they may not admit to having personal problems and may want to see abusers of other chemicals jailed. However, a large number have sought and received treatment through such effective after-care treatment modalities as Alcoholics Anonymous, an organization that uses group and individual interaction, including ex-alcoholics, as its primary treatment modality.

Alcohol is socially sanctioned and retailed in this country at an annual rate of over 350 million gallons of hard liquor, in addition to several billion gallons of beer and wine. The companies responsible for this supply have never advertised the debilitating effects of their products, and few Americans even realize that alcohol is a dangerous drug.

---

*Becker, C. E., Roe, R. L., and Scott, R. A.: Alcohol as a drug: a curriculum on pharmacology, neurology and toxicology, New York, 1974, Medcom Press.

Fewer still are aware that alcohol is more harmful than heroin to the mind and body. It should also be stressed that alcohol interacts with a variety of other drugs. This interaction, as described in great detail by Coleman and Evans,* is not confined just to other sedative-hypnotics, but rather to a whole series of drugs prescribed for totally different reasons.

Because of this public ignorance, most people take their first drink in a social setting under pressure from their peer group to do so. Alcohol is used primarily as a social and medicinal agent, by adult and young Americans alike. Some drink beer and wine at gatherings and rarely become intoxicated. Yet others begin to abuse the compound by drinking only to deaden their senses and cope with anxiety.

Inhalants—volatile hydrocarbons[12]

Substitutes for drugs that pose a serious threat to the health of young people are the halogenated and unhalogenated hydrocarbons found in petroleum distillates, including cleaning fluids, model airplane cement or glue, and carbon tetrachloride. If inhaled in sufficient quantities, these compounds can exert a sedative-hypnotic-general anesthetic effect by depressing the CNS. Their use can lead to liver damage, bronchial inflammation, chemical pneumonia, and potentially fatal illnesses such as aplastic anemia, a condition characterized by bone marrow depression with subsequent reduction in certain blood cells that results in tachycardia, excessive bleeding, and lassitude. The hydrocarbons can also cause physical addiction, as evidenced by those recorded cases in which people have become addicted to gasoline.

Glue

The most common glue sniffed is a form of plastic cement prepared for the construction of model airplanes and purchasable in most drug, novelty, hobby, and grocery stores throughout the country. Plastic cements vary

---

*Coleman, J. H., and Evans, W. E.: Drug interaction with alcohol, Alcohol, Health and Research World, Winter 1975-1976.

in chemical composition, depending on the formula used by the manufacturer, but all contain volatile organic solvents such as hexane, benzene, acetone, toluene, carbon tetrachloride, chloroform, ethyl alcohol, and ethyl acetate—substances considered in industry to be relatively safe when inhaled in low vapor concentrations, but toxic when inhaled over a period of time in high concentrations.

The glue sniffer first experiences a tingling sensation in his head, a lightness, and an exhilaration known to him as a jag. If he continues to inhale the substance, he will experience a state comparable to alcoholic intoxication. He will feel dazed and may repeatedly lose contact with reality in periods he refers to as "blackouts" or "flash-outs." His speech will likely be slurred and his walk unsteady. If inhalation is prolonged after this stage, he may become disoriented, commit irresponsible acts, and ultimately lapse into a coma.

The solvents present in glue cause a temporary depression of the CNS and affect the mucous membranes of the nose and the throat, causing them to become swollen and inflamed. There is also evidence of the development of temporary blood abnormalities, including anemia, among glue sniffers.

Certain of the organic solvents present in plastic cements are capable of damaging the brain, of affecting liver and kidney action, and of interfering with the bloodforming function of the bone marrow. There is evidence that habitual glue sniffing leads to the development of tolerance and psychic dependence. Whereas one tube may suffice to produce a mild intoxication in the beginner, it may take several tubes to produce comparable results in the experienced sniffer who has developed a tolerance. In one case a 19-year-old youth admitted sniffing from 15 to 20 tubes a day. In the words of another glue sniffer, "Once you start, it's hard to lay off; you shake and shiver at night when you're off the stuff."

The extent of the practice of glue sniffing is difficult to determine. Glue is not classified as a narcotic or as a dangerous drug. Hence the statistics on narcotic and drug arrests do not include those of glue sniffing. Children who sniff glue to the point of acute intoxication are typically from lower socioeconomic groups and often show symptoms of emotional disturbance. Many youngsters apparently inhale fumes from paint, paint thinner, and lacquer, in addition to glue.

Gasoline

The hydrocarbons in gasoline, notably butane, hexane, and pentane, affect the CNS, causing symptoms of intoxication that range from mild to severe, depending on the susceptibility of the individual and the volume of gasoline fumes inhaled. Mild symptoms resemble those of alcoholic intoxication; in extreme cases, delirium, coma, seizures, and death may occur. Symptoms appear rapidly and are exaggerated upon exposure to fresh air. The practice of gasoline sniffing in the cases reported appears not to have resulted in permanent organic damage, although some potentially serious initial symptoms were found. It is likely that prolonged sniffing can lead to permanent brain impairment.

Nonintoxicating solvents probably will eventually replace those now present in airplane glue. It is not likely, however, that the intoxicating volatile solvents will ever be eliminated from gasoline, kerosene, lighter fluid, paint and lacquer thinners, marking pencil fluid, and innumerable similar substances available to the general public. Injudicious use of any of these substances is potentially dangerous; deliberate misuse is an ever-present possibility.

Marijuana[22,26]

Among all the current drugs of abuse, marijuana has drawn the most public attention. Endless controversy, much hysteria, and much plain misinformation have revolved around this substance. Nevertheless, the facts are largely known. The essential pharmacological and sociological findings arrived at by armies of researchers demonstrate that marijuana, by and large, is a mild drug.

Many persons believe that marijuana is, in fact, like LSD. We disagree with this grouping and concur with Dr. Frederick Meyers[17] that it is properly classified as a sedative-hypnotic. The closest pharmacological equivalent to marijuana would not be LSD or heroin, but rather nitrous oxide, or laughing gas.

Dr. Bertram Brown, director of the National Institute of Mental Health, has summed up the findings: "For the bulk of smokers, marijuana does not seem to be harmful—but it may be for some."[5] He cautioned that information is still unclear, especially about the long-term effects of marijuana.

The purpose of our discussion here is to try to provide for the health educator as reasonable an answer as can currently be framed to the question: what are the health implications of marijuana use? As we examine the drug in its various natural and synthetic forms, however, it becomes evident that this deceptively simple question is highly complex. Marijuana is not a single, simple substance of uniform type. It consists of varying mixtures of different parts of the plant *Cannabis sativa*, with psychoactive properties ranging from virtually nonexistent to decidedly hallucinogenic in its stronger forms and larger doses. Unfortunately much of the discussion in lay and scientific forums ignore this basic and important fact. The experience of most Americans has been limited to the widespread, relatively infrequent use of a weak form of marijuana. Early research dealing with the drug is inevitably faulted by the fact that it is difficult to be certain just what the potency of the material involved was, what the dose level was, and in what form the drug was consumed.

Patterns of use

The extent of marijuana use by schoolchildren has rapidly increased over the last few years. It is virtually certain that in some high schools and colleges a majority of students have tried it.

Subjective effects

As is true of other drugs, the effects of marijuana are related to its amount and strength. There is general agreement that at the usual levels of social usage the typical subjective effects are alteration of time and space perception; sense of euphoria, relaxation, well-being, and disinhibition. At higher doses dulling of attention, fragmentation of thought, impaired immediate memory, an altered sense of identity, exaggerated laughter, and increased suggestibility may appear. Other less common effects are dizziness, a feeling of lightness, nausea, and hunger. At very high doses more pronounced thought distortions may occur, including a disrupted sense of one's own body, a sense of personal unreality, visual distortions, sometimes hallucinations, and paranoid thinking. The more marked distortions of reality or psychotic-like symptoms become increas-ingly common if the dosage used becomes extremely large.

In addition to the amount of the drug that is consumed, the set and setting of use are important factors in determining marijuana's subjective effects. Set refers to the attitudes, mood, expectations, and beliefs that the individual brings to the drug-using experience. A situation in which the individual is depressed or apprehensive about the drug's effects differs markedly from one in which the user is more sanguine and looks forward to the drug experience with eager anticipation. The degree of personality integration, psychological rigidity, and the presence or absence of psychopathology are all important contributors to one's subjective re-

TABLE 4-8. *Cannabis sativa**

Cannabis drug terms	Location	Potency	Method of administration	Duration of action	Actual content
Charas	India	Most potent form	Usually smoked	6-8 hr	Unadulterated resin
Ganja	India	Quite potent	Usually smoked; sometimes confections, beverages	4-6 hr	Top leaves, some resin
Bhang	India	Low potency	Usually beverage	4 hr	Top leaves, uncultivated inferior plant
Hashish	Middle East	Most potent form	Usually smoked	6-8 hr	Powdered sifted form of Charas
Kif	N. Africa (Morocco)	Usually highly potent	Usually smoked	4-8 hr	Variable preparations
Dagga	S. Africa	Usually highly potent	Usually smoked	4-8 hr	Variable preparations
Marijuana	U.S., Latin America	Potent	Usually smoked	4-6 hr	Leaves, flowers, mostly dried

Legitimate medical uses (present and projected)—Treatment of depression, tensions, loss of appetite, sexual maladjustment, and narcotic addiction
Potential for psychological dependence—Moderate
Potential for tolerance leading to increased dosage—No
Potential for physical dependence—No
Overall potential for abuse—Moderate
Usual short-term effects—Relaxation; euphoria; increased appetite; some alteration of time perception; possible impairment of judgment and coordination; probably CNS depressant; vomiting as side effect
Usualy long-term effects—Usually none; possible diversion of energy and money
Forms of legal regulation and control—Unavailable (although permissible) for ordinary medical prescription; possession, sale, and cultivation prohibited by state and federal narcotic or marijuana laws; severe penalties; extensive illicit traffic

*Pharmacologically not a narcotic; obtained from flowering tops of female plants and resinous excretion from clusters and upper leaves.

actions to marijuana or other psychoactive drugs.

All of these psychological aspects also play a role in what is often referred to as the "placebo effect," that is, the response to the substance based not on its pharmacological activity but on the totality of *expectations* brought about by the set and setting of use.

Toxicity

We define a toxic reaction to marijuana as any effect that may result in physical or psychological damage unpleasant to the user, or that produces significant interference with his socioeconomic functioning. We specifically exclude the relaxed euphoric effect the user describes as being high or stoned from the definition of a toxic reaction. There is little evidence of physical damage with the use of marijuana, except for occasional cases of bronchial irritation in individuals who use the drug excessively, that is, from 2 to 10 marijuana cigarettes ("joints") per day. Almost all of these individuals also smoke tobacco cigarettes, so that it is impossible to determine the relative contribution of cannabis smoke inhalation to bronchial irritation. However, there is a threat to highway safety on the part of higher potency and greater frequency users.

Acute adverse psychological reactions do occur periodically with marijuana, as with any psychoactive drug. Their incidence ranged from approximately 8% in our study of college freshmen at a midwestern major university to 33% in the heavy drug-using population seen at the Haight-Ashbury Free Clinic.* By far the vast majority of these reactions consisted of nausea, some dizziness, and occasional confusion. With experienced marijuana-using groups who had adopted the drug as their primary social agent, these ad-

*The primary setting for this research has been the Haight-Ashbury Free Clinic, which has seen over 400,000 patients in 10 years of operation, over 90% of whom have had varying degrees of experience with marijuana. In addition, we have conducted surveys and interviews in the San Francisco Bay Area, with primary emphasis on high school students and students from selected college campuses across the country.

verse reactions were similar to those resulting from drinking too much alcohol. There was very little evidence of residual hangover or depression after these acute marijuana reactions. They seemed, in fact, to be less destructive to the individual than a similar alcohol overdose experience. This lack of "morning after" adversity seemed to be a significant factor in the adoption of marijuana as a social drug by many of the individuals interviewed. For example, one young adult said, "The reason I switched from alcohol to marijuana is that you don't have a hangover."

Effects of long-term chronic use and amotivational syndrome

Certain individuals, primarily adolescents and young adults, attempting to deal with both internal and external psychosocial confusion, use marijuana at high doses on a long-term daily basis. They smoke from 2 to 10 marijuana cigarettes a day and, as a consequence of excessive sedation and chronic intoxication, there is substantial deterioration in their performance and psychosocial functioning. Virtually all of these patients had adjustment problems prior to their heavy use of marijuana. When excessive use of marijuana was stopped, changes produced by the drug were, for the most part, reversed. Unfortunately the public and various professionals, in their determination to overstate the case against marijuana, have implied that even the experimental or social use of marijuana produces an impairment in motivation. It is the logical equivalent of saying that everybody who uses alcohol is an alcoholic. Nationally published statistics indicate that out of every 10 persons who use alcohol, one abuses it. Our data indicate that out of every 100 who use marijuana, only one abuses it. Thus, as marijuana is used in the United States, it has a lower potential for chronic abuse than does alcohol, the social drug whose patterns of use most closely approximate those of cannabis.

The vast majority of individuals who use marijuana do not develop psychopathology, nor do they perceive acute adverse marijuana reactions as a medically treatable condition. There is no question that we should have great concern about the use of psychoactive drugs by adolescents as they go through their crucial stages of adolescent maturation. However, it has not been demonstrated that making the use or the user of marijuana criminal will in any way prevent adolescent experimentation. In fact, it appears that more often than not just the opposite has happened. Our war on marijuana and the dishonest "killer weed" educational philosophy have tended to glamorize the drug and created the mystery of forbidden fruit in growing numbers of adolescents. Educators must recognize that the primary reasons most youth begin experimenting with marijuana are curiosity and peer-group pressure, and that by making the drug criminal we have helped create drug subcultures that are quite appealing to alienated youths who are going through identity crises.

Birth defects

A basic concern with any drug substance coming into wide use is the possibility that it may affect fetal mortality or fetal development (may be teratogenic) in such a way as to bring about abnormal offspring of pregnant users. It may also conceivably affect unborn generations by causing chromosomal changes (may be mutagenic) that persistently alter the genetic heritage. There is no evidence to suggest that marijuana use in humans affects fetal development. Despite the absence of such evidence, it is obviously unwise for anyone to use any drug of unknown teratogenic or mutagenic properties during the child-bearing years. Use during pregnancy is particularly unwise.

Relationship to drugs of higher abuse potential

It is often stated that the primary reason to maintain the criminality of marijuana use in American society is that marijuana leads to more serious drugs of abuse, particularly to heroin. The origin of this argument seems to have come from heroin addicts who stated

that they started on their road to heroin through the use of marijuana. One wonders why they picked marijuana as the first step of the often quoted stepping stone theory, when in fact studies have indicated that over 90% of those heroin addicts had their first psychoactive drug experience with alcohol.

It is generally conceded that marijuana use does not necessarily lead directly to the use of other drugs. On a worldwide basis there is little evidence of a progression from the use of marijuana to that of opiates or hallucinogens. However, those who study the use of other drug substances note that those drugs chosen may be popular among the peer group. These may include stronger hallucinogens, amphetamines, and the opiates. Although it is true that a high percentage of heroin addicts have used marijuana as well, most marijuana users both here and abroad do not appear to be attracted to the use of heroin.

What is the relationship between marijuana and heroin? It is primarily a social relationship, in that marijuana and heroin coexist in the same criminal culture. Naive young marijuana users must enter into this criminal subculture to purchase their drug and are very often exposed to a variety of pressures to experiment with drugs of higher abuse potential. The only relationship of marijuana to heroin with a nonpsychopathological user is by association, and that link could be broken by removing marijuana from this criminal subculture.

Summary and social policy recommendations

The current policy of making the use of marijuana a criminal act has contributed substantially to the toxicity of the drug and has forged the only link between marijuana and drugs of higher abuse potential. However, despite the destructive contributions of existing social policy, it appears that marijuana, at worst, is no more harmful to the individual or to society than its evolving social equivalent—alcohol. In addition, those of the emerging young generation who have adopted marijuana as their new social drug perceive the marijuana laws to be arbitrary, hypocritical, and discriminatory. (See Chapter 5.) Dishonest presentations about marijuana have severely damaged the credibility of much-needed drug education and drug abuse prevention programs. The current policy of maintaining the criminality of marijuana use has contributed to the alienation of many young persons from traditional social institutions as well as from our system of government.

PSYCHEDELIC DRUGS (HALLUCINOGENS)[23,25]

The psychedelics are a number of compounds from different pharmacological classes that are able to disorganize nerve and ego functions and thereby induce a toxic psychosis or acute brain syndrome. The word "hallucinogenic" is most commonly used to describe their effects, but the terms "psychotomimetic" and "psychedelic" have also been employed.

The mechanism by which the psychedelics work is not clearly understood. Their effects are mostly indirect, releasing or inhibiting particular chemicals that in turn alter the transmission of neural impulses in the brain. This has an effect on the brain's screening and organizational processes.

LSD

LSD was isolated from the ergot fungus of rye in 1938 by Albert Hofmann, a chemist at Sandoz Laboratories in Switzerland. In 1943 he accidentally ingested some of the substance and took the first acid trip in history, which he later vividly described. LSD is an extremely potent substance, causing pharmacological effects in doses as low as 10 to 30 micrograms. By weight it is about 3 million times more potent than crude marijuana. It is postulated that LSD may act by blocking the effect of serotonin at the nerve synapse, but as yet its actual mechanism of action is unknown. As little as 100 micrograms of LSD can produce stimulative and hallucinogenic effects that are 300 times more powerful than those resulting from a much larger dose of mescaline.

As a sympathomimetic agent, LSD causes an increase in blood pressure, a dilation of the pupils, a relaxation of the bronchial muscles, and other peripheral actions. These effects last as long as 12 hours and serve as the prototype of hallucinogenic or psychedelic drug experience.

Individuals under the influence of LSD may have vivid perceptual alterations, including illusions or auditory perceptions of musical compositions never before heard. Frequently there is a crossing of one sensory perception into another, called synesthesia. Music may be seen as colored lights, a pin prick becomes an explosion of light, or twinkling lights become tinkling bells.

Users rarely lose consciousness and can often recollect the entire content of their experience. But their thinking, their capacity for making judgments, and their coordination are likely to be impaired. Thoughts seem to move much faster during the hallucinogenic intoxication than they do under normal consciousness, and they appear in neither a logical nor a causal way. Phenomena that are usually perceived as being opposite can therefore suddenly coexist; good and bad may appear equal, and persons may feel light and heavy at the same moment. Most important, space and time orientations are frequently distorted much more than they are with marijuana, allowing past and future to merge with the present. Those using the drugs seem to desire this state of timelessness more than any other effect and prefer to avoid anything that detracts from its intensity. Many other individuals who take or have taken the drugs feel that they experience a form of protoplasmic consciousness that is so pronounced that they seem to lose their personal identities. This can produce the feeling of being an integral part of the universe, of being in union with the rest of the world and with whatever power exists behind the world, and of finally resolving all dichotomies. A feeling of rapture or ecstasy may occur. Conversely, the drugs may cause paranoia, sensations of death or nonexistence, and panic reactions of a bad trip.

TABLE 4-9. Psychedelics

Brand or common name	Generic name or components	Slang name	Usual single adult dose	Duration of action
LSD	d-Lysergic acid diethylamide	"A," acid	100 μg or greater	12 hr
Psilocybin		Magic mushroom	25 mg	8 hr
DET	Diethyltryptamine		0.7 mg/kg	
DMT	N,N-Dimethyltryptamine	The businessman's trip	0.7 mg/kg	½-2 hr
MDA	2,3-Methylenedioxyamphetamine		100 mg	12 hr
STP	2,5-Dimethoxy-4-methylamphetamine	Serenity, tranquility, and peace	3.2-10.0 mg	6-24 hr
Peyote	Mescaline	Cactus	½-¾ oz or 6-12 buttons, 500-800 mg	14 hr
Ditran, JB 329	N-Ethyl-3-piperidyl phenylcyclopentylglycolate			
Serynl (PCP)	Phencyclidine	Peace pill		
THC*	Tetrahydrocannabinol	Synthetic grass, "THC"		
K2,* "THC," hog	Benactyzine, Sernyl, various barbiturates			
Morning glory seeds	LSD-like components		300-400 seeds	
Baby wood rose seeds	Lysergic acid monoethylamide	Woodies	10-18 seeds	
Sominex†	Contains atropine-like compound			

Method of administration—Chewing plant; swallowing liquid, capsules, and pills; I.M. or I.V. injection
Legitimate medical uses (present and projected)—Experimental study of mind and brain function; treatment of alcoholism, neurosis, psychosis, psychosomatic disorders, and vomiting
Potential for psychological dependence—Minimal
Potential for tolerance leading to increased dosage—Yes (rare)
Potential for physical dependence—No
Overall potential for abuse—Moderate
Usual short-term effects—Production of visual imagery; increased sensory awareness; anxiety; nausea; impaired coordination; sometimes consciousness expansion
Usual long-term effects—Usually none; sometimes precipitates or intensifies an already existing psychosis; more commonly can produce a panic reaction when person is improperly prepared
Form of legal regulation and control—Available only to a few medical researchers or to members of the Native American Church; other manufacture, sale, or possession prohibited by state dangerous drug laws or federal drug laws; moderate to severe penalties, extensive illicit traffic

*Synthetically produced marijuana is presently being used in research in various parts of the country and supposedly is being sold on the streets. Preliminary analysis of samples of the "THC" being sold on the streets show it to be benactyzine, Sernyl, or a combination of several barbiturates. Sernyl was encountered in December 1967 in the form of the "peace pill." Market for this veterinary anesthetic was virtually destroyed in Haight-Ashbury by a one-page flier published by the clinic explaining its composition and lack of treatment. Now it and PCP are coming back under the names of Hog, THC, and K2. Presently no true THC is being sold on the street.
†Use of Sominex is currently on the rise. When used in dangerously high doses, hallucinations will occur. These are caused by the scopolamine found in Sominex. Sominex overdose should be treated in the same manner as an overdose of scopolamine, that being use of Librium and chloral hydrate.

Such dissolution can cause a terrifying feeling of unreality, with messianic delusions. It can also result in depression and periodic flashbacks or perceptual distortions months after the hallucinogenic experience. In certain cases individuals can be so panicked by these adverse reactions that they renounce the drug. In others, the toxic hallucinogenic psychoses seem to trigger more permanent disturbances. Adverse reactions are greatly dependent on the mood of the individual, the setting in which the drug is taken, and the availability of someone to give support and reality orientation to avert bad trips.

Long-term LSD aftereffects may be seen, such as a recurrence of drug-related symptoms with anxiety or a paranoid feeling at times of stress. These are commonly called flashbacks and generally fade away as the use of hallucinogens is discontinued. There have been many reports concerning the potential of LSD to cause chromosomal breaks, perhaps leading to birth defects, but as yet this is unproved.

NARCOTIC DRUGS[11]

The natural alkaloids of opium and their derivatives are classified pharmacologically as CNS modifiers because they manifest both depressant and excitory effects on the nervous system. They are categorized also as narcotics because they can induce sleep, and as narcotic analgesics because they are employed for the relief of pain.

Opium and heroin

Morphine, codeine, and some 20 other alkaloids occur naturally in the seed pods of the opium poppy, *Papaver somniferum*, which is indigenous to Asia Minor. The alkaloids are extracted from a gum that is exuded from the plants and then is used directly or modified to produce such semisynthetic derivatives as dihydromorphinone hydrochloride (Dilaudid) and dihydrohydroxycodeinone (Percodan) or converted by a simple and illegal process into heroin, which is approximately twice as potent as morphine in its central effects and is known chemically as diacetylmorphine.

The natural alkaloids and their equivalents have marked peripheral actions, the most immediately noticeable is a constriction of the pupils to pinpoint size. The drugs suppress coughing, cause a warm, flushed skin because of their dilating effect on surface blood vessels, and depress respiration and the heart rate in large doses. They also depress the secretion of gastric acid and liver bile, decrease urine flow, and reduce the propulsive contractions of the intestines, exerting a constipating effect.

More pronounced is the opiates' mixed stimulative and depressant effect on the CNS. Their essential central effect is to relieve pain not by blocking impulse transmission in the nervous system, but by altering the perception and psychological reaction to pain. This analgesia occurs before and often without sleep when the chemicals are administered in small or moderate doses, that is, in amounts from 5 to 10 milligrams. Pain is relieved regardless of its origin and intensity, and euphoria is frequently achieved.

Narcotics, more than any other drugs, can suppress those instinctual drives that usually motivate people to assuage hunger, seek sexual gratification, and respond to provocation with anger. They thus produce a state of drive satiation and a feeling of nurturance that is comparable to that enjoyed by fortunate children in early infancy. These compounds do not induce the sense of protoplasmic consciousness associated with hallucinogens, the general depression of barbiturates, the general stimulation of amphetamines, or the delirium of such parasympatholytic agents as atropine. But if taken intravenously, narcotics bring about an orgasmic rush that is as powerful as that of amphetamines. This feeling is followed by a toxic numbness and insulation that one addict has described as "death without permanence—life without pain."

The greatest danger from prolonged use or abuse of the opiates is the psychological dependence and physical addiction that occur because the drugs alter the body's chemistry

TABLE 4-10. Narcotics

Brand or common name	Generic name	Slang name	Usual single adult dose	Method of administration	Duration of action
Opiates					
Opium		"O," op	1-2 "pipes" per single evening	Smoking, inhalation	4 hr
Heroin		"H," horse, Harry, hairy, joy power, smack, skag, junk, shit, jive	Spoon, bag, paper, or balloon of 5%-10% heroin	I.M. or I.V. injection	4 hr
Analgesics					
Dilaudid	Hydromorphone hydrochloride		2 mg	Swallowing pill, I.M. or I.V. injection	4 hr
Morphine	Morphine sulfate	Miss Emma, white stuff, MS	15 mg	Swallowing pill, I.M. or I.V. injection or subcutaneously	4 hr
Codeine	Codeine sulfate	Fours	30-65 mg	Swallowing pill, I.M. or I.V. injection	4 hr
Percodan	Oxycodone		1 tablet	Swallowing tablet	4 hr
Demerol hydrochloride	Meperidine hydrochloride		50-100 mg	Swallowing pill, I.M. or I.V. injection	4 hr
Dolophine hydrochloride	Methadone hydrochloride		5-10 mg	Swallowing pill, I.M. or I.V. injection	4 hr
Cough syrups Romilar, Robitussin A-C, terpin hydrate elixir, terpin hydrate with codeine, Cheracol, Hycodan			2-4 oz for euphoria; however, not recommended; 1 oz for cough	Swallowing liquid	2-4 hr

Legitimate medical uses (present and projected)—Treatment of severe pain, diarrhea, and cough; prevention of withdrawal symptoms

Potential for psychological dependence—High

Potential for tolerance leading to increased dosage—Yes

Potential for physical dependence—Yes

Overall potential for abuse—High

Usual short-term effects—CNS depressants; sedation; euphoria; relief of pain; impaired intellectual functioning and coordination

Usual long-term effects—Constipation; loss of weight and appetite; temporary impotency or sterility; habituation and addiction with unpleasant and painful withdrawal illness

Form of legal regulation and control—Available by special narcotics medical prescriptions; some (except opiates) available by ordinary prescription or over the counter; other manufacture, sale, or possession prohibited under state and federal narcotics laws; severe penalties; extensive illicit traffic in such a way that normal metabolic functioning becomes impossible if they are withdrawn. Two hundred thousand Americans were estimated to be addicted to legal and illegal narcotics in 1969. In 1977 the number is 500,000.

Experimental narcotics use usually begins by smoking opium, sniffing, or snorting heroin, or taking heroin and other compounds orally. Users may proceed from this point to skin popping, in which they inject the drugs under the skin. The next step is intravenous injection, or "mainlining," which is alleged to be desirable both because of the attendant rush and because of the self-feeding implications of the needle. Most users are known as junkies at this point in their addiction. Others consider themselves "chippers," or occasional users, and insist, perhaps euphemistically, that they can regulate their consumption through self-control.

Such occasional use is complicated by the fact that tolerance to the effects of narcotics develops more rapidly and to a much greater extent than tolerance to other drugs. Persons given repeated and progressively larger doses over a 6- to 8-week period are soon able to tolerate many multiples of the original dose and may consume as much as 300 milligrams of morphine or heroin in several doses each day. In this process they develop a cross-tolerance to other narcotics.

For most addicts, then, the acquisition of opiates becomes an extremely expensive procedure. A kilogram of morphine costing $350 in Vietnam or Turkey is worth more than $250,000 after it is converted into heroin, passed through upper-level distributors, and sold on the street in fifteen-cent ($15) and quarter ($25) balloons or glassine bags containing from 300 to 400 milligrams of white or brown powder. The 30 to 40 milligrams of heroin in these containers is generally mixed with procaine, quinine, or milk sugar. Because of the small percentage of heroin (East coast heroin, 5 to 10%; West coast heroin, 3 to 5%) in its composition, many addicts develop such a tolerance to street smack that they are soon shooting from 3 to 15 quarter bags a day. Most become trapped in an addictive pattern that leads them to depend on opiate dealers, who are called connections, or pushers, as they might depend on a doctor for medical care. The addicts develop hustling skills to pay for their medication and engage in such criminal practices as petty theft, forgery, prostitution, and burglary.

Assuming that each of the 200,000 narcotics addicts in the United States had a $100-a-day habit, the total cost to society from their thefts, robberies, and related offenses exceeded $6 billion in 1969 (and is considerably higher today). This figure included relatively few crimes of violence, for opiate addicts are characteristically unaggressive, especially while stoned. Unlike amphetamines, barbiturates, and alcohol, narcotics per se seem to inhibit aggression; it is the need for them, rather than their pharmacological action, that motivates the user to criminality. The drugs also have few debilitating effects on the mind and body, so that addicts should be able to live as long as nonaddicts. The fact that they do not is related less to the chronic action of narcotics than to the drugs' illegality and to the dangers that accompany their abusers' life-style.

These dangers are comparable to, although more intense than, those associated with all underground drugs. Narcotics addicts run a regular risk of being poisoned if they have untrustworthy connections. They stand a good chance of being beaten up or arrested by the police or of being burned by competitors when they try to cop, or acquire, chemicals. They are subject to malnutrition because they rarely eat while intoxicated. They often overlook their physical condition because of the analgesia they experience from opiates. They are exposed to the high disease rates of their environment and are particularly prone to such problems as abscesses, septicemia, tetanus, bacterial infections, and serum hepatitis from unclean needles. They may die from acute opiate toxicity following an overdose. Overdose difficulties are sometimes related to impurities in street heroin, but are caused most often by uncommonly pure preparations that impose too great a demand on the user's constantly fluctuating tolerance.

The character and severity of withdrawal symptoms depend on several factors, including the kind and amount of opiates taken, the interval between doses, the duration of usage, the tolerance developed, and the health and personality of the patient involved. In cases of morphine or heroin addiction, withdrawal symptoms usually occur 6 or more hours after the final dose and persist for 48 hours or longer, the duration being shorter and more intense in the case of methadone.

The first withdrawal symptoms are anxiety and hyperexcitability; these occur shortly before the time of the next scheduled dose. Excessive yawning, sweating, tearfulness, and rhinorrhea, or nasal discharge begin at this point and may lead to a restless sleep known as the "yen," from which patients awake even more anxious than before. Their pupils then dilate widely, the hair on their skin stands up in a gooseflesh pattern, and the skin becomes cold, resembling that of a plucked turkey. This condition accounts for the term "cold turkey," applied to any form of abrupt or nonmedically assisted withdrawal.

Contractions may pass over the stomach a few hours after the onset of cold turkey, causing an explosive vomiting. Abdominal pain also increases as the intestines contract and the previously constipated bowels are suddenly voided. Weakness becomes prominent, the heart rate is elevated, and marked chilliness alternating with skin flushes and sweating may occur. So may the muscle spasms and kicking motions that are the basis of the often heard expression "kicking the habit." Convulsions and delirium tremens, however, do not occur.

As these conditions persist, patients usually become emaciated and dehydrated because they cannot eat or drink during withdrawal. They may improve, but they remain weak and often suffer from lingering diarrhea. These and other symptoms will disappear if narcotics are adminis-

tered, so physicians often use methadone to ease the pain and remission rate of withdrawal.

Methadone—a chemical approach to heroin addiction[15,16]

Methadone is a long-acting, orally administered narcotic possessing chemical characteristics that provide a blockage for the effects of heroin as well as eliminating the addicts' narcotic hunger. It compensates for the chemical imbalance created by long-term heroin usage.

Despite the fact that the use of methadone is substituting one drug dependency for another, experts are convinced that no other presently available therapy offers comparable promise for the many thousands of heroin addicts who are seeking help. The American Medical Association endorses methadone as the drug of choice for heroin withdrawal and detoxification. However, a number of problems have emerged indicating that methadone may not be as effective as expected. People are overdosing, dying from injection of the substance and increased alcohol use while on a maintenance schedule.

The technique of methadone maintenance was developed and used with great success in New York by Dr. Vincent Dole and Dr. Marie Nyswander.[7] They have reported a heroin-free, crime-free, success rate of over 83% with 3000 hard-core addicts. Methadone has proved to be effective with some persons who had been addicted as long as 10 years and who had failed with other treatments.

The effectiveness of methadone as a type of immunization against further heroin usage results from its ability to block the euphoriant effects of heroin and to eliminate the craving for the opiate without heroin's deleterious physical and mental effects. Given as a tablet or predissolved in orange juice, the drug allows the patient to function with neither sedation nor euphoria, and with no impairment of vigilance, reaction time, or intellectual processes. This effect is specific for opiate-type drugs and does not help patients using other psychoactive drugs such as barbiturates, amphetamines, hallucinogens, or alcohol.

The dosage of methadone required by a patient to avoid abstinence symptoms during the initial treatment phase depends on how much heroin or other opiates he has been taking. Once on a regular methadone schedule, he returns to the hospital or clinic for a daily dose. He leaves a daily urine specimen for drug analysis. In many programs, supplementary social services such as vocational and social counseling are made available to him. The patient will continue receiving his daily dose as long as the attending physician considers it necessary. Social adjustment and rehabilitation over a long period of time should permit the addict eventually to become drug-free. The advantages of administering a stabilization dose of methadone are that the patient has to receive only one dose daily, he feels no need to supplement the dose with heroin, he feels no narcotic hunger or euphoria, and he is able to work at a socially useful job or to go to school.

Narcotic antagonists[10]

A technique is now being tested to implant narcotic antagonists under the skin of the user. A narcotic antagonist is any drug such as nalorphine (Nalline) that antagonizes or blocks the effects of any narcotic. Such chemicals occupy sites in the brain cells and stop the action of heroin. If a narcotic user later takes a fix, he will feel no high. Research is being conducted on "second generation" antagonists that can be embedded in body tissue and released slowly and constantly over a period of days or weeks.

Investigation also is being carried on to develop viable immunization not only to heroin but to a variety of drugs of abuse. By coupling a psychoactive chemical molecule with certain proteins it may be possible to prepare vaccines whose action with respect to a specific drug or to a wide range of substances would be similar to a vaccination against measles. The body would release antibodies to destroy the drug before it acted in the brain centers.

Nonchemical treatment approaches to addiction

Groups for addicts, such as Synanon, that use no drugs are generally opposed to methadone (and other chemical blocking agents), which they claim are chemical crutches to carry a drug-dependent individual along without his having to deal with the inner person who craves such drugs. Despite the fact that methadone programs have high success rates, those of a more psychotherapeutic bent insist on changing the user's drug-using style of life, social environment, and ways of dealing with himself and others by nondrug means.

Many drug treatment specialists are convinced that Synanon and Synanon-like groups are the solution to drug addiction. Such programs typically offer a living-in community. Treatment specialists often are ex-users themselves who insist on embarrassingly frank personal intercommunications. Within the therapeutic community, there is intense verbal attacking of personal habits and character traits that are considered "drug oriented." To treat means to focus as a group on the habit, traits, and emotions that drive the addict to drugs.

Such "reality" type therapy is considered to reach the underlying motivational level that creates the need, the weakness, for drugs. Therapeutic communities have sprung up all over the United States and have become a major treatment modality, along with methadone. Unfortunately these projects usually receive very little financial support and are severely limited in capacity to handle the thousands of new, young addicts who are being created every week.

TRANQUILIZERS AND ANTIDEPRESSANT DRUGS

Tranquilizers such as Thorazine (chlorpromazine) are drugs useful in medicine for the treatment of people with psychosis. There are periodic cases of acute overdose and rare cases of chronic abuse.

Antidepressants such as Elavil (amitryptaline) are substances used by psychiatrists in the treatment of individuals with depression.

TABLE 4-11. Tranquilizers

Brand name	Generic name	Usual single adult dose*	Duration of action
Thorazine	Chlorpromazine hydrochloride	10-25 mg	4-6 hr
Compazine	Prochlorperazine dimaleate	10 mg	4-6 hr
Stelazine	Trifluoperazine dihydrochloride	2 mg	4-6 hr
Serpasil	Reserpine	1 mg	4-6 hr

Method of administration—Swallowing pill or liquid and sometimes I.M. and I.V. injection
Legitimate medical uses (present and projected)—Treatment of anxiety, tension, alcoholism, neurosis, psychosis, psychosomatic disorders, and vomiting
Potential for psychological dependence—Minimal
Potential for tolerance leading to increased dosage—No
Potential for physical dependence—No
Overall potential for abuse—Minimal
Usual short-term effects—Selective CNS depressants; relaxation, relief of anxiety-tension; suppression of hallucinations or delusions; improved functioning
Usual long-term effects—Sometimes drowsiness, dryness of mouth, blurring of vision, skin rash, tremor; occasionally jaundice, agranulocytosis
Form of legal regulation and control—Same as for the barbiturates except not usually included under the special federal or state drug law; negligible illicit traffic

*Institutional dose often greater.

TABLE 4-12. Antidepressants

Brand name	Generic name	Slang name	Usual single adult dose	Duration of action
Tofranil	Imipramine hydrochloride	Antidepressant	25-75 mg	4-6 hr
Elavil	Amitryptaline	Antidepressant	25-75 mg	4-6 hr
Nardil	Phenelzine		15 mg	4-6 hr
Parnate	Tranylcypromine		10 mg	4-6 hr

Method of administration—Swallowing pills or capsules
Legitimate medical uses (present and projected)—Treatment of moderate to severe depression
Potential for psychological dependence—Minimal
Potential for tolerance leading to increased dosage—No
Potential for physical dependence—No
Overall potential for abuse—Minimal
Usual short-term effects—Relief of depression (elevation of mood); stimulation
Form of legal regulation and control—Same as tranquilizers

There is occasional chronic abuse and overdose, usually in suicide attempts.

OVER-THE-COUNTER DRUGS

The discussion of these drugs is found in Chapters 1 and 2. For more detailed information obtain the latest edition of *Handbook of Non-Prescription Drugs* by contacting:

American Pharmaceutical Association, 2215 Constitution Avenue, N.W., Washington, D.C. 20037.

GENERAL PHARMACOLOGICAL CLASSIFICATION OF DRUGS
CNS STIMULANTS

Amphetamines (Table 4-2)
  Benzedrine—amphetamine sulfate
  Dexedrine—dextroamphetamine sulfate
  Methedrine—methamphetamine hydrochloride
  Desoxyn—methamphetamine hydrochloride
Amphetamine equivalents
  Ritalin—methylphenidate
  Preludin—phenmetrazine

Cocaine—coca (Table 4-3)
Minor stimulants
   Nicotine—tobacco (Table 4-4)
   Caffeine—coffee, tea, cocoa, cola drinks (Table 4-5)

CNS DEPRESSANTS—SEDATIVE-HYPNOTICS, GENERAL ANESTHETICS

Alcohol—alcoholic beverages (Table 4-7)
Barbiturates (Table 4-6)
   Amytal—amobarbital
   Nembutal—pentobarbital sodium
   Luminal—phenobarbital
   Seconal—secobarbital
   Doriden—glutethimide
   Pentothal sodium—thiopental sodium
Nonbarbiturates (Table 4-6)
   Librium—chlordiazepoxide
   Valium—diazepam
   Miltown—meprobamate
Cannabis sativa—marijuana (Table 4-8)
Volatile hydrocarbons—inhalants, deliriants
   airplane glue—toluene
   gasoline, kerosine, paint thinner
Sernyl (PCP)—phencyclidine
Hog—benactyzine; antipsychotic tranquilizer
Nitrous oxide

PSYCHEDELICS—HALLUCINOGENS (Table 4-9)

Psychomimetic amphetamines—DOM, MDA, MMDA
LSD—*d*-lysergic acid diethylamide
DMT—mescaline-like substance
Peyote—mescaline
Psilocybin—magic mushrooms

NARCOTICS (Table 4-10)

Opiates—natural derivatives
   Opium
   Morphine
Semisynthetic opiates
   Heroin (from morphine)
   Codeine
   Dilaudid
Synthetic opiates
   Dolophine—methadone
   Demerol—meperidine

TRANQUILIZERS, ANTIDEPRESSANTS, AND MISCELLANEOUS PSYCHOACTIVE AGENTS (Table 4-11)

Major tranquilizers—phenothiazines
   Thorazine—chlorpromazine hydrochloride
   Compazine—prochlorperazine dimaleate
   Stelazine—trifluoroperazine
Antidepressants (Table 4-12)
   Elavil
   Includes the category of amphetamines
Miscellaneous
   Atropine—scopolamine in Sominex, Compoz
   Jimson Weed—Dr. Shifman's Asmodor
   Loco-weed—atropine-like compound

OVER-THE-COUNTER DRUGS— NONPRESCRIPTION (Chapter 2)

Nonnarcotic analgesics (pain relief)
   Salicylates (in aspirin)
   Phenacetin
Sleep aids—Sominex
Sedatives—Compoz
Stimulants—NoDoz (caffeine)
Cold remedies—Contac, antihistamines

REFERENCES

1. Batiste, C. G., and Yablonsky, L.: Synanon: a therapeutic life style, Calif. Med. **114:**90-94, 1971.
2. Becker, C. E., Roe, R. L., and Scott, R. A.: Alcohol as a drug: a curriculum on pharmacology, neurology and toxicology, New York, 1974, Medcom Press.
3. Becker, C. E.: The fetal-alcohol syndrome, California Society for the Treatment of Alcoholism and Other Drug Dependencies Newsletter 3(1): January 1976.
4. Blum, R. H., and others: Society and drugs, San Francisco, 1969, Jossey-Bass, Inc., Publishers.
5. Brown, B.: Statement made at press conference releasing Marihuana and health, second annual report, Washington, D.C., Feb. 11, 1972, Department of Health, Education and Welfare.
6. Coleman, J. H., and Evans, W. E.: Drug interaction with alcohol, Alcohol, Health and Research World, Winter 1975-1976.
7. Dole, V., and Nyswander, M.: Speech presented at the fourth annual Methadone Maintenance Conference, San Francisco, Jan., 1972.
8. Goodman, L. S., and Gilman, A.: The pharmacological basis of therapeutics, ed. 4, London, 1971, The Macmillan Co.
9. Hammond, A. L.: Narcotic antagonists: new methods to treat heroin addiction, Science **173:**503-506, 1971.
10. Hammond, E. C.: The scientific background: world costs of cigarette smoking in disease, disability, and death, World Conference on Smoking and Health, New York, 1967, National Interagency Council on Smoking and Health.
11. Harris, R. T., and others, editors: Drug dependence, Austin, 1970, University of Texas Press.
12. Kitzinger, A.: Narcotics and dangerous drugs: a manual of basic information for teachers, Sacramento, 1964, California State Department of Education.
13. Kumagai, H.: Drug abuse in Japan, paper presented at the Conference on Psychotropic Drugs in Ottawa, Canada, Sept., 1971.
14. Lewin, L.: Phantastica: narcotic and stimulating drugs; their use and abuse, London, 1931, Kegan Paul, Trench, Trubner & Co.
15. Methadone in the management of heroin addiction, Med. Lett. Drugs Ther. **14:**13-15, 1972.
16. Methadone, 1972, Connection, Jan.-Feb., 1972.
17. Meyers, F. H., and Smith, D. E.: Pharmacologic

effects of marijuana, J. Psychedel. Drugs 2:31-36, 1968.

18. Practical criteria for the diagnosis of alcoholism in hospital practice, California Medical Association Position Paper, West. J. Med. 120:348-349, May 1974.

19. Public Health Service: Cigarette smoking and health characteristics, July 1964-June 1965, Washington, D.C., 1967, Public Health Service Publication no. 1000, series 10, no. 34, U.S. Government Printing Office.

20. Ray, O. S.: Drugs, society and human behavior, St. Louis, 1972, The C. V. Mosby Co.

21. Report on cigarette smoking, New York, 1971, American Cancer Society.

22. Smith, D. E., editor: Current marijuana issues, J. Psychedel. Drugs 2:1, 1968.

23. Smith, D. E., editor: Psychedelic drugs and religion, J. Psychedel. Drugs 1:2, 1967-68.

24. Smith, D. E., editor: Speed kills: a review of amphetamine abuse, J. Psychedel. Drugs 2:2, 1969.

25. Smith, D. E., editor: Drug abuse papers, ed. 2, San Francisco, 1969, University Extension, University of California at Berkeley.

26. Smith, D. E., and Bentel, D. J.: Drug Abuse Information Project, the fifth annual report to the legislature, San Francisco, 1971, University of California San Francisco Medical Center.

27. Smith, D. E., and Gay, G. R.: "It's so good, don't even try it once." Heroin in perspective, Englewood Cliffs, N.J., 1972, Prentice-Hall, Inc.

28. Smith, D. E., and Luce, J.: Love needs care, Boston, 1971, Little, Brown & Co.

29. Smith, D. E., and Wesson, D. R. Community approaches to drug abuse treatment and rehabilitation, J. Psychedel. Drugs 6(2): April-June, 1974.

30. Smith, D. E., and Wesson, D. R.: Diagnosis and treatment of adverse reactions to sedative-hypnotics, Rockville, Md., 1974, National Clearinghouse for Drug Abuse Information.

31. Smith, D. E., and Wesson, D. R.: Uppers and downers, Englewood Cliffs, N.J., 1973, Prentice-Hall, Inc.

32. Smoking and health facts, Washington, D.C., 1972, American Association for Health, Physical Education and Recreation.

33. Smoking and health, report of the Advisory Committee to the Surgeon General of the Public Health Service, Washington, D.C., 1964, Public Health Service.

34. U.S. Department of Health, Education and Welfare: Chartbook on smoking, tobacco, and health, Washington, D.C., 1969, U.S. Government Printing Office.

35. White Paper on Drug Abuse. A Report to the President from the Domestic Council Drug Abuse Task Force, Washington, D.C., September 1975, U.S. Government Printing Office.

36. Wesson, D. R., and Smith, D. E.: Barbiturate use, misuse and abuse, New York, 1977, Human Sciences Press.

37. Wilder, J.: Paradox reactions to treatment, N.Y. State J. Med. 57:3348-3352, 1957.

5
The role of the community in the drug problem

The magnitude of the drug problem is such that it does not limit itself to certain economic, social, educational, intellectual, or ethnic groups of people. Rather it involves the total community, including the home, school, church and religious groups, governmental and nongovernmental service, professional and voluntary organizations and agencies, and industry. All must participate in a variety of programs in terms of prevention, including education, control, rehabilitation, and treatment. There is need for different types of programs and approaches, many of which have not yet been developed. Without the multimodality concept approach and without community action on the part of a broad spectrum of individuals and groups in coordinated endeavors, the attack on the drug problem in society will be limited and probably ineffectual.

It is the purpose of this chapter to identify (1) the possible and current approaches to treatment and rehabilitation, (2) the governmental agencies developing leadership for action, (3) selected legal provisions for control, (4) illustrations of activities or programs, and (5) suggestions for community action. Occasional reference only will be made to schools, since this book emphasizes the school's role. This information is not meant to be prescriptive nor all-inclusive, but merely illustrative. Many new approaches, activities, and programs are constantly

emerging and being developed. The comments presented should not be construed as guidelines or models for community action, but rather as suggestions to receive consideration for local application.

TREATMENT AND REHABILITATION

In this discussion of treatment programs, we want the reader to be aware of the crucial difference between "civil commitment," forced commitment, and voluntary entry. To be helped away from drugs, the user must *want* very much to be helped, and he must want very much the *type* of help being offered. Our use of the term "voluntary" means just that—treatment without applying negative or criminal sanctions to encourage the user to volunteer for treatment.

For example, the prevailing law enforcement model of arresting the addict or drug user and forcing him into treatment must be seriously questioned. We believe that people create the market for drugs by demanding them in order to deal with both the *internal* and *external* chaos of their lives. Effective programs must not only be voluntary but must also help people to resolve their life problems.

Multimodality concept

We must first explain what we mean by a "multiple modality" approach to treatment, and why we feel this is important for the educator to understand. The causes of drug abuse and drug addiction are not well understood, and we are uncertain as to the *cures* of the problem as well. One likely reason for this uncertainty is that the term "drug abuse" embraces a wide variety of divergent behavior, and that, even in the narcotic addict population, there is marked heterogeny with many relevant variables.

Those who make up what is referred to as the "soft drug" or "hard drug" using populations as well as the multiple drug abusers exhibit widely differing reasons for initiating their use, engage in widely varying patterns of use, and are involved in widely differing psychosocial relationships, even within each population subgroup. Clearly a heterogeneous group such as drug abusers requires a number of highly differentiated treatment and rehabilitative approaches. For example, Synanon[7] is a well-known treatment program for narcotic drug addicts. But the Chicano or Mexican-American addict typically adjusts poorly to Synanon-type programs because of the disjunction from the family to which he is traditionally tied. He often fails to develop a usable, new group identity. Other programs seem better suited to his needs.

Not only is the phenomenon we loosely refer to as drug abuse constantly in a state of flux (the only thing constant about drug abuse is constant change), but it also requires a number of treatment and rehabilitative approaches. There is also great diversity among the available resources of any one community. Therefore rather than selecting one program or approach to the exclusion of others, the multimodality treatment concept allows all community groups to participate.

Besides being heterogeneous, drug users also appear to have some common characteristics. A population of drug-involved or drug-dependent persons seems to generally be divided into a number of identifiable types and subgroups. Such divisions, as Van Dusen[21] observes, fall along age lines (teenagers as against college-age youths), along racial lines, and include persons with particular life-styles who normally relate to each other exclusive of their drug involvement. Thus when a drug subgroup functions as a cultural entity, approaches to the group as a whole are possible as long as some treatment provision is *acceptable* to that group, and will be effectively utilized by it. However, the addict housewife or professional person who belongs to no drug subculture and may identify with no group must be treated individually.

Treatment for drug abusers today is in a state of monumental flux and transition, with new approaches still evolving. Mandell[8] draws the interesting analogy between drug treatment today and the treatment of pneumonia during the early part of this century. Before the discovery of antibiotics and modern chemotherapy, wide diversity of opinion existed among medical experts as to proper treatment—the appropriate temperature of the sick person's room, either regular or intermittent use of mustard plasters, etc. Such arguments are irrelevant and seem ridiculous in the light of our present knowledge, just as certain drug abuse treatment methods will seem ridiculous to future generations.

One may conclude, however, that whatever the evolution of medical treatment, spirited, antagonistic, and polarized positions as to the one appropriate strategy will always arise. Mandell states, "when human suffering combines with professional ignorance and the expectation of expertise by the patient, there inevitably arises superstition and politicized organization of the so-called body of knowledge within which the delivery of health care . . . must go on."[8]

As viewed through the perspective of the medical model, drug abuse is a complex disease process. Presently, instead of a single expedient protocol, one must select among multiple treatment strategies—if they are available—and a community should utilize or provide as many as possible. A multimodality treatment system, if it is financially feasible, is the preferred choice. As Mandell states, a multimodality treatment system may be developed within a single administrative structure in order to reduce or eliminate entirely much of the inefficiency and destructive rivalries between various treatment programs. The multimodality concept, Mandell believes, is defensible; it brings together doctors, mental health professionals, indigenous groups, community organizations, and government in a potentially constructive way.

Procedures

To begin dealing with treatment requires that we first identify the three conventional treatment functions, that is, crisis intervention, detoxification, and aftercare. These are important because the first time the drug user interacts with the treatment facility, a crisis may result or may have resulted.

Crisis intervention

Crisis intervention occurs either when a patient first arrives at a treatment facility, or, closer to the school situation (Chapter 8), when a student becomes ill or disturbed and needs assistance.[21]

In order to appropriately handle a crisis involving drug abuse, someone with *first-hand knowledge* must accurately assess the severity of the problem and make a diagnosis. This assessment is particularly important in such situations as handling the frantic phone calls from parents asking where they should take their youngster for treatment, or responding to the crisis created by an acutely disturbed student. No queries should be answered nor advice given until someone close to the problem has carefully assessed the nature of the youngster's drug-taking behavior.

The assessment of all significant persons involved in the crisis situation is important for the resolution of the problem. The attitudes, the behavior, the level of knowledge and sophistication about drugs and drug abuse, the communication skills, the degree of rapport with the youngster, and the maturity and emotional health of the parents must be considered in determining recommendations for the alleviation and elimination of the crisis.[3]

After disposition is made of the precipi-

tating crisis, the severity of the individual's drug problem should be determined. The drug use per se may be the primary factor or even the cause of personality disturbances; here treatment must be directed at the drug use pattern or at the life-style of the individual involved. But it must be remembered that the *drug use* itself or the acute medical-psychiatric crisis that it has created may be *secondary factors*, and long-term treatment should be focused on the fundamental psychological difficulties that may be the source of the drug-using behavior.

The "bad trip." Arising out of an extremely complex drug scene involving multiple drugs, unknown compounds, adulteration, contamination, and some of the unknown potentials of "homegrown" psychedelic agents is the bad trip. All the reactions of all psychedelic drugs cannot ever be known, since an ever-increasing list of new drugs leads to drug fads and indiscriminate usage as the popularity of one street drug gives way to another.

Threatening or moralizing approaches, although sincere, create stress at an inappropriate time and work detrimentally. They have no place in the short-term attack on the problem. The best aspects of a helped-helping relationship can be of value. This is highlighted by Dr. David E. Smith, Medical Director of the Haight-Ashbury Free Medical Clinic: ". . . remember that the patient has probably come reluctantly. To him, you represent the dominant culture that nearly all drug users—whether initiates or confirmed addicts—are somewhat at odds with, and he expects disapproval. *Try to make him feel as comfortable as possible. Show him by your manner as well as your words that you're concerned, that you're not just pumping him but trying to get information that will help you to help him.*"[14]

Protection of the individual from dangerous behavior to himself or to others should be of primary concern. The patient in a disturbed state should be provided with a quiet place, but *never* left entirely alone.

The comatose patient. Although the patient using psychedelic and other drugs and experiencing an acute toxic reaction ("freaking out") may appear to be a more difficult, demanding case, the comatose patient actually represents the most difficult of diagnostic and treatment problems. Whenever a student collapses into unconsciousness, you are dealing with a dangerous situation where prompt and *proper* therapy is essential and may be literally lifesaving. The airway should be cleaned and mouth-to-mouth resuscitation with closed chest cardiac massage initiated if necessary, while a physician or nurse is called.*

Time is essential. If the emergency has to proceed through the administrative chain of command (student courier is sent to the vice-principal's office, where the school nurse is summoned, who then calls a doctor, who must drive to the school from somewhere across town), precious minutes will be lost and the patient may suffer irrevocable damage or die. This has happened many times. An immediate response to this possibility should be planned with someone readily available who is experienced in handling such emergencies.

A school located in the inner city should establish specific procedures for overdose. Arrangements may be made with the county medical society or with a city hospital to have personnel other than a physician trained and available to intervene in a life-threatening situation. A paramedic who can give first aid to the drug victim may be a great asset to many schools. Schools should anticipate drug problems of a serious nature and make provisions for rapid, practical, and effective first aid and care (Chapter 8).

Freaking out. The other situation that we briefly mentioned earlier, freaking out, concerns the student who is disoriented and disturbed after taking psychedelic drugs.[2,17] Behavior may range from aimlessness, incoherence, and unresponsiveness (being "spacey" or "spaced") to screaming hysteria ("freak out"). These reactions occur particu-

larly with LSD; one moment the person is experiencing a pleasant or even exhilarating "dream" and the next instant, a horrifying nightmare. Both situations can be unnerving to the teacher or administrator and can create considerable classroom disturbance. There are two important points to remember in dealing with these experiences: (1) do not become drawn into the person's hysteria and confusion and (2) remember that this situation is generally manageable through patience and comforting. With these two guidelines, the educator should be able to cope with either of the two extremes encountered in psychedelic drug use.

An hysterical, confused person seems to create confusion and hysteria in others. The educator must act calmly and confidently with the knowledge that he or she can handle the situation if certain procedures are followed. Otherwise the confusion is infectious and only amplifies an already stressful situation beyond all manageable limits.

Because freaking out *is* generally manageable, the person's bad trip can be turned into a good one by patient suggestion and comfort. The remedy typically applied by people experienced with this situation is *not medicinal.* The worst procedure is to forcibly restrain the disturbed person and inject him with a tranquilizer. The results of this approach may include permanent psychic damage. The experienced approach is to lead the person calmly to a quiet room or a calm environment where paranoia, fear, and suspicion can be removed and the person talked down into a more relaxed frame of mind. The patient can usually be talked out of his bad trip and will calm himself to the point of becoming once again quite rational and cooperative. In his disoriented state the patient desperately needs a sympathetic, compassionate person to help him deal with his hysteria.

In most instances of freaking out *hospitalization will not be required*, since sympathetic reassurance, coupled with the appropriate use of medication, will tide the patient over the acute aspects of his experience. This is especially true when such aid can be

---

*Smith, D. E., and Wesson, D. R.: Diagnosis and treatment of adverse reactions to sedative-hypnotics, Rockville, Md., 1974, National Clearinghouse for Drug Abuse Information.

given in a quiet room under adequate but subdued lighting, with no noise or extraneous stimuli, and in the presence of, or with the help of, a friend who can assist in establishing rapport with the patient. Physical contact, such as a reassuring arm around the shoulder, may be of help, but care must be taken to prevent misinterpretation by the patient, making him fearful of possible harm.

The successful use of verbal, nonpharmacological techniques to treat a bad trip requires qualities such as sympathy, empathy, and friendliness on the part of the therapist. Reassurance should be provided to abort spiraling anxiety and loss of control on the part of the patient. The simple use of the phrase, "This is just a bad drug reaction and the effects will soon be over," and the changing of the subject foremost in the patient's thoughts to a neutral or pleasant topic, such as music or an attractive object in his visual environment, can bring a patient back to reality (Chapter 8). Teachers who feel uncomfortable in such a role can utilize others for this purpose, and may learn how to do a "talkdown" from more experienced persons, often youths, who have mastered the technique. Friends of the patient may have a role here. Although controlled observations have not been reported, physicians who have treated bad trips generally concede that the patient's interests are best served by attempting a talkdown before considering the use of any drugs.

Detoxification

Although a modality such as detoxification is primarily medical and requires medical expertise, we want to include just enough specifics to provide the educator with guidelines and some familiarity with what is involved.

Detoxification is a technical-medical term that simply means the elimination of drug substance from the user's system. In most cases this involves nothing more than providing a drug-free environment where the user's body will metabolize and eliminate the foreign chemical without outside intervention. While under the influence of a certain drug, another drug may have to be administered to counteract its effects.

As an example, a patient acutely intoxicated with an overdose of heroin or a morphine base compound would be injected with Nalline, a chemical antagonist, to diminish the drug's effect or cancel it out. This, of course, is done only by a physician and is not without some danger. Most drug ingestion, like drunkenness, should be allowed to *run its course under careful supervision.* We expect to "sleep it off" and sober up after a night of heavy drinking. The drug user must be treated in much the same way. Pills, including sedatives and tranquilizers, and injections are too often administered to bad effect. The main exception to this, noted in this chapter, is the comatose or unconscious person. Here, drastic emergency measures may need to be taken, including maintenance of cardiopulmonary function, as described by Smith and Wesson, and the patient needs to be hospitalized.

Once the individual is drug free, he is ready for the next stage in his rehabilitation to a non-drug-dependent person, treatment, which may involve a variety of techniques and procedures.

Aftercare

When a narcotic addict has been detoxified (is drug free), the long, hard job of rehabilitation begins. Rehabilitation means many things to many people. Perhaps "aftercare" is a less ambiguous term. No doubt the most important factor here is what the term means to the ex-addict himself.

There are several rehabilitative approaches currently available to the addict who seeks— or who is compelled—to kick his habit. These include the classic psychiatric hospital approach offered at the federal hospitals at Lexington, Kentucky and Fort Worth, Texas, established in the late 1930s to provide continuity of treatment in an environment removed from the addict's old haunts and lifestyle; mutual help communities such as Synanon, Daytop Village, Phoenix House, and Awareness House; religion-oriented programs such as Teen Challenge; narcotic antagonists therapy; and methadone maintenance. We shall briefly discuss each of these in turn to familiarize the educator with the barest essentials of the types of treatment.

Four approaches to drug abuse treatment, or aftercare, exist—the pharmaceutical, the psychiatric, the psychosocial, and the religious. Each is strikingly different and is supported by a highly vocal, dedicated group of treatment experts, each of whom claims that *his* treatment system is superior to the others.

Long-term treatment by chemicals, or synthetics, such as methadone (a long-acting narcotic) and cyclazocine (a long-acting narcotic antagonist), is called the pharmaceutical approach to addiction. This method of treatment is aimed primarily at the drug addict (narcotic drug user) and was found by the innovators of methadone treatment, Dr. Dole and Dr. Nyswander of New York.[15] The rationale is that addiction is not a moral or ethical issue but largely a *chemical* one. The person's body chemistry has changed once he becomes addicted, they claim. The answer then, say Dole and Nyswander (and now thousands of other treaters), is to provide a *chemical substitute* until the user's own body chemistry can be changed back—a task requiring maybe 20 years.

In contrast to this position is the classical psychiatric approach, which basically excludes the use of drugs in treatment and believes that only a long-term, fundamental restructuring of the patient's ego structure and outlook will alter his drug-using behavior.

The therapeutic community approach believes that drug use problems are largely incidental to problems of personal lifestyle and values. Many communities are modeled after a family with "big brothers and big sisters" who guide novices through the program. Such communities usually reside in one house or dormitory and typically insist that *no* drug of any kind, including coffee and cigarettes, be used. Later we shall discuss the therapeutic community approach to rehabilitation further and provide two examples.

Finally, the religious approach involves, or invokes, reference to something, or someone, supernatural or beyond the natural.

Pharmaceutical approaches. Within recent years, experimentation in the use of synthetic drugs to treat persons addicted to narcotics has been conducted in various institutions. The results of this experimentation have provided two techniques in particular— treatment with cyclazocine, a narcotic antagonist, and methadone—that have received the greatest amount of attention both in the literature and in their actual use.

Cyclazocine—a narcotic antagonist.[11] It has been proposed that the regular administration of cyclazocine, a long-acting narcotic antagonist, might be useful in the treatment of highly motivated, ambulatory patients to avoid relapse to the compulsive use of narcotics. When cyclazocine is given in appropriate doses, it reduces the subjective and physiological effects of any morphinelike drug even when such a drug is used frequently. The regular use of cyclazocine reduces or prevents the development of physical dependency on morphinelike drugs, thereby stabilizing the patient and allowing the process of rehabilitation to be more rapid and efficient.

However, treatment through the use of cyclazocine does not appear to provide the patient with the opportunity to be completely abstinent. The "narcotics hunger" still exists and the patient may stop taking the antagonist and return to narcotic use. Individuals may reduce their use of drugs from full addiction to occasional use and may resort to irregular shots of narcotics because they no longer fear the danger of addiction. Studies have shown that the use of cyclazocine alone is ineffective in the rehabilitation process and that individual and group helping services are needed as well.

Research for an additional drug that will have the same effect as cyclazocine but with longer lasting application is now being conducted. This new synthetic would last for 7 to 10 days and would alleviate the necessity for daily maintenance. In addition, longer maintenance would remove the temptation on the part of the individual to use other drugs.

Methadone.[9,10] The synthetic drug used for therapeutic purposes receiving the greatest amount of attention and generating the most controversy has been a synthetic addicting opiate called methadone. Research begun in 1964 by Dr. Vincent Dole and Dr. Marie Nyswander at Rockefeller University in New York indicates that methadone, when administered appropriately, blocks the action of heroin, eliminates the drug craving that drives many detoxified addicts to resume heroin use, and produces neither euphoria nor other distortions of behavior.

Methadone was brought to the United States from Germany after World War II. It was administered as a synthetic pain killer during the war when the Germans were in short supply of opiate derivatives. Since the war it has been used in Europe as an analgesic. The experimentation of Dole and Nyswander was among the first directed at employment of the drug in the treatment of heroin addiction.

The methadone program. Dole and Nyswander attribute drug addiction to a metabolic deficiency and tend to question psychological factors. They designed their experimental program into two phases. During phase 1 the patient undergoes an initial 6-week inpatient period during which oral doses of methadone dissolved in orange juice are administered. The doses are increased until a stabilizing dosage is reached. If the medication is given in proper doses, euphoria or undesirable side effects during the stabilization period should be nonexistent. In phase 2 of the program the patient is allowed to return to his community setting but is required to report to the clinic each day to take his supervised oral dose of methadone. Patients give daily urine samples to be analyzed for traces of illicit drugs. Eventually, if warranted by good conduct, patients are provided with several days' dosage at a time, and return once or twice a week for urinalysis and other tests.

Withdrawal from methadone is not, as of now, a part of the treatment process, except in a few experimental programs. Indications are that once withdrawn from methadone, patients experience a recurrence of the narcotic hunger and revert to the use of heroin. During each phase of the program, patients are provided with supportive services to aid in their rehabilitation. These supportive services are in the form of psychological, social, and vocational support. A wide array of therapists in each of these disciplines assist the patient. One of the problems with methadone maintenance is that it blocks only the effects of narcotics. Unfortunately, an increasing number of patients on such programs are abusing other drugs, particularly alcohol.

Opposition to methadone. Despite the positive reaction regarding methadone maintenance in treating opiate drug addiction, there exists much opposition to its use on social, medical, and legal grounds. Former addicts who have chosen to become totally abstinent from the use of drugs via the cold turkey approach have voiced strong opposition to any treatment method that uses synthetic drugs to maintain an addict. These opponents see more worth in halfway houses such as Phoenix House, Synanon, and Daytop Village where, by living with other former addicts in a structured setting, one is kept drug free. They reason that addicts maintained on methadone will be deprived of the opportunity to ever be drug free.

It is also believed that the same modality of treatment is not desirable for all addicts. Those who were addicted to drugs but were rehabilitated with methadone should not be denied the right to choose the method of treatment best suited for them.

Psychiatric approach. The psychiatric approach is characterized by individual counseling in a psychiatric hospital. Counseling involves an intense, long-term, personal, one-to-one dialogue with a psychiatrist. This means that whereas the addict picks up his methadone and goes home or to work, the patient of a classical psychiatrist is typically committed as an ambulatory or bed patient to a traditional psychiatric hospital. The cost of psychiatric treatment on the one-to-one model, with the "treater" playing "expert professional" and the patient acting as "passive submitter" to treatment, is therefore much higher than that of methadone, which can be administered cheaply to thousands of patients.

Clinical Research Center. The prototype of the psychiatric approach was the federal hospital for narcotics addiction treatment opened in 1935 in Lexington, Kentucky.[23] It was first called the United States Narcotics Farm, but within a year the name was changed to the United States Public Health Service Hospital. The institution was essentially a medical prison with barred windows and locked wards, "volunteer" admission being an alternative to an even longer sentence in a federal prison.

In 1967 the hospital joined the National Institute of Mental Health and became the Clinical Research Center; since then the Center has undergone changes in its treatment, philosophy, program procedures and rationales, operational structure, and physical facilities.

New patients receive physical examinations, undergo methadone detoxification, and then are assigned to wards. Individual and ward treatment teams consist of a physician, a social worker, and nurses. Most residents participate in group therapy; individual therapy is provided when it is both desirable and feasible. Patients engage in part-time work assignments related to maintaining the Center; residents who refuse to work are denied rewards and privileges. The education and training sections offer vocational training courses in bookbinding, shoe repair, alteration, dry cleaning and pressing of men's clothing, barbering, plastic laminating, auto ignition, microfilming, and the polishing, repairing, and waxing of dentures. Interested patients may also attend clases teaching paramedical or business-related subjects and Negro history and culture. Charm, beauty culture, and fashion design courses are available in the Women's Service.

Patients are given opportunities to control their own behavior and improve their environment. Increased freedom, visits to the city, special social and recreational functions, choice of rooms, and vocational guidance opportunities are incentives for mature behavior, productivity, and progress in therapeutic activities. Male and female patients eat their meals together and attend social hours, picnics, dances, and religious services together. Patient government maintains an ethics committee and a representative council. Residents have been appointed to task forces to revamp the Center's structure and have surveyed the patient population to find areas of need and interest for future education.

To maintain a drug-free environment, the Center conducts routine random urine tests. Within each unit, residents who temporarily require restraint are given intensive therapy in a locked ward. Unacceptable behavior is dealt with therapeutically rather than punitively, in accordance with the goal of conveying knowledge and principles without dogmatism. As patients are released, the Center refers them to Narcotic Addicts Rehabilitation Act (NARA) aftercare agencies, the Salvation Army, Greenwich House Counseling Center, and welfare agencies.

Psychosociological approaches. The term "psychosociological" is applied to treatment methods and practitioners who do not believe maintenance with synthetic drugs is an effective means of treating drug addiction but who advocate instead the use of structured settings, specific therapeutic techniques, and other methods of treatment to effect the rehabilitation process.

There are those who contend that drug addicts suffer from *character disorders* that cause them to express their conflicts by behavioral manifestations. Individuals of this description present complex, enduring problems and an extreme degree of social pathology in all their familial and community relationships. In recognition of this, it has been suggested that only limited goals be set in the treatment and rehabilitation of addicts and that primary emphasis be placed on allowing the addict to develop the means for limiting and curing his acting-out behavior.

Therapeutic communities. An almost total-living alternative to the addict's or drug user's former street life is available. The therapeutic community is specifically designed to counter all the styles of personal interaction and hustling of the professional drug user with an acceptable alternative. Although such living communities do produce "graduates" who typically become outstanding treatment personnel, the number of those who complete the specified period of rehabilitation is small. Many novices are simply unable to adjust to the new life and "split" after a few days or a few weeks. Such treatment is not applicable to a large number of addicts. The programs themselves are not able to accommodate very many persons. Yet they represent an important innovation in drug treatment.

The expectation on entering a therapeutic community is prompt and complete renunciation of heroin. Traditionally this meant cold turkey, but many current therapeutic communities have somewhat relaxed their treatment ideology to permit detoxification with methadone or nonnarcotic therapeutic medication over the first 5 to 7 days of initial treatment.

One noticeable aspect of initiation into a therapeutic community is the benign nature of the withdrawal syndrome which, when occurring in a hostile setting, such as a jail or a hospital, can be severe. Passivity and regression, typically created in the patient by a more hostile setting, are not encouraged in the therapeutic community. The novice is nursed through his cold turkey or withdrawal, but at the same time expected to perform his share of the work. He is assigned housekeeping chores and is expected to actively participate in the social life of the house. The role expected of the new community member is critical for future rehabilitation because psychological set and psychosocial reinforcement, or the lack of it, are always relevant variables in drug-related behavior.

A prospective patient must be able to live in the therapeutic community for 1 to 2 years of 24-hour a day, 7-day a week involvement with the "dynamics" of the house where he

lives. All habits and relationships—past, present, and future—are subject to group inspection and evaluation. A patient has to prove his ability to be independent because a central part of the treatment philosophy of therapeutic communities is the view that the heroin addict is a dependent child who does not have the ability to be honest about property or feelings. Treatmet is seen as a total resocialization process in which direct, honest communication is practiced with respect to all aspects of the addict's new life. If the addict can adjust to the experience (and it is clear that many cannot), he or she experiences tremendous support from his membership in the group.

Humor, tenderness, and affirmation begin to be felt as real experiences. The addict learns that negative feelings do not necessarily destroy the possibility of future warmth and he begins to learn effective social responses. These trusting and relating experiences are often totally contradictory to those experiences of his former life-style as a hustling street junkie.

One negative aspect is that the "reborn" addict may find himself as psychologically dependent on the new community as he was on the old. Most experts in the field of drug abuse treatment feel that therapeutic communities are of unquestioned value for some patients, but that such a community does not constitute an approach that is applicable to large numbers of persons. Charles Dederick, creator of the first therapeutic community (Synanon), is quoted as stating that he feels that his community was suitable for only one out of ten addicts.[1] The addict who is married, has children, and has a steady job is usually not disposed to want or to accept treatment in a therapeutic community. The single, more dependent, younger addict is more likely to want to do so.

Most therapeutic communities are organized around more or less identifiable steps in which increments of trust, status, and power in the group are acquired. These steps can be thought of as roughly similar to the various rites (such as confirmation or bar mitzvah) utilized by social groups in the "straight" world to mark various stages of maturation. Therapeutic communities have not institutionalized these basic steps, but the underlying process is the same.

Subcommunity settings. The advent of structured community settings such as Daytop Village[4] and Synanon as a means for treating and rehabilitating drug addicts has come about as the result of the conviction that the most effective way to rid an individual of his addiction to drugs is through a combination of abstinence and supportive therapy. Control of the individual's behavior, including his use of drugs, is achieved by the fact that he lives within a subcommunity created for the exclusive purpose of treating and rehabilitating drug addicts. The use of any drug is forbidden while the individual is a member of the subcommunity and he may actually be excluded from the community if he does not abstain.

Supportive therapy in the treatment process is usually labeled "encounter therapy." In encounter therapy a specific treatment relationship is used to promote the personal growth of all the individuals involved. A definition of a treatment relationship has been offered by Casriel, who has stated: "A treatment relationship is any situation in which two or more persons encounter each other as equal human beings with a sense of challenge, and with responsible concern rather than indulgence."[4] The need to submit to the comments of others regarding one's own behavior and to encounter or challenge the behavior of these others is a necesary ingredient of any therapeutic relationship if an individual is to grow and understand his own behavior and eventually control it in more socially acceptable ways. Any treatment that evolves from sessions involving one or more persons demands a more human kind of involvement from the therapist and leads ideally to a fuller, more mature kind of growth for the individuals concerned.

Any person who accepts the responsibility for the treatment of drug addicts by means of encounter therapy must be willing to be open to challenges concerning changes in his own behavior. He must accept a relationship with drug addicts that reflects their dignity as human beings. He must not see their addiction or general behavior as a reflection of weakness, but must perceive the patient as an individual who is capable of achieving his aspirations and reducing his failures. In addition, this form of therapy is contraindicated for the severely mentally disturbed or psychotic polydrug abuser, as it may precipitate a psychiatric crisis leading to a suicide attempt.

The success of these programs and their form of therapy has been questioned. The main consensus is that whatever success these methods may have achieved has been confined to the subcommunity setting in which the patient lives. Reintegration of the patient into the general community has not always been as successful.

Synanon: prototype of a therapeutic lifestyle. Founded in California in 1958 by Charles E. Dederick, Synanon is the foremost therapeutic community in the country for drug rehabilitation. The organization has pioneered an alternative life-style involving thousands of people, most of whom have stopped their former drug use patterns. The Synanon model has been copied in many parts of the country, especially in New York.

Few people interested in the problem of drug abuse take neutral positions with regard to Synanon. Apart from Synanon's enormous direct impact in helping to solve the drug problem, the element of controversy about the organization and its life-style has evoked a considerable amount of highly significant and valuable dialogue.

The dictionary definition of Synanon, "a private organization assisting those who wish to be cured of drug addiction," refers to only one dimension of the overall Synanon system. The organization has steadily moved beyond the work of treating drug addiction and crime. Dederick, chairman of the Board of Regents at Synanon, has repeatedly stated that Synanon is not primarily interested in curing drug addiction, but that this seems to occur as a side effect of an individual's participation in Synanon's life-style.

Synanon's overall program encompasses (1)

a new kind of group therapy; (2) an approach to racial integration; (3) a humane solution to some facets of bureaucratic organization; (4) a different way of being religious; (5) a humanistic method of encounter therapy; (6) an unusual kind of communication; and (7) an exciting, fresh approach to the cultural arts and to philosophy. One side effect of intense participation in these diverse human experiences is that those participants who were criminal addicts have found a new existence and now lead constructive lives.

A drug user with a past history of institutionalized treatment of another kind generally finds himself in a new situation in Synanon. In most standard treatment programs a patient or inmate subculture usually develops within the overall approach. This tends to produce a "we-they" conflict and a split between the professional personnel and the "clients." The "client society" tends to be underground and to develop norms, patterns of behavior, and goals different from and, more often than not, in conflict with the "treatment establishment." This is partly due to the fact that most clients have had severe difficulties with authority for a good part of their lives. Synanon does not have a "we-they" caste system where the client is relegated to a lower position in the organization. It provides instead an open-ended stratification situation. A full possibility for upward mobility is available in the organization. There is not only upward social mobility in Synanon, but healthy status seeking is encouraged.

Synanon assumes, with some supportive evidence, that a person's position in its hierarchy is a correlate of social maturity and mental health. An old Synanon adage is "character is the only rank." Since the development of character is related to success in the organization, certain behavior is encouraged, such as speaking out in a Synanon game when someone feels or observes a wrong. This is encouraged regardless of the wrongdoer's status in the organization. In fact, to be silent in the face of injustice carries with it the moral condemnation of the group. Unlike the code of the streets, "copping out" on each other for behavior that is

either self-destructive or harmful to the group is both condoned and actively fostered. This does not occur in the usual institutional "we-they" atmosphere.

The most important widely and continually used group process in Synanon is "the game." All members participate in its process at least several times a week. In part it is an intimate group interaction situation in which a member can openly express his problems, fears, and hostilities to his fellow members. He can expect a response that enables him to see his personal truths in a new and exciting perspective. The game also enables members to express what they really think of each other without fear of retribution. Members can often solve the confusions and conflicts of their occupational and interpersonal relationships. A participant in a game can be as spontaneous, creative, rigid, angry, loud, or passive as he chooses with no authority rules save one, the proscription of physical violence.

The game frequently helps to regulate behavior in Synanon. Transgressions are often prevented by the knowledge that the next time the game is played a member's deviance will rapidly and necessarily be brought to the attention of the Synanon community. The participant is living in a community where others know about and, perhaps more importantly, care about his behavior.

Another major impact of the Synanon game is its ability to convey to each member a sense of responsibility and its corollary, a sense of personal value and significance. To persons who have suffered from chronic feelings of weakness or helplessness and who characteristically see themselves as victims, the game becomes very meaningful because they are shown that their behavior can have a direct effect on other people and that is is within their power to change the overall society in a positive way.

Some of the more recent activities of Synanon include (1) Synanon game group interaction sessions; (2) a challenging and involving educational system; (3) business activities that help finance the operation; (4) a human research and development center at Tomales

Bay, California, where plans are being made for a model city; (5) a black social, cultural, and educational program; (6) a group program for the parents of residents; and (7) a continuing series of marathon trips (some lasting 24 and 48 hours) and educational and emotional experiences that have produced positive results.

Daytop village.[5] The provision of a residential or community setting in which the addict can live in order to overcome his need for drugs and to be rehabilitated is also the premise on which Daytop Village functions. Originating in New York City, where three facilities are now able to help some 450 persons at a time, Trenton, New Jersey, has become the site of the first such "village" outside of New York City.

Anyone who shows a sincere desire to be helped is accepted. The only demands made are the following: no chemicals, drugs, or alcohol may be used and no violence or even threat of violence is allowed. An individual's degree of sincerity is measured by the staff, all ex-addicts, who feel they can tell when someone is insincere about wanting to be helped because they have been in that position themselves.

The process of treatment includes withdrawal, work, and therapy. Before an addict is accepted he must agree to free himself of drugs. When asked about the withdrawal process, Jim Halloram, the director of the program, has commented: "Withdrawal is not that bad. It's no worse than a case of the flu, and they go through it right here with everyone around them." Withdrawal is followed by a short period in which the prospective resident assists in maintaining the facility in which the center is located and participates in discussions. Once eligible for residency, the patient is accepted into one of the residential facilities.

During his tenure as a resident, usually about 20 months, the individual is assigned menial jobs initially, followed by other assignments as his degree of responsibility increases. During this time, therapy is provided by all enrolled in the program and by the staff through the means of periodic group sessions. Peer-group acceptance is empha-

sized at Daytop and with it the hope that each ex-addict will gain a sense of responsibility to himself and to others.

Religious approach. Last of all, the religious approach should be mentioned. The most effective examples that we have observed are fundamentalist groups called "Jesus freaks," who inculcate a whole Christian way of living and meaningful service to others. Some of these groups have almost no use of drugs among their teenagers and have proved effective in turning off ordinarily nonreligious drug users. Usually these fundamentalist groups are closely knit and have a warm emotional interchange and a rewarding life of public service. Teen Challenge is one such organization. Young persons in these church groups are usually drug resistant, in contrast to average teenagers who have few or no mores against drugs.

Within the domain of what might be called spiritual or religious approaches to drug abuse treatment is the approach used by Alcoholics Anonymous. Emphasis in these groups is on testimonials from those who have struggled with a debilitating addiction, and who meet regularly to plan and discuss the importance of abstinence. AA relies on developing a quasi-religious community whose salvation is working together to lick their common affliction—alcoholism. Many persons who for 20 or 30 years were not able to develop the willpower "to stay off alcoholic beverages" were able to do so for the first time after they joined AA. There is also a "Tobacco Anonymous."

GOVERNMENT PROGRAMS AND RESOURCES

The programs available to help combat the drug abuse problems at the federal, state, and local levels are numerous. This section will make brief reference to such programs.

National programs

There are thousands of treatment and rehabilitation programs[22] in the United States and its territories. They offer a variety of types of services that include the following: detoxification, methadone maintenance, crisis intervention, educational counseling, psychotherapy, family counseling, religious counseling, recreational counseling, social services, encounter groups, self-awareness groups, job placement, vocational preparation and guidance, and medical-surgical treatment. Information on these ever-changing federal programs can be obtained from ADAMHA (Alcohol Drug Abuse and Mental Health Administration), the umbrella agency for the NIAAA (National Institute on Alcohol Abuse and Alcoholism), NIDA (National Institute on Drug Abuse), and NIMH (National Institute on Mental Health), all located in the Washington, D.C., area or in the respective single state agencies on alcohol and drug abuse located in state capitals.

State level

Each state has its own organizational arrangement for handling drug problems. Single state agencies on alcohol and drug abuse have been established in state capitals to be responsible for coordinating the efforts of such departments as health, mental health, education, and law enforcement as well as other community activities in terms of prevention, control, treatment, and research. An advisory committee comprising a variety of community representatives may be appointed to render assistance and guidance. In addition, individual departments may employ specialists to deal with problems unique to that department.

Civil addict program

In 1961 California established the Civil Addict Program to provide compulsory inpatient and aftercare treatment and control for opiate users. Addicts are civilly committed by a California superior court. The proceedings under which the addict may be committed can be initiated in three ways: (1) The addict, a relative, or some other responsible person may approach the county district attorney, who may then petition the court for consideration of the addict's commitment. No criminal charge is involved. When necessary, provisions are available to detain the alleged addict for medical exami-

nation. (2) If any person is convicted of any crime in a superior court of law and is believed by the judge to be an addict, the proceedings shall be adjourned or the judge may suspend the imposition of sentence. (3) Any person convicted of a felony (with certain exceptions) may, if the judge believes he is an addict, be referred to another superior court to determine the issue of his addiction after he is convicted and the original criminal proceedings are suspended.

All commitments are for the same technical and legal reason—addiction or "imminent danger" of addiction—regardless of the basis for referral. The criminal matter, if any, becomes irrelevant, remaining in suspended status with the court. Whether the addict is committed voluntarily or not, he is bound for a definite period of treatment. The law provides a maximum 2½-year commitment for volunteers and a 7-year commitment for others. This term is to include both inpatient and aftercare treatment. On an original commitment a minimum of 6-months' inpatient treatment is required; however, for a returnee there is not limit on length of stay for treatment.

Inpatient care consists of intensive interaction in community living groups, small group work, academic and vocational instruction, recreation, work therapy, physical fitness and religious programs. The inpatient phase of the treatment process may be terminated after the minimum time has elapsed and when the professional staff of the institution feels that the person has made sufficient progress. The suggestion for termination is referred for certification to the Narcotic Addict Evaluation Authority, which acts in cases of release, return, and discharge. Upon transfer from the inpatient treatment center to the state-wide outpatient program, the individual is supervised by a specially trained field agent who works only with releasees from one of the centers.

The Civil Addict Program offers close supervision, antinarcotic testing, group therapy, job placement service, and halfway houses. Abstention from the use of narcotics for 3 consecutive years may permit the releasee to be discharged from his commitment and the criminal charges against him, if any, may be dismissed by the judge.

Specific provisions of the program, compulsory inpatient treatment, close and continuing supervision in the community, and antinarcotic testing are means by which the former addict is forced to continue treatment. The results of these efforts have been fruitful.

Local level

Organizational patterns for handling drug problems in communities differ throughout the United States. These patterns probably relate to state level arrangements in which there may be an advisory committee and a coordinator. In California, legislation has mandated drug coordinators at the county level, thereby completing the federal, state, local agency interactions.

LEGAL PERSPECTIVE
Federal laws regarding narcotics and drugs[17]

Since 1914 numerous federal laws have been passed concerning the distribution of narcotics and other drugs. The principal statutes are designed to ensure an adequate supply of narcotics for medical and scientific needs, and at the same time to curb the abuse of narcotic drugs and marijuana. What we consider to be the most important of these laws are summarized here and presented in chronological order.

Harrison Narcotic Act (1914). The Harrison Narcotic Act set up the machinery for the distribution of narcotic drugs within the country and initiated a policy that is still the basis of present drug control programs. Enacted as a revenue measure, the Treasury Department was designated as the enforcement agency. Under this law, all persons who imported, manufactured, produced, compounded, sold, dealt in, disposed of, or transferred narcotic drugs had to register annually and pay a graduated occupational tax of $1 to $24 per year. They were required to keep records, make them available to law officers, and file returns specified by the Secretary of the Treasury. The tax was placed on the following narcotic drugs: opium, isonipecaine, coca leaves, and opiates; compounds, manufactures, salts, derivatives, or preparations of the foregoing; and substances chemically identical to the foregoing.

Traffic in narcotic drugs without registration was a separate offense, independent of failure to register. Thus the transportation of narcotic drugs in interstate commerce by persons not registered was prohibited except for employees and agents of registrants within the scope of their employment.

Narcotic Drugs Import and Export Act (1922). The passage of the Narcotic Drugs Import and Export Act of 1922 extended the prohibition against opium imports (set in 1909) to other narcotics, including morphine, coca leaves, and their derivatives. The amount of narcotics that could be lawfully imported was limited to such amounts as the Commissioner of Narcotics found necessary for legitimate medical and scientific uses. Manufactured drugs and preparations could be exported under a rigid system of controls to assure that the drugs were used for medical needs only in the country of destination.

The penalty for unlawfully importing, receiving, facilitating transportation, or sale under this act was imprisonment for not less than 5 nor more than 20 years and a maximum fine of $20,000. Subsequent offenses were punishable by a minimum sentence of 10 years and a maximum sentence of 40 years, plus a $20,000 fine. A similar penalty was provided for smuggling marijuana.

Marijuana Tax Act (1937). The Marijuana Tax Act required all persons who imported, manufactured, produced, compounded, sold, dealt in, dispensed, prescribed, administered, or gave away marijuana to register and pay a graduated occupational tax ranging from $1 to $24 per year. No commodity tax was imposed on this drug. Transfer of marijuana was limited to that made on the authority of official order forms.

A 1969 Supreme Court decision removed two of the federal government's major legal weapons against marijuana traffic in holding that the Marijuana Tax Act is unenforceable when the accused claims the Fifth Amendment privilege against self-incrimination. The Court also declared unreasonable the law's presumption that a person with marijuana in their possession knows that it was imported illegally, thus violating due process of law.

Federal Food, Drug, and Cosmetic Act (1938). The pertinent drug sections of the Federal Food, Drug, and Cosmetic Act of 1938 may be summarized as follows:

1. Proper labeling is required and the statement, "WARNING—May Be Habit Forming," must be attached to a drug that is for use by man and that contains any quantity of narcotic or hypnotic substance, alpha eucaine, barbituric acid, beta eucaine, bromal, cannabis, cabromal, chloral, coca, cocaine, codeine, heroin, marijuana, morphine, opium, paraldehyde, peyote, sulfonmethane, or chemical derivates of the foregoing.

2. Prescription is required for the dispensing of a drug intended for use by man that (a) contains certain narcotic or other substances designated by regulation as habit forming; (b) is not safe except under the supervision of a licensed practitioner because of its potentiality for harmful use; or (c) is limited to use under the professional supervision of a licensed practitioner under procedures for the introduction of new drugs into interstate commerce.

3. No new drugs may be introduced into interstate commerce unless an application filed with the Secretary of Health, Education and Welfare is in effect with respect to such drug.

4. Annual registration is required of establishments that manufacture, compound, or process drugs and that wholesale or distribute any depressant or stimulant drug. The 1962 Drug Act established registration requirements. The depressant stimulant drug registrations were added by the Drug Abuse Control Amendments of 1965, which established special federal controls over these and hallucinogenic drugs.

The Federal Food, Drug, and Cosmetic Act as amended in 1962 and 1965 enumerates prohibited acts as follows:

1. Introduction or delivery into interstate commerce of adulterated or misbranded foods, drugs, devices, or cosmetics

2. Their adulteration or misbranding in interstate commerce

3. Their receipt and delivery in adulterated or misbranded state

4. The introduction or delivery into interstate commerce of any article in violation of temporary permit controls (applicable to food) or in violation of procedures for the introduction of new drugs

5. Refusal to permit access to records of interstate shipments of food, drugs, devices, or cosmetics, or to make the records or reports required under procedures for the introduction of a new drug

6. Refusal to permit entry and inspection of certain establishments in which foods, drugs, devices, and cosmetics are manufactured or held

7. Manufacture of adulterated or misbranded foods, drugs, devices, and cosmetics

8. The giving of certain false guarantees regarding good faith in receiving or delivering such articles

9. Certain false use of identification devices required under law, doing of certain acts that cause a drug to be counterfeit, or the sale, dispensing, or holding for sale or dispensing of a counterfeit drug

10. Misuse of trade secret information

11. Certain acts resulting in adulteration or misbranding of foods, drugs, devices, or cosmetics in interstate commerce

12. Representing or suggesting in labeling or advertising that approval of a new drug application is in effect or that the drug complies with new drug introduction procedures

13. Violation of laws governing the coloring of margarine

14. The use in sales promotion of any reference to a report or analysis furnished under inspection procedures
15. In the case of prescription drugs, failure of the manufacturer, packer, or distributor to maintain or transmit to requesting practitioners true and correct copies of all printed matter required to be included in the drug package
16. Failure of drug manufacturers and processors and depressant or stimulant drug wholesalers, jobbers, or distributors to register with the Secretary of Health, Education and Welfare
17. Relative to stimulant or depressant drugs: manufacturing, processing, or compounding, except by registered drug firms for legal distribution; distributing such drugs to persons not licensed or authorized by law; failure to prepare, obtain, or keep required records and to permit inspection as authorized; and filling or refilling prescriptions for these drugs in violation of law

Imprisonment for not more than 1 year or a fine of not more than $1000 or both is the penalty for violation of any of these prohibitions. If the violation is committed after a previous conviction has become final, or is made with intent to defraud or mislead, the violator is subject to imprisonment for not more than 3 years or a fine of not more than $10,000 or both.

Opium Poppy Control Act (1942). Production of the opium poppy in the United States except under license of the Secretary of the Treasury, was prohibited by the Opium Poppy Control Act of 1942. No license has ever been issued under this statute.

Harrison Narcotic Act Amendment (1946). This amendment to the 1914 Harrison Narcotic Act was made to include synthetic substances having addiction-forming or addiction-sustaining qualities similar to cocaine or morphine.

Boggs Amendment (1951). The 1951 legislation known popularly as the Boggs Amendment increased penalties for persons vio-

lating federal narcotic and marijuana laws, precluded suspension of sentence or probation on second and subsequent offenses, and made conspiracy to violate the narcotic laws a special offense. It substituted for the old maximum sentences a series of sentences for repeated offenders as follows:

First offense—not less than 2 nor more than 5 years
Second offense—not less than 5 nor more than 10 years with probation and suspension excluded
Subsequent offenses—not less than 10 nor more than 20 years with probation and suspension excluded

Narcotic Control Act (1956). As the result of 1955 congressional investigations of the illicit narcotic traffic, the Narcotic Control Act of 1956 increased and made more inflexible the penalties for narcotic offenders. Parole was excluded in cases of a selling offense and second or subsequent possession offenses. The penalties were as follows:

First possession offense—not less than 2 nor more than 10 years, with probation and parole permitted
Second possession or first selling of narcotics or marijuana—not less than 5 nor more than 20 years, with probation, suspension, and parole excluded
Third possession or second selling and subsequent offenses—not less than 10 nor more than 40 years with probation, suspension, and parole excluded

These penalties carried, in addition, a maximum $20,000 fine. Exclusion of drug offenders from federal parole laws means that they must serve two thirds of their sentence. Most other federal prisoners are eligible for release under supervision after serving one third of their sentences.

This act also banned the possession of heroin and required persons possessing heroin to surrender it to the Secretary of the Treasury within 120 days.

Narcotics Manufacturing Act (1960). A system for licensing manufacturers to produce narcotic drugs was developed in the Narcotics Manufacturing Act of 1960. It also set manufacturing quotas for the basic classes of narcotic drugs, both natural and synthetic, ensuring that an adequate supply of each drug would be available for medicine and science.

Under this and other federal laws, the Secretary of the Treasury is the cabinet officer charged with responsibility for investigating offenses and regulating lawful imports and exports. He acts through the Commissioner of Narcotics, who is the chief officer of the Federal Bureau of Narcotics, and is required to cooperate with the states in the suppression of the abuse of narcotic drugs in their respective jurisdictions.

Drug Abuse Control Amendments (1965). In January 1963 President Kennedy established a President's Advisory Commission on Narcotic and Drug Abuse. The Commission made 25 recommendations, the influence of these being reflected in the Drug Abuse Control Amendments of 1965.

Three groups of dangerous drugs—depressants, stimulants, and hallucinogens—are controlled by the Drug Abuse Control Amendments to the Federal Food, Drug, and Cosmetic Act passed in 1965 and amended in 1968. These amendments provide for stronger regulations in manufacture, distribution, delivery, and possession and strong criminal penalties against persons who deal in these drugs illegally. All registered manufacturers, processors, and their suppliers, wholesaler druggists, pharmacies, hospitals, clinics, public health agencies, and research laboratories must take an inventory, keep accurate records of receipts and sales of these drugs and make their records available to Bureau of Narcotics and Dangerous Drugs agents for examination. No prescription for a controlled drug older than 6 months can be filled nor can refills be made more than five times in the 6-month period.

The Drug Abuse Control Amendments of 1965 impose more stringent controls on stimulant, depressant, and hallucinogenic drugs. The new law, which became effective in 1966, begins with a declaration by Congress that these drugs need not move across state lines to be subject to its regulations. The law notes that "in order to make regulation and protection of interstate commerce in such drugs effective, regulation of intrastate commerce is also necessary" because of the difficulties of determining place of origin and consumption and because regulation of interstate but not intrastate com-

merce "would discriminate against and adversely affect interstate commerce in such drugs."

The amendments add to the body of law a definition of a depressant or stimulant drug as follows:

1. One that contains barbituric acid or its salts or a derivative therefrom which has been designated under federal law as habit forming
2. One that contains amphetamine or its salts or a substance designated as habit forming by the Secretary of Health, Education and Welfare because of its stimulant effect on the central nervous system
3. One containing a substance designated by regulations as having a "potential for abuse" because of its depressant or stimulant effect on the central nervous system or its hallucinogenic effect. (Narcotic drugs are specifically excluded.)

Lysergic acid and lysergic acid amide are drugs covered by the amendments of 1965, along with mescaline and its salts, peyote, and psilocybin. The act also prohibits the possession of depressant or stimulant drugs except by seven classes of persons who can be generally described as manufacturing or doing research upon the drug.

Further changes in the Drug Abuse Control Amendments to the Federal Food, Drug, and Cosmetic Act of 1965 were made in 1968. These changes increased the penalties for anyone who illegally produced, sold, or disposed of dangerous drugs, and imposed a misdemeanor penalty for possession.

Narcotic Addict Rehabilitation Act (1966). A significant effort toward the treatment and rehabilitation of narcotic addicts was enacted in 1966 with the signing of the Narcotic Addict Rehabilitation Act. The legislation, effective February 1967, provided for civil commitment in lieu of prosecution (Chapter 4).

Comprehensive Drug Abuse Prevention and Control Act (1970). In 1969 President Nixon delivered before Congress a ten-point message calling for a new federal drug law that would consolidate over 50 public drug-related laws promulgated by the federal government since 1914. On October 27, 1970, President Nixon signed into law the Comprehensive Drug Abuse Prevention and Control Act of 1970 (P.L. 91-513). Thus all federal dangerous drug, narcotic, and marijuana laws are consolidated into one comprehensive act designed to control the legitimate drug industry and to curtail importation and distribution of illicit drugs throughout the United States.

Controlled Substances Act (1971). With the passage of the Controlled Substance Act, effective May 1, 1971, the control of narcotics and dangerous drugs was transferred from the Treasury Department, Internal Revenue Service, to the Department of Justice, Bureau of Narcotics and Dangerous Drugs (BNDD).

Many items not previously restricted are now included on the list of controlled substances, and stricter requirements for obtaining and handling such substances have been established. Five schedules of controlled substances have been defined.

Schedule I substances. Drugs in this schedule are those that have no *currently* accepted medical use in the United States. Some examples are heroin, marijuana, LSD, peyote, mescaline, psilocybin, tetrahydrocannabinol, morphine, methylsulfonate, and nicocodeine.

Schedule II substances. The drugs in this schedule have a high abuse potential with severe psychic or physical dependence liability. Most Schedule II substances have been known in the past as Class A narcotic drugs. One narcotic group is currently included in this schedule, the amphetamines, including methamphetamines (Syndrox, Desoxyn, Methedrine). Some examples of Schedule II narcotic substances are opium, morphine, codeine, dihydromorphinone (Dilaudid), methadone (Dolophine), pantopium (Pantopon), meperidine (Demerol), cocaine, and oxycodone (Percodan).

Schedule III substances. The drugs in this schedule have an abuse potential less than those in Schedules I and II and include those drugs formerly known as Class B narcotics,

and, in addition, nonnarcotic drugs such as glutethimide (Doriden), phenmetrazine (Preludin), methyprylon (Noludar), methylphenidate (Ritalin), nalorphine, and barbiturates (except phenobarbital, methylphenobarbital, and barbital). Paregoric is now listed in this schedule.

Schedule IV substances. The drugs in this schedule have an abuse potential less than those listed in Schedule III and include barbital, phenobarbital, methylphenobarbital, chloral hydrate, ethchlorvynol (Placidyl), ethinamate (Valmid), and meprobamate (Equanil and Miltown).

Schedule V substances. The drugs in this schedule have an abuse potential less than those listed in Schedule IV and consist of those preparations formerly known as *exempt narcotics*, with the exception of paregoric (camphorated tincture of opium).

• • •

It must be stressed, however, that federal drug abuse strategy changes quite rapidly. For example, in November, 1976, the Strategy Council on Drug Abuse presented the following federal strategy for drug abuse prevention, listing six key points:

1. Total elimination of drug abuse is unlikely but governmental actions can contain the problem and limit its adverse effects. The federal government recognizes that drug abuse is a long-term problem and requires a long-term commitment.
2. All drugs are not equally dangerous and all drug use is not equally destructive. Enforcement efforts should therefore concentrate on drugs which have a high addiction potential, and treatment programs should give priority to those individuals abusing high-risk drugs and to compulsive users of any drugs.
3. Efforts to reduce the supply of and the demand for drugs are complementary and interdependent, and federal programs should continue to be based on a balance between these two concepts.
4. Existing programs aimed at supply and demand reduction must be broadened.

In supply reduction, greater emphasis should be given to regulatory and compliance activities aimed at curtailing diversion from legitimate production and a higher priority should be given to increasing international cooperation in preventing the illicit production of drugs. In demand reduction, increased attention should be given to prevention, early intervention, and vocational rehabilitation.

5. Program management must be improved to ensure the maximum return from resources committed to drug programs. Better interagency coordination and stronger intra-agency management are required. More attention should be paid to the setting of priorities, with federal law enforcement efforts focused on high-level traffickers and federal treatment resources focused on habitual users of high-risk drugs such as heroin, amphetamines, and barbiturates.

6. The federal government should provide leadership in the national drug abuse prevention effort, but it cannot do the job alone. The support and cooperation of state and local governments, private businesses, and community organizations are essential if we are to contain drug abuse and minimize its costs to the individual and society.

It is quite obvious that this summary differs dramatically from federal drug abuse strategies developed from previous decades, and the reader should maintain an awareness of the changing laws and federal approach to drug abuse prevention.[6]

Table 5-1 lists the present federal marijuana penalties.

State laws

Criminal penalties for the use of illegal drugs vary from state to state. Classifications of violation differs, as do the lengths of sentences for transporting, selling, or using different drugs, the laws affecting treatment, parole practices, and so on. The teacher or counselor whose responsibilities include working with drug users should know the laws as they apply in his particular state. Many municipalities also have specific ordinances regarding marijuana, narcotics, and dangerous drugs, and these also may be consulted.

However, it must be stressed that state drug laws also change frequently as legislative and public attitudes towards drug abuse and related problems change. For example, Table 5-2 identifies eight states which, as of 1976, have decriminalized personal possession of marijuana. Just a short time ago such possession would have been a *felony* and theoretically could again be made a felony in the future. Further, there is still great variation in individual state drug laws with some drugs receiving more strict penalties and others receiving less severe penalties. Table 5-3 illustrates the differing state penalties for possession of marijuana. It is important to understand that review of *current* drug laws in the various states is necessary in order to be up to date at a particular place and time, in this complex area. The single state agency in each state can provide this information.

Drug abuse treatment and the laws of the state of California*

The legislature of this state has made the treatment of a narcotics addict by a physician in private practice extremely difficult, if not impossible. The law provides that no person shall treat an addict for addiction except in a county jail, state prison, state hospital, county hospital, county-operated mental health center, or an institution approved by the Board of Medical Examiners. In 1970 the legislature amended the law to provide that methadone in the continuing treatment of narcotic addiction shall be used only in those programs approved by the California Research Advisory Panel. The Research Advisory Panel was originally set up to encourage research into the nature and effects of marijuana and hallucinogenic drugs. Physicians are prohibited from issuing prescriptions to

---

*Modified from Blake, R. L.: A short summary of drug laws, Santa Clara, Calif., 1971, Catholic Social Service.

Text continued on p. 127.

TABLE 5-1. Federal marijuana penalties (all fines represented as maximum amounts possible)

Offense	First offense	Second offense	Subsequent offense
Simple possession	0-1 yr and/or $5,000*	0-2 yrs and/or $10,000	Same
Possession with intent to distribute	0-5 yrs and/or $15,000	0-10 yrs and/or $30,000	Same
Sale or distribution	0-5 yrs and/or $15,000†	0-10 yrs and/or $30,000	Same
Sale or distribution to a minor	0-10 yrs and/or $30,000	0-15 yrs and/or $45,000	Same

NOTE: These penalties are contained in the Federal Controlled Substances Act of 1970, 21 U.S.C. Sec. 801 *et seq.*
*For first offenders, the court has discretionary authority to defer proceedings and place the defendant on probation, which if successfully discharged, avoids an adjudication of guilt. For offenders under 21, the court has further discretionary authority to completely expunge the records.
†Distribution of a "small amount of marijuana for no remuneration" is treated the same as simple possession.

TABLE 5-2. Summary chart of eight state decriminalization laws

State	Maximum fine imposed	Maximum amount possessed	Criminal or civil violation	Effective date
Oregon	$100	1 oz	Civil	Oct. 5, 1973
Alaska	$100	Any amount in private for personal use or 1 oz in public	Civil	Sept. 2, 1975
Maine	$200	Any amount* for personal use	Civil	Mar. 1, 1976
Colorado†	$100	1 oz	Class 2 petty offense; no criminal record	July 1, 1975
California†	$100	1 oz	Misdemeanor; no permanent criminal record	Jan. 1, 1976
Ohio†	$100	100 gm (approx. 3½ oz)	Minor misdemeanor; no criminal record	Nov. 22, 1975
South Dakota	$ 20	1 oz	Civil	April 1, 1977
Minnesota†	$100‡	1½ oz	Civil	April 10, 1976

*There is a rebuttable presumption that possession of more than 1½ oz is with an intent to distribute.
†Distribution of marijuana by gift, or for no remuneration, is treated the same as possession in four states: California (for up to 1 oz), Colorado (up to 1 oz), Ohio (up to 20 gm), Minnesota (up to 1½ oz).
‡Only Minnesota provides for increased penalties for second offense: 0-90 days in jail and/or a $300 fine.

TABLE 5-3. State penalties for possession of marijuana (all fines represented as maximum amounts possible)

State	Amount†	First offense	Second offense	Subsequent offense
Alabama	Any amount	0-1 yr and/or $1,000	2-15 yrs and/or $25,000	Same
Alaska‡	Any amount in private for personal use, or up to 1 oz in public	$100 fine only	Same	Same
	More than 1 oz in public	0-1 yr and/or $1,000	Same	Same
	Any amount while driving a motor vehicle	$1,000 fine only	Same	Same
Arizona	Any amount	0-1 yr in county jail and/or $1,000; or 1-10 yrs in state prison and/or $50,000	2-20 yrs and/or $50,000	5 yrs-life and/or $50,0000
Arkansas*	Any amount§	0-1 yr and/or $250	0-2 yrs and/or $500	2-5 yrs
California	Up to 1 oz	$100 fine only	Same	Same‖
	More than 1 oz	0-6 mos and/or $500	Same	Same
Colorado	Up to 1 oz	$100 fine only	Same	Same
	More than 1 oz	0-1 yr and/or $500	0-2 yrs and/or $500-$1,000	1-14 yrs and/or $1,000-$2,000
	Public display or consumption of up to 1 oz	0-15 days and mandatory $100 fine	Same	Same
Connecticut	Up to 4 oz	0-1 yr and/or $1,000	0-5 yrs and/or $3,000	Same
	More than 4 oz	0-5 yrs and/or $2,000	0-10 yrs and/or $5,000	Same
Delaware*	Any amount	0-2 yrs and/or $500	0-7 yrs and/or $500	Same
Florida*	Up to 5 gm	0-1 yr and/or $1,000	0-3 yrs and/or $1,000	Same
	More than 5 gm	0-5 yrs and/or $5,000	0-10 yrs and/or $5,000	Same
Georgia	Up to 1 oz	0-1 yr and/or $1,000	Same¶	Same
	More than 1 oz	1-10 yrs	Same¶	Same

*Conditional discharge authorized for first offense possession. This permits judges to release defendants, generally without an adjudication of guilt, on condition that they satisfy certain requirements, such as participation in a drug education program. If the conditions of the program are satisfied, the criminal case will then be dismissed. Some states authorize the expungement (physical destruction) of the criminal records after the case has been dismissed.

†Many state laws provide for different penalties for possession of different amounts of marijuana. Some of these statutes distinguish by ounce (oz) weights, and others by gram (gm) weights. For comparative purposes: 1 oz = 28.35 gm; 1 lb = 453.59 gm; 2.2 lbs = 1 kg.

‡In 1975, the Supreme Court of Alaska held that the constitutional Right of Privacy protects the possession of marijuana for personal use in the home by adults. *Ravin* v. *State*, 537 P.2d 494(1975). This decision invalidates the $100 fine for simple possession in the home.

§There is a rebuttable presumption that possession of more than 1 oz is with an intent to distribute.

‖If the person charged with possession of up to 1 oz of marijuana was previously convicted of this offense three times within a 2-year period, that person will be diverted to an educational or treatment program in lieu of the fine, but if no suitable program can be found, the fine will be imposed.

¶This statute's general multiple-offender provision provides that if the person was sentenced to a term in prison for the first offense, the maximum penalty must be given for subsequent offenses. It is presently being litigated whether this general provision applies to marijuana offenders.

TABLE 5-3. State penalties for possession of marijuana (all fines represented as maximum amounts possible)—cont'd

State	Amount	First offense	Second offense	Subsequent offense
Hawaii*	Up to 1 oz	0-30 days and/or $500	Same	Same
	1 oz-2.2 lb	0-1 yr and/or $1,000	Same	Same
	More than 2.2 lb	0-5 yrs and/or $5,000	Same	Same
Idaho*	Up to 3 oz	0-1 yr and/or $1,000	0-2 yrs and/or $2,000	Same
	More than 3 oz	0-5 yrs and/or $15,000	0-10 yrs and/or $30,000	Same
Illinois*	Up to 2.5 gm	0-30 days and/or $500	Same	Same
	2.5-10 gm	0-6 mos and/or $500	Same	Same
	10-30 gm	0-1 yr and/or $1,000	1-3 yrs and/or $10,000	Same
	30-500 gm	1-3 yrs and/or $10,000	1-10 yrs and/or $10,000	Same
	More than 500 gm	1-10 yrs and/or $10,000	1-20 yrs and/or $10,000	Same
Indiana* (effective July 1, 1977)#	Up to 30 gm	0-1 yr and/or $5,000	Same	Same
	More than 30 gm	2-4 yrs and/or $10,000; or 0-1 yr and/or $5,000	Same	2-34 yrs
Iowa*	Any amount	0-6 mos and/or $1,000	0-18 mos and/or $3,000	Same
Kansas*	Any amount	0-1 yr and/or $2,500	0-10 yrs and/or $5,000	Same
Kentucky*	Any amount	0-90 days and/or $250	Same	Same
Louisiana*	Any amount	0-6 mos and/or $500	0-5 yrs and/or $2,000	0-20 yrs, with or without hard labor
Maine	Any amount** for personal use	$200 fine only	Same	Same
Maryland*	Any amount	0-1 yr and/or $1,000	0-2 yrs and/or $2,000	Same
Massachusetts*	Any amount	0-6 mos and/or $500	0-2 yrs and/or $2,000	Same
Michigan*	Up to 2 oz	0-1 yr and/or $1,000	0-2 yrs and/or $2,000	Same
	More than 2 oz	0-4 yrs and/or $2,000	0-8 yrs and/or $4,000	Same
Minnesota	Up to 1½ oz	$100 fine only	0-90 days and/or $300††	Same
	More than 1½ oz	0-3 yrs and/or $3,000	0-6 yrs and/or $6,000	Same
	More than .05 oz while driving a motor vehicle	0-90 days and/or $300	Same	Same
Mississippi*	Up to 1 oz	0-1 yr and/or $1,000	0-2 yrs and/or $2,000	Same
	More than 1 oz	0-3 yrs and/or $3,000	0-6 yrs and/or $6,000	Same
Missouri	Up to 35 gm	0-1 yr and/or $1,000	0-5 yr and/or $1,000	Same
	More than 35 gm	0-5 yrs and/or $1,000	5 yrs-life	10 yrs-life

These provisions are contained in P.L. 148 Sec. 7, Acts of 1976, effective July 1, 1977. Until that date, possession of up to 30 gm was subject to 0-1 yr and/or $500 for first offense, 0-2 yrs and/or $1,000 for second offense. Possession of more than 30 gm was subject to 1-10 yrs and/or $1,000 for first offense, 1-20 yrs and/or $2,000 for second offense.

**There is a rebuttable presumption that possession of less than 1½ oz is for personal use and possession of more than 1½ oz is with an intent to distribute.

††A second violation within a 2-year period is subject to 0-90 days and/or $300 and participation in a diagnostic examination for chemical dependency.

Continued.

TABLE 5-3. State penalties for possession of marijuana (all fines represented as maximum amounts possible)—cont'd

State	Amount	First offense	Second offense	Subsequent offense
Montana	Up to 60 gm	0-1 yr and/or $1,000	0-3 yrs and/or $1,000	Same
	More than 60 gm	0-5 yrs	Same	Same
Nebraska	Up to 1 lb	0-7 days and/or $500	0-14 days and/or $1,000	Same
	More than 1 lb	0-6 mos in county jail or 1 yr in state prison and/or $500	0-1 yr in county jail or 2 yrs in state prison and/or $1,000	Same
Nevada*	Any amount by person over age 21	1-6 yrs and/or $2,000	1-10 yrs and/or $2,000	1-20 yrs and/or $5,000
	Up to 1 oz by person under age 21	0-1 yr and/or $1,000	1-6 yrs and/or $2,000	1-10 yrs
New Hampshire	Up to 1 lb	0-1 yr and/or $1,000	0-7 yrs and/or $2,000	Same
	More than 1 lb	0-7 yrs and/or $2,000	0-15 yrs and/or $2,000	Same
New Jersey*	Up to 25 gm	0-6 mos and/or $500	Same	Same
	More than 25 gm	0-5 yrs and/or $15,000	Same	Same
New Mexico*	Up to 1 oz	0-15 days and/or $50-$100	0-1 yr and/or $100-$1,000	Same
	1-8 oz	0-1 yr and/or $100-$1,000	Same	Same
	More than 8 oz	1-5 yrs and/or $5,000	Same	Same
New York*	Any amount	0-1 yr and/or $1,000	Same	Same
	¼ oz or more; 25 cigarettes or more	Same as above, or 0-7 yrs	3-7 yrs (must serve half of sentence)	Same
	1 oz or more; 100 cigarettes or more	Same as above, or 1-15 yrs	6-15 yrs (must serve half of sentence)	Same
North Carolina*	Up to 1 oz	0-6 mos and/or $500	0-2 yrs and/or $2,000	0-5 yrs and/or $5,000
	More than 1 oz	0-5 yrs and/or $5,000	5-10 yrs and/or $10,000	10-30 yrs and/or $30,000
North Dakota*	Any amount	0-1 yr and/or $1,000	0-2 yrs and/or $2,000	Same
Ohio	Up to 100 gm	$100 fine only	Same	Same
	100-200 gm	0-30 days and/or $250	Same	Same
	200-600 gm	6 mos-5 yrs and/or $2,500	1-10 yrs and/or $5,000	Same
	More than 600 gm	1-10 yrs and/or $5,000	2-15 yrs and/or $7,500	Same
Oklahoma*	Any amount	0-1 yr	2-10 yrs	Same
Oregon	Up to 1 oz	$100 fine only	Same	Same
	More than 1 oz	0-10 yrs and/or $2,500	Same	Same
Pennsylvania*	Up to 30 gm	0-30 days and/or $500	Same	Same
	More than 30 gm	0-1 yr and/or $5,000	Same	Same
Rhode Island	Any amount	0-1 yr and/or $500	0-2 yrs and/or $1,000	Same
South Carolina*	Up to 1 oz	0-3 mos and/or $100	0-6 mos and/or $200	Same
	More than 1 oz	0-6 mos and/or $1,000	0-1 yr and/or $2,000	Same

TABLE 5-3. State penalties for possession of marijuana (all fines represented as maximum amounts possible)—cont'd

State	Amount	First offense	Second offense	Subsequent offense
South Da-kota (effective: April 1, 1977)‡‡	Up to 1 oz	$20 fine only	Same	Same
	1 oz-1 lb	0-1 yr and/or $1,000	Same	Same
	More than 1 lb	0-2 yrs and/or $2,000	Same	Same
Tennessee	Any amount	0-1 yr and/or $1,000	1-2 yrs	2-3 yrs
Texas*	Up to 2 oz	0-6 mos and/or $1,000	30 days-6 mos and/or $1,000	Same
	2 oz-4 oz	0-1 yr and/or $2,000	90 days-1 yr and/or $2,000	Same
	More than 4 oz	2-10 yrs and/or $5,000	2-20 yrs and/or $10,000	Same
Utah*	Any amount	0-6 mos and/or $299	0-1 yr and/or $1,000	0-5 yrs
Vermont	Any amount	0-6 mos and/or $500	0-2 yrs and/or $2,000	Same
Virginia*	Any amount	0-1 yr and/or $1,000	Same	Same
Washington	Up to 40 gm	0-90 days and/or $250	Same	Same
	More than 40 gm	0-5 yrs and/or $10,000	0-10 yrs and/or $10,000	Same
West Virginia*	Any amount	90 days-6 mos and/or $1,000	Same	Same
Wisconsin*	Any amount	0-1 yr and/or $250	0-2 yrs and/or $500	Same
Wyoming*	Any amount	0-6 mos and/or $1,000	Same	0-5 yrs and/or $5,000
District of Columbia	Any amount	0-1 yr and/or $100-$1,000	0-10 yrs and/or $500-$5,000	Same

‡‡These provisions are contained in the South Dakota criminal code revision, Senate bill No. 29, which was approved on February 29, 1976, and became effective on April 1, 1977. Until that date, possession of up to 1 oz was subject to 0-1 yr and/or $500, and possession of more than 1 oz was subject to 0-5 yrs and/or $5,000 for first offense.

TABLE 5-4. State penalties for possession with intent to distribute and sale of marijuana (all fines represented as maximum amounts possible)

State	Possession with intent to distribute		Sale	
	First offense	Second offense	First offense	Second offense
Alabama	2-15 yrs and/or $25,000	4-30 yrs and/or $50,000	2-15 yrs and/or $25,000	4-30 yrs and/or $50,000
Alaska	0-25 yrs and/or $20,000	0-life and/or $25,000	0-25 yrs and/or $20,000	0-life and/or $25,000
Arizona	2-10 yrs and/or $50,000	5-15 yrs and/or $50,000	5 yrs-life and/or $50,000	5 yrs-life and/or $50,000
Arkansas*	3-10 yrs and/or $15,000	3-20 yrs and/or $30,000	3-10 yrs and/or $15,000	3-20 yrs and/or $30,000

*There is a rebuttable presumption that possession of more than 1 oz of marijuana is with an intent to distribute.

Continued.

TABLE 5-4. State penalties for possession with intent to distribute and sale of marijuana (all fines represented as maximum amounts possible)—cont'd

State	Possession with intent to distribute		Sale	
	First offense	Second offense	First offense	Second offense
California (effective: July 1, 1977)†	16 mos, 2 yrs, or 3 yrs	Same	2, 3, or 4 yrs	Same
Colorado	1-14 yrs and/or $1,000	Same	3-14 yrs and/or $10,000	5-30 yrs and/or $10,000
Connecticut	0-7 yrs and/or $1,000	0-15 yrs and/or $5,000	0-7 yrs and/or $1,000	0-15 yrs and/or $5,000
Delaware	0-10 yrs and $1,000-10,000	3-15 yrs and $1,000-10,000	0-10 yrs and $1,000-10,000	3-15 yrs and $1,000-10,000
Florida	0-5 yrs and/or $5,000	0-10 yrs and/or $5,000	0-5 yrs and/or $5,000	0-10 yrs and/or $5,000
Georgia	1-10 yrs	Same‡	Same	Same‡
Hawaii	No such offense	Same	Up to 2 ozs, 0-1 yr and/or $1,000; more than 2 ozs, 0-5 yrs and/or $5,000	Same
Idaho	0-5 yrs and/or $15,000	0-10 yrs and/or $30,000	0-5 yrs and/or $15,000	0-10 yrs and/or $30,000
Illinois	Less than 2.5 gm, 0-6 mos and/or $500; 2.5-10 gm, 0-1 yr and/or $1,000; 10-30 gm, 1-3 yrs and/or $10,000; 30-500 gm, 1-10 yrs and/or $10,000; More than 500 gm, 1-20 yrs and/or $10,000	Same	Less than 2.5 gm, 0-6 mos and/or $500; 2.5-10 gm, 0-1 yr and/or $1,000; 10-30 gm, 1-3 yrs and/or $10,000; 30-500 gm, 1-10 yrs and/or $10,000; More than 500 gm, 1-20 yrs and/or $10,000	Same
Indiana (effective: July 1, 1977)§	Up to 30 gm, 0-1 yr and/or $5,000	Same	Same	Same
	More than 30 gm, 2-4 yrs and/or $10,000; or 0-1 yr and/or $5,000	Same	Same	Same

†These penalties are contained in S.B. 42, adopted August, 1976, effective July 1, 1977. The judge will select a fixed term of imprisonment from the three alternatives set out above. The middle sentence must be imposed unless there are aggravating circumstances (the higher penalty will then be imposed) or mitigating circumstances (the lower penalty will then be imposed). Until S.B. 42 took effect, possession with intent to distribute was subject to 2-10 yrs, up to life for third offense, and sale was subject to 5 yrs-life.

‡This statute's general multiple-offender provision provides that if the person was sentenced to a term in prison for the first offense, the maximum penalty must be given for subsequent offenses. It is presently being litigated whether this general provision applies to marijuana offenders.

§These provisions are contained in P.L. 148, Sec. 7, Acts. of 1976, effective July 1, 1977. Until that date, possession with intent to distribute or sale of up to 30 grams was subject to 0-1 yr and/or $500 for first offense, 0-2 yrs and/or $1,000 for second offense. Possession with intent to distribute or sale of more than 30 grams was subject to 1-20 yrs and/or $2,000 for first offense, 1-40 yrs and/or $4,000 for second offense.

TABLE 5-4. State penalties for possession with intent to distribute and sale of marijuana (all fines represented as maximum amounts possible)—cont'd

State	Possession with intent to distribute		Sale	
	First offense	Second offense	First offense	Second offense
Iowa‖	5 yrs mandatory and/or $1,000	5-15 yrs and/or $3,000	5 yrs mandatory and or $1,000	5-15 yrs and/or $3,000
Kansas	0-10 yrs and/or $5,000	Same	0-10 yrs and/or $5,000	Same
Kentucky	0-1 yr and/or $500	1-5 yrs and/or $3,000-5,000	0-1 yr and/or $500	1-5 yrs and/or $3,000-5,000
Louisiana	0-10 yrs and/or $15,000	0-20 yrs and/or $30,000	0-10 yrs and/or $15,000	0-20 yrs and/or $30,000
Maine¶	0-1 yr and/or $500	Same	0-1 yr and/or $500	Same
Maryland	0-5 yrs and/or $15,000	0-10 yrs and/or $30,000	0-5 yrs and/or $15,000	0-10 yrs and/or $30,000
Massachusetts	0-2 yrs and/or $5,000	2-5 yrs and/or $10,000	0-2 yrs and/or $5,000	2-5 yrs and/or $10,000
Michigan	0-4 yrs and/or $2,000	0-8 yrs and/or $4,000	0-4 yrs and/or $2,000	0-8 yrs and/or $4,000
Minnesota	0-5 yrs and/or $15,000	1-10 yrs and/or $30,000	0-5 yrs and/or $15,000	1-10 yrs and/or $30,000
Mississippi	0-10 yrs and/or $15,000	0-20 yrs and/or $30,000	0-20 yrs and/or $30,000	0-40 yrs and/or $60,000
Missouri	No such offense	Same	5 yrs-life	10 yrs-life
Montana	0-20 yrs #	Same	1 yr-life	Same
Nebraska	0-6 mos in county jail or 1-5 yr in prison and/or $2,000	0-12 mos in county jail or 2-10 yrs in prison and/or $4,000	0-6 mos in jail or 1-5 yrs in prison and/or $2,000	0-1 yr in jail or 2-10 yrs in prison and/or $4,000
Nevada	No such offense	Same	1-20 yrs and/or $5,000	0-life and/or $5,000
New Hampshire	No such offense	Same	0-15 yrs and/or $2,000	Same
New Jersey	0-5 yrs and/or $15,000	0-10 yrs and/or $30,000	0-5 yrs and/or $15,000	0-10 yrs and/or $30,000
New Mexico	1-5 yrs and/or $5,000	2-10 yrs and/or $5,000	1-5 yrs and/or $5,000	2-10 yrs and/or $5,000
New York	0-7 yrs	3-7 yrs (must serve half of sentence)	1-15 yrs	6-15 yrs (must serve half of sentence)
North Carolina	0-5 yrs and/or $5,000	5-10 yrs and/or $10,000	0-5 yrs and/or $5,000	5-10 yrs and/or $10,000
North Dakota	0-10 yrs and/or $10,000	0-20 yrs and/or $20,000	0-10 yrs and/or $10,000	0-20 yrs and/or $20,000

‖An essential element of the possession with intent to distribute and sale offenses is that they must be committed with an intent to profit, rather than as an accommodation. If this is not proven, the defendant will be sentenced under the simple possession penalties.
¶There is a rebuttable presumption that possession of more than 1½ oz is with an intent to distribute.
#Must possess 1 kg or more.

Continued.

TABLE 5-4. State penalties for possession with intent to distribute and sale of marijuana (all fines represented as maximum amounts possible)—cont'd

State	Possession with intent to distribute		Sale	
	First offense	**Second offense**	**First offense**	**Second offense**
Ohio	No such offense	Same	Up to 200 gm, 6 mos-5 yrs and/or $2,500; 200-600 gm, 1-10 yrs and/or $5,000; over 600 gm, 2-15 yrs (6 mos mandatory) and/or $7,500	Up to 200 gm, 1-10 yrs and/or $5,000; 200-600 gm, 2-15 yrs and/or $7,500; over 600 gm, 2-15 yrs (1 yr mandatory) and/or $7,500
Oklahoma	2-10 yrs and/or $5,000	4-20 yrs and/or $10,000	2-10 yrs and/or $5,000	4-20 yrs and/or $10,000
Oregon	0-10 yrs and/or $2,500	Same	0-10 yrs and/or $2,500	Same
Pennsylvania	0-5 yrs and/or $15,000	0-10 yrs and/or $30,000	0-5 yrs and/or $15,000	0-10 yrs and/or $30,000
Rhode Island	0-30 yrs and/or $50,000	0-60 yrs and/or $100,000	0-30 yrs and/or $50,000	0-60 yrs and/or $100,000
South Carolina	0-5 yrs and/or $5,000	0-10 yrs and/or $10,000	0-5 yrs and/or $5,000	0-10 yrs and/or $10,000
South Dakota (effective: (April 1, 1977)**	No such offense	Same	Up to 1 oz, 0-1 yr and/or $1,000; 1 oz-1 lb, 0-2 yrs and/or $2,000; 1 lb or more, 0-5 yrs and/or $5,000	Same
Tennessee	Up to ½ oz, 0-1 yr and/or $1,000; more than 1 oz, 1-5 yrs and/or $3,000	Up to ½ oz, 1-2 yrs; more than ½ oz, 1-10 yrs and/or $6,000	Up to ½ oz, 0-1 yr and/or $1,000; more than ½ oz, 1-5 yrs and/or $3,000	Up to ½ oz, 1-2 yrs; more than ½ oz, 1-10 yrs and/or $6,000
Texas	No such offense	Same	2-10 yrs and/or $5,000	2-20 yrs and/or $10,000
Utah	0-5 yrs and/or $5,000	Same	0-5 yrs and/or $5,000	Same
Vermont	More than ½ oz or 25 cigarettes, 0-2 yrs and/or $2,000; more than 2 oz or 100 cigarettes, 0-5 yrs and/or $5,000	Same	0-5 yrs and/or $10,000	10-25 yrs and/or $25,000

**These provisions are contained in the South Dakota criminal code revision, Senate Bill No. 29, which was approved on February 29, 1976, and became effective on April 1, 1977. Until that date, the penalties for possession with intent to distribute and sale were as follows: 0-10 yrs and/or $5,000 for first offense; 0-15 yrs and/or $10,000 for second offense.

TABLE 5-4. State penalties for possession with intent to distribute and sale of marijuana (all fines represented as maximum amounts possible)—cont'd

State	Possession with intent to distribute		Sale	
	First offense	Second offense	First offense	Second offense
Virginia	5-40 yrs and/or $25,000	Same	5-40 yrs and/or $25,000	Same
Washington	0-5 yrs and/or $10,000	0-10 yrs and/or $20,000	0-5 yrs and/or $10,000	0-10 yrs and/or $20,000
West Virginia	1-5 yrs and/or $15,000	1-10 yrs and/or $30,000	1-5 yrs and/or $15,000	1-10 yrs and/or $30,000
Wisconsin	0-5 yrs and/or $15,000	0-10 yrs and/or $30,000	0-5 yrs and/or $15,000	0-10 yrs and/or $30,000
Wyoming	0-10 yrs and/or $10,000	0-20 yrs and/or $20,000	0-10 yrs and/or $10,000	0-20 yrs and/or $20,000
District of Columbia	No such offense	Same	0-1 yr and/or $100-1,000	0-10 yrs and/or $500-5,000

an addict or habitual user of narcotics, not in the normal course of professional treatment, but for the purpose of providing the user with narcotics sufficient to keep him comfortable by maintaining his customary use. A physician is also prohibited from prescribing, administering, or furnishing a narcotic to or for any person who is not under his treatment for a pathology or condition other than narcotic addiction. The requisites for addiction are as follows:

1. Emotional dependence on the drug in the sense that the user experiences a compulsive need to continue its use
2. A tolerance to its effects that leads the user to require larger and more potent doses
3. Physical dependence so that the user suffers withdrawal symptoms if he is deprived of his dosage.

There is an exception allowing the treatment of an addict by the use of narcotics during emergency treatment. No definition is given as to what "emergency treatment" covers.

It should also be stressed that in many states there is a growing trend toward diversion of drug abuse from the criminal justice system into the community-based drug treatment and education facilities. This has an important advantage in that the individual is not criminalized for his drug involvement and has an opportunity to participate in an educational or treatment approach to his difficulty. One of the most innovative of these diversion programs, dealing with peer education, was developed in Minnesota by Sandra Valle and associates. The program, "Peer Education and Health Resources Developed by the Teenage Health Consultants," focuses on health education and peer counseling for young people who become involved with alcohol and drug abuse and have difficulty with the law.*

COMMUNITY ACTION

Previous chapters have cited many resources and techniques for community action. However, it is often difficult for parents to admit that they may have a drug problem within their own family; a community may be equally reluctant to face up to its drug problem.

Too often the people in a community are unwilling to admit that there is a problem until something drastic happens. Resistance to a drug program occurs unless there al-

*Information on this peer education and health resource program can be obtained from Ms. Sandra Valle, 1600 Partland Avenue, St. Paul, Minnesota 55104.

ready has been a serious drug confrontation in a community. For many "pillars of the community," it is much more convenient to sweep the problem under the rug or to pretend that it does not exist—not in *their* community! The truth is that even if only *one* child in the community is involved with drugs, that community has the beginning of a drug problem. Use by one child may be highly symptomatic of the approaching use by many others. There are going to be communities that are going to say that they really do not have a drug problem. Denial is the first line of defense for most communities, unfortunately, even when the situation is obvious to an outsider.

It is true that any search for a solution indicates that there is a problem. Once a community considers the possibility of a drug program, it is admitting the necessity for such a program or confessing that some of the area's residents are involved with drugs.

Once a community is able, calmly and objectively, to face the fact that drugs are now within its boundaries and affecting its citizens, what can be done? How, in detail, can responsible, concerned persons in the community take positive action? Admitting that there are no simplistic, overnight answers, *can* teachers and parents band together and accomplish much, if anything at all; can the segments of the community marshall their efforts toward a unified attack? *Yes*, if they go about it rationally. It is imperative, however, that community resources for prevention, control, and treatment be developed and coordinated for effective action.

Objectives

In general there is too much isolation and not enough mutual problem solving and sharing between families in any community. There has to be a much more interrelated and integrated approach. Programs must be a total community effort and should be based on the following objectives:

1. Research and community involvement to determine what the problem is and to set up the machinery to develop and coordinate a program
2. Education of children, parents, and teachers
3. Treatment via clinics, rehabilitation centers, hot lines, and therapy in school and by private professionals
4. Law enforcement to spell out the laws, to alert parents, and to locate drug sources

Coordination by a drug abuse council

Who takes the bull by the horns? Any responsible person in a community—a doctor, a teacher, a minister, a real-estate salesman, or a stockbroker—can take the first step. It simply means accepting the fact that there *is* a drug problem in the community and reaching the conclusion that *something* has to be done about it. Many communities have set up what are, in essence, drug advisory councils, composed of concerned, open-minded persons within the community who are attempting to set up antidrug programs tailored to the specific needs of their communities. The membership comprises a variety of community people; there is no set organizational pattern. Such councils, working closely with the schools, law enforcement, and governmental and nongovernmental agencies, are primarily concerned with how best to educate in a predrug abuse program and how to treat those who are already abusers. It is their responsibility to enlist community support, coordinate the overall community program, and raise whatever funds are necessary.

It is also up to these councils to lead in an effort to educate the community. Their efforts can assist the teacher or school administrator. Some communities have initiated weekly town meetings during which area doctors, psychologists, law enforcement people, and the like discuss various aspects of the drug problem.

In some ways the job of educating the community has already begun. Representatives from various antidrug groups as well as former addicts are constantly speaking at community meetings. The National Institute of Mental Health has spot announcements on television to transmit information about drugs. It seems clear that all the tools—community groups, television, radio, literature, and local service agencies—should be utilized to spread the message in a steady, ongoing program.

In any community approach to drug abuse, some individuals feel that one of the major errors made is total *failure to get youth involved in the planning stage*. We have seen it happen over and over again. Community leaders all too often sit around, come to "meaningful" decisions, and pass them along to the young people. Although the decisions may be perfectly good ones, they will not have much meaning unless they are validated by young people. This kind of "we-they" thinking is not nearly as effective as a true dialogue.

Any valid, community-based approach must be a *balanced effort between law enforcement, research, education, and treatment*, even if this means confrontation and disagreement. The administration of such a program or series of programs cannot simply be turned over to health or education "professionals"; it has to have the active backing as well as the participation of the legal and educational establishment, influential citizens, and young people from the communities in which the problem first developed. Youth must be part of the solution rather than just part of the problem. Involving the youth is the key to success of any community.

One authority thinks that young people should have a right to be involved with designing programs that are going to have a direct relationship to them and their lives. Various people believe that many students are beginning to assume leadership when they are given the chance. They are striving to bring the school back into the total society, so that the school is an integral part of life and not just some place young people go for 6 or 7 hours before returning to the real world.

There is no doubt that students could be of value in helping to establish a drug education program merely by their aid in deciding what information should be furnished and how it should be presented. Some educators feel that young people could even take on some of the research themselves, such as determining how widespread the problem is in their own community. Such an evaluation has always been difficult to obtain, but perhaps the young people, talking to each other, could arrive at a more accurate estimate of the situation. On the basis of their findings a realistic program might emerge.

Another function of the drug advisory council should be the matter of locating financial support. Some communities have handled this particular concern by soliciting voluntary contributions. In other communities there is often local money available from such sources as state and local health departments and mental health departments.

Particularly important now is the massive federal funding through programs in the Office of Education and the National Institute of Mental Health. Many types of grants are available for counties and individual communities, even individual school districts, to support the development of training and educational programs.

It has been observed that the only communities in which the treatment, prevention, and educational programs achieved a substantial amount of success were those wherein all the elements worked together to seek mutual solutions for the betterment of their most valuable resource—their own children.

Such groups as constitute the community council should consist of two types of persons. First, community leaders who hopefully do not have a vested interest in any one modality should include minority groups, the city mayor and his council, business leaders, clergy, and students. The other group of persons consists of agency heads who do not have vested interests and should include law enforcement officials, such as the chief of police; the head of a hospital, clinic, or local health service; local business heads; city and county administrators; city educators, superintendent of schools, etc.; researchers; government administrators (of program monies, etc.); and parents.

Such cooperating groups ought to include the *involved children themselves*. Too often such collaborations achieve merely escalated confrontation with those of school age rather than cooperation. An unhappy split occurs, separating the "we" from the "they" group.

There will always be differences of opinion as to just how such cooperative ventures should function and on whose terms. Drug abuse is intimately linked with human social values. About these values people differ strenuously. That which involves our social values touches upon the most sensitive part of the whole human social system. Certainly attitudes toward drugs center more around personal value systems than on one's knowledge of pharmacy. Large differences in educational emphasis, approach, and ideology, then, will occur from participant to participant, from school to school, and even from community to community.

Unfortunately such conflicts of values rapidly become translated into controversy— easily the most dreaded, threatening aspect of any group venture. A compromise is often achieved by importing a commercial "packaged" program that will hopefully serve the needs of everyone. Such commercially prefabricated efforts toward drug education show a great deal of resourcefulness on the part of their promoters and sometimes benefit from widespread public and private endorsement. They are likely, however, not to meet the needs of individuals involved in personal crises and of group processes unique to the various communities in which they occur. As has been stated before, drug abuse is not so much a problem of pharmacology as one of human needs and values. No single program will meet the needs of all. Drug use, its nature, and the life-style of its different types of users vary widely from city to city and even within the communities of a single city.

Certainly some basic information on the psychopharmacology of drugs as well as the peculiarities of their various uses is a practical and necessary adjunct to any compre-

hensive educational curriculum. Beyond that the peculiar abuse pattern of each area, modified by the conditions unique to that area, must be dealt with by a concerned public at that time and place. Styles and habits of use are in constant flux. Ambitious programs geared to one style of abuse may rapidly become obsolete.

Role of law enforcement

Our experience has demonstrated that, whatever problem is contemplated for a community, it is essential to bring the police in at the *planning stage*. Do not wait until the program is set up and trouble develops. Ensuring the cooperation, even the *neutrality*, of local law enforcement in the operation of a drug program is vital to its success. If law enforcement personnel are ignored, their hostility to any drug program can almost be guaranteed, and as a consequence of that alone, the program may be doomed to failure.

Community programs and facilities

We need to look at community programs and how they can best be utilized. Basically there are two types of programs: (1) an urban or ghetto-type program and (2) a small town or suburban program. In each case the needs, although similar in some respects, must be approached differently. One stresses treatment; the other is concerned with prevention. One operates with the isolated individual; the other considers him as part of the family unit.

Haight-Ashbury Free Medical Clinic

In the various urban programs available, one of the most common resources is the free clinic, such as the Haight-Ashbury Free Clinic in San Francisco. There are now over 500 free clinics nationwide, and in the Haight-Ashbury,* as in certain sections of other cities, a drug culture has evolved, the

---

*Smith, D. E.: The role of the free clinic in America's changing health care delivery system, J. Psychedelic Drugs 7(1):January-March, 1975; and Smith, D. E.: The free clinic movement in the United States: a ten year perspective (1966-1976). In press.

young people have been totally alienated from their parents, and drug problems tend to be much more severe than in suburban areas. Here drug prevention education is not the major issue, although a task force of workers may spread out through the district to try and steer experimenters away from heavy drug involvement. For the most part, these young people are not concerned with the decision of *whether* to use drugs, but rather with the question of "what kind of drugs will it be this time?"

Young persons are viewed as candidates for medical and psychological treatment rather than as criminal or deviant drug abusers. At the Clinic there is a medical section, a women's needs center, a rock medical section, which delivers medical services to young people at music concerts, a dental section, a drug treatment section, a psychiatric section, and a vocational rehabilitation section. The medical section staff deals with general adolescent medicine—abscesses, hepatitis, malnutrition, infections, breakdown of blood vessels, etc. The drug section is equipped to deal with acute drug detoxification and heroin withdrawal. The dental clinic is important because so many drug abusers have poor oral hygiene. Dental pain is one of the reasons people return to heroin use. The psychiatric section works with those patients who have "flipped" or who require long-term therapy, and the vocational rehabilitation section attempts to train and find work for ex-addicts outside the drug culture.

The Haight-Ashbury Free Clinic is a comprehensive medical facility for drug abusers and for other neighborhood people who cannot find adequate health care elsewhere. In 10 years of operation the clinic has seen over 400,000 patients. Seeing a large number of patients means that most can be worked with for only a short period of time. An attempt is then made to refer them to other programs that have long-term treatment modalities, such as metadone maintenance programs or a therapeutic community. A certain number of patients are kept in long-term treatment using the multiple modality approach and trying a variety of different techniques

with different persons. For example, non-drug approaches such as acupuncture are being used to detoxify heroin addicts and compared in effectiveness with standard medication approaches.

Extensive use is made of ex-addicts in working with the more compulsive drug users. An outpatient psychiatric clinic works with the psychological problems of the individuals on a one-to-one basis. There is vocational counseling and, at the present time, a small residential facility. There are, in fact, many young drug abusers in a long-term treatment, but the majority of the work is short-term crisis intervention, diagnosis, and referral, since about 150 patients are seen each day.

The phases of treatment are outlined as follows:

Phase 1: detoxification. The patient is provided with medication, supportive counseling, and housing while going through withdrawal. Referrals may be made to other existing aftercare drug treatment facilities.

Phase 2: group house—self-help program. Certain patients who have passed through detoxification will be admitted to one of the six group residence homes for a stay of 3 to 6 months, as needed. Each residence will be limited to a maximum of ten persons. In a homelike atmosphere, members will share responsibilities for operating and supporting the house and remaining drug free. Therapy will be provided through encounter groups, sensitivity training, and weekly meetings, as well as through special activities designed to expand social and personal experiences.

Phase 3: group treatment. Group treatment will be provided on a regular weekly basis.

Phase 4: job counseling and placement. Since this is a most important aspect of rehabilitation, a full-time employment counselor provides personal guidance and referrals for testing, training, and placing individuals in temporary, part-time, and full-time work. The intention is to expand job placement relations with community businesses in addition to working through the usual community agencies. Contact is made with vocational training programs as well as with the Department of Rehabilitation, the State Department of Employment, and other job placement and training agencies.

Phase 5: street workers. A mobile team of four ex-users is employed to circulate freely with the street people and provide assistance and guidance if needed.

Phase 6: family and community education. This phase provides a crucial bridge between the users, their families, and the community. It will involve (1) group sensitivity training for parents of users and other interested individuals; (2) community education and lecture series; and (3) publication of drug-related literature.

Teen or drop-in center

Community resources can be utilized in the development of a teen or drop-in center on campus or off campus. Within this framework the school can be innovative and develop its own approach. For example, the school might provide an open clubroom or locale where students can sit around and talk, or the community may provide such a service and make it available to schools (Chapter 8).

Teen-agers will *come* to a place with a relaxing atmosphere that allows them to be themselves. Pot smoking or drugs might become problems, but they are already problems. An on-campus teen center where students make their own rules to keep drugs out is likely to have more effect in shaping the nucleus of an antidrug culture than strict surveillance by the school.

Such a locale might also be a place where the bad tripper can be cared for. The availability of quick emergency care from a staff of volunteer ex-drug users with clinic medical support as an available backup seems an ideal situation.

The point we are trying to make is that the services, including the school health services, existing on the campus should be *made more responsive to student needs* (Chapter 8). Make the school respond to the need and be relevant in its educational approach is the slogan that might express this position.

Community facilities

Let us again briefly touch upon the question of facilities and personnel available to communities or already there. The particular treatment facility established must of necessity depend on the community involved. The urban approach can stress prevention as well as different treatment programs. Urban treatment centers often have to deal with hardcore addiction, whereas suburbia is concerned with soft drug abuse. Basically, however, these treatment facilities may be categorized as follows:

1. Crisis centers. These may be part of a clinic, part of a college medical group, or a special section of a hospital. The main purpose of a crisis center is to provide immediate onsite help and long-range support for the drug abuser as well as treatment of acute drug toxicity.

2. Clinics. In addition to being able to handle acute drug toxicity, the clinics concentrate on overall medical treatment, including deleterious drug-caused side effects and long-term therapy.

3. Hot lines. In many parts of the country, groups of young persons, often ex-drug abusers or addicts, are manning round-the-clock hot lines to answer calls from either curious or drug-disturbed youngsters. Often, under the guidance of a psychologist or other drug expert, these anonymous counselors can provide information, talk down a bad trip on LSD, inform medical authorities of dangerous symptoms, and provide a full range of therapeutic resources and emergency medical treatment centers.

4. Ongoing groups. Informal meetings should be held where adolescents have an opportunity to participate in honest discussions without fear of being arrested. One example is the Sunrise House in Salinas, California, an off-campus meeting place for youth where counselors and psychologists are available to answer any and all questions.

5. Self-help groups. One of the most hopeful treatment methods revolves around the so-called "self-help" groups. Usually staffed for the most part by ex-addicts and abusers and operating out of storefronts, offices, or coffeehouses, these rehabilitation centers are

springing up around the country. They document the increasing public awareness of the need for alternative health care systems.

An example of cooperative, unified community action. Guidelines and support from local, state, and federal sources may provide vital initiative. However, drug abuse is specific for any given area and should be handled at its source. For example, there is great variation between urban and rural communities, and therefore the community plan should vary as community needs vary. However, we have listed one community example to serve as a *general* guideline for community action.

Awareness on the part of Center City citizens (fictitious) of the chronic use of drugs by their children came several years ago almost accidently with the publishing of a series of articles in the local newspaper. Two reporters had been routinely assigned to cover the local marijuana situation because big news had been lagging for several days. They found that a great deal more than marijuana was being distributed and consumed by local high school and junior high school children. The reporters spent several days talking with students and collected a large sample of assorted stimulants and depressants, including LSD, DMT, and some mysterious unknowns. They even engaged two local college students to make a study of local drug use, including a sample poll of the attitudes of young persons of various communities in the city toward drug use.

The reporters found additionally that, although the drugs were easily attainable and many of the students had developed serious habits of use, the local, flourishing drug scene had very *low visibility* to both adults and police. Increasing incidents of students falling asleep in class were explained by teachers as due to the all-night beer busts and other social gatherings of students excited because summer and graduation were only a month away. Clearly most of the adult community was out of touch with its youth.

But students, once queried about what was happening, were extremely candid about their drug use. They said that for just a couple of bucks you could buy handfuls of assorted pills from just about anybody. It seemed to be true. Everybody was using just about everything, they said, and everything about the drug business was "kind of loose."

The city was shocked by these disclosures. Over the next several months, community interest and concern, as well as the expected hysteria, slowly mounted. Local response, though, was more or less fractionated. Various concerned citizen groups joined together for discussion and local law enforcement activity against drug users and sellers mounted sharply. Law officers began to pose as local hippies to infiltrate the local scene. Almost immediately children from some of Center City's most respected families were arrested. The community became galvanized into action almost overnight. There was a drug crisis in Center City. Something had to be done and done soon.

The Center City police department, which had reported only 38 total arrests of youth and adults on drug charges during the past year and only one arrest during the previous year, now reported that 44 youths had been arrested in the past 3 months.

These reports culminated in a mass meeting on November 17. Over 1000 people from the community attended the meeting held in the high school auditorium, to hear a panel discussion on the local drug problem. The panel included a speaker from Synanon, a police sergeant, a probation officer, a doctor, a judge, a high school teacher, several self-confessed users, and the student body president of the local high school.

The mood of the meeting was serious but not vindictive. Everyone agreed that there was a serious drug problem among all the school-age youth and that some kind of substantial action had to be taken. As one might expect, opinions on what to do ranged from "harsh laws won't solve the problem" (judge), "we can't handle every kind of problem here in our classes" (one teacher), to "if you see someone using drugs, you're really saving a life when you snitch on him" (Synanon speaker).

But the idea of community unity, of cooperation without factionalism in educating both the students and the community at large to the problem of youth and drugs easily carried the day. On that point there was almost unanimous agreement. The specific projects and programs that were a result of this meeting clearly reflected the community's orientation; education for the total community is the real key to solving the "November drug crisis."

Residents opened a drug information center on January 20 to provide information to the general public about the danger of drugs, their use, and their effects. Films, literature, and lists of prominent speakers were solicited from the state and other communities to round out the program. These materials were made available at cost to all contingents of the city. Other salient features of the new community drug center included a 24-hour a day referral service, a "troubled parents" talk session, and a regular teen-age rap session.

A second, dovetailing program was being run at the same time by the local high schools. High school students were selected and sent to the elementary and junior high schools to speak to younger students. The emphasis was on what was really happening, not on how young persons should behave. In short, the youth-to-youth programs were totally reality oriented; or, as they put it, "where it's really at with drugs." Although admittedly the programs may have lacked something in sophistication and even in total accuracy of presentation, the difference was more than made up for by the fact that the students themselves were doing their own program and were personally involved in its outcome.

A third aspect of the community's action response to drug use was also educationally oriented. It involved talks with industrial employees at Center City companies. Local industry requested this service because their own employees had developed a drug problem that started with the night shift crews taking pep pills to stay awake.

A final program, and perhaps the most innovative and helpful in this community, was the "Our Family" halfway house rehabilitation project. The program was a continuation of an innovative state hospital rehabilitation program for narcotic addicts. The halfway house established in Center City was a final, decisive step in an almost totally integrated program, inasmuch as one is possible in any large urban center. It provided the needed transition for ex-drug users returning to a useful life as part of the community.

The halfway house served two functions. First, it provided rehabilitated addicts with work at the center or at an outside job, returning them to community life. Second, the center provided its own drug abuse information and education program. It recruited its own rehabilitated addicts to give presentations in Center City and other adjacent communities.

The "Our Family" project offered free weekly counseling for concerned parents and weekly open house meetings where insiders and guests could discuss their handicaps and hang-ups about drugs. Counseling was also scheduled on an individual basis. The Center City Police Department had taken a supporting role and assumed responsibility for the program.

At a recent meeting in a continuing series of the Center City Citizens Committee on Drug Abuse, everyone agreed that things had improved considerably. Where they had not, at least the prospects for the future looked considerably brighter. The name Center City is fictional. But the community and its services really exist.

SUMMARY

This brief and sketchy description of the role of the community in the drug abuse problem should provide information and suggestions about the community resources available for action programs. Programs of treatment, rehabilitation, control, and education should be initiated and carried out on local levels using guidelines and models developed elsewhere, but modified to fit the particular needs of the locale where they are put to use.

Community action includes coordination at all levels of all agencies and organizations, including the schools, for an effective attack on the drug problem. Finally, community approaches must be flexible—for the only constant about the drug scene is that it will change.

REFERENCES

1. Batiste, C. G., and Yablonsky, L.: Synanon: a therapeutic life style, Calif. Med. **114**:90, 1971.
2. Benforado, J. M.: A guide to the medical management of acute mind-altering drug reactions, ed. 2, Madison, Wis., 1972, Charitable, Educational and Scientific Foundation of the State Medical Society of Wisconsin.
3. Berman, R.: An introduction to crisis counseling: making the best use of the "dangerous opportunity," Los Angeles, 1970, Los Angeles County Superintendent of Schools Office.
4. Casriel, D. H.: The family physician and the narcotics addict, Panorama, Feb., 1970.
5. Drug abuse: escape to nowhere, Philadelphia, 1969, Smith, Kline & French Laboratories.
6. Federal Strategy Drug Abuse Prevention. Prepared by the Strategy Council on Drug Abuse, Superintendent of Documents, Washington, D.C., November 1976, U.S. Government Printing Office.
7. Garrett, D. L.: Synanon: the communiversity, Humanist **25**:184-189, 1965.
8. Mandell, A. J.: The sociology of a multi-modality strategy in the treatment of narcotics addicts. In Blackly, P., editor: Drug abuse, Springfield, Ill., 1971, Charles C Thomas, Publisher.
9. Methadone in the management of heroin addiction, Med. Letter Drugs Ther. **14**:13-14, 1972.
10. Methadone, 1972, Connection, Jan.-Feb., 1972.
11. Narcotic antagonists: new methods to treat heroin addiction, Science **173**:503-506, 1971.
12. Smith, D. E.: The free clinic movement in the United States: A ten year perspective (1966-1976). J. Drug Issues, Part I, **7**:343-355, Fall, 1977.
13. Smith, D. E.: The role of the free clinic in America's changing health care delivery system, J. Psychedelic Drugs **7**(1): January-March 1975.
14. Smith, D. E.: Speech at Michigan Physician's Conference, Ann Arbor, Mich., Nov., 1970.
15. Smith, D. E., and Bentel, D. J.: Drug Abuse Information Project, The third annual report to the legislature, San Francisco, 1969, University of California San Francisco Medical Center.
16. Smith, D. E., and Bentel, D. J.: Drug Abuse Information Project, the fourth and fifth reports to the legislature, San Francisco, 1970 and 1971, University of California San Francisco Medical Center.
17. Smith, D. E., and Gay, G. R.: Office and emergency room care of the new drug scene, Unpublished paper, San Francisco, 1971, Haight-Asbury Free Medical Clinic.
18. Smith, D. E., and Wesson, D. R.: Community approaches to drug abuse treatment and rehabilitation, J. Psychedelic Drugs **6**(2): April-June, 1974.
19. Smith, D. E., and Wesson, D. R.: Diagnosis and treatment of adverse reactions to sedative-hypnotics, Rockville, Md., 1974, National Clearinghouse for Drug Abuse Information.
20. Taylor, R. L., and others: Management of "bad trips" in an evolving drug scene, J.A.M.A. **213**: 422, 1970.
21. Van Dusen, W.: Treatment approaches to drug subcultures, Unpublished monograph, Fort Bragg, Colo., 1969.
22. Watson, D.: National directory of drug abuse treatment programs, Washington, D.C., 1972, National Clearinghouse for Drug Abuse Information.
23. Watson, D., and Sells, G. B.: Directory of narcotic addiction treatment agencies in the United States, Fort Worth, Tex., 1970, National Institute of Mental Health.

PART THREE

THE ROLE OF THE SCHOOL

6
The school drug program

. . . programs which address the broad developmental needs of children and youth are the most effective in preventing and reducing drug abuse and other forms of self-destructive behavior . . .

The demand reduction program is intended to: 1) dissuade the nonuser from experimenting with drugs; 2) deter the occasional user or experimenter from progressing to the abuse of drugs; 3) make treatment available for abusers of drugs who seek it; and 4) help the former abuser regain his place as a productive member of society.

White House Paper on Drug Abuse
1975[20]

. . . There are no recipes for effective drug education programs.

HELEN NOWLIS[13]

Efforts continue in the areas of law enforcement, rehabilitation, and treatment to control and reduce the drug abuse problem, but such efforts by themselves are not adequate, do not reach people at the most appropriate times, nor are they sufficient in themselves to prevent or reduce the problem. Society is turning to educational institutions for help, and the emphasis is being placed on a preventive approach to the problem. The National Institute on Drug Education has focused its efforts on primary prevention. The school is expected to act as society's officially designated primary educational agent despite the lack of appropriate guidelines and model programs.

Much confusion continues to exist regarding the role of the school in the drug misuse and abuse problem in the United States. It has been mentioned (Chapter 1) that this dilemma is due to a number of factors: (1)

the lack of clarity in definitions of drug education and drug prevention, (2) the lack of understanding of the nature and extent of drug use and nonuse, (3) the belief that the school's responsibility is solely educational and can be developed and conducted in isolation from the social problems of young people and the community, (4) the confusion as to whether or not educational objectives should emphasize turning off students to drug use, reduce the incidence of drug use, or to emphasize effective education, and (5) the objection to the sordid image of the addict, the street pusher, and the youthful abuser (long hair, dirty, lazy), stereotypes that some people believe relate to student drug experimentation and drug abuse, among other forms of deviance. Thus drug education has been labeled as a controversial subject for inclusion in the curriculum. In addition, the information available today does not provide simple or complete answers to the drug problem. Nor are there easy or single solutions. Adequate ways for schools to help solve the problem do not exist despite the many excellent efforts and constructive activities that have occurred in recent years and that are now taking place. Despite the many positive programs that have emerged in recent years, schools continue to develop partial, incomplete, and uncoordinated programs that frequently produce ineffectual results.

Schools alone cannot solve the drug problem now confronting society. However, they have a unique and special role to play in its resolution. However, there is no one best, effective school program in operation today. Nor are there clear guidelines to define or identify the nature of an adequate or complete program. Is it any wonder that schools are criticized for ineffective programs? The forces in society tell schools to take action and yet the schools must explore and experiment with a variety of ways to find solutions because they are not provided with the needed parameters. When schools fail in their efforts, they are subject to criticisms that are often unjustified. This book has been prepared in order to help in this dilemma. An attempt will be made to provide guidelines that will give the clarity and direction that schools so desperately need. The proposals are not meant to be prescriptive, since there is no single model or single program that is usable, or useful, in all schools. Each school or school district must devise and determine its own program to meet local needs. Programs for the minorities need different emphases than those for middle-class Caucasians. The material contained in this book will provide directions and practical suggestions that can be utilized in developing suitable and appropriate school programs. There is sufficient diversity so that schools can be innovative and creative in resolving local problems.

Before identifying the conceptual model of the school drug program there are important fundamental principles usable in its development that must be identified.

PRINCIPLES

An effective preventive school drug program must give consideration to the following basic principles:

1. The nature and extent of the drug problem (Chapter 1) in each school and school district must be identified, and attention must be given to the variety of physical, psychological, social, and spiritual needs of the users and nonusers of drugs. Although the majority of pupils are nonusers of the illegal drugs, there are a substantial number who are experimenters, a considerably smaller number of periodic and infrequent users, and a very small group of so-called compulsive users. This student distribution may vary according to area and to type of drug.

2. The school program must include more than just education. Students who are periodic, compulsive, and relapse users and abusers of drugs will need special counseling, guidance, and assistance that cannot be provided in the usual formal educational program.

3. Drug misuse and abuse must be viewed as symptomatic in nature and as illustrative behavior. Drug use provides alternatives that help young persons satisfy such needs as excitement or thrills, avoidance of pressures, escape from boredom, escape from certain environmental conditions, attainment of identity, definition of self-image, development of values, success experiences, security, peer challenge, affection, independence, and equality of opportunity. Drug abuse unquestionably is related to such social and spiritual factors as war, violence and destruction, bias and prejudice, stress on materialism, dichotomies in values and morals in terms of beliefs as opposed to practices, the search for life's meaning, and the influence of the mass media. Thus the basic deterrents to drug misuse and abuse are not related directly to drugs themselves but to (a) social environment, (b) provision for a variety of necessary social and spiritual considerations and arrangements, (c) encouragement and improvement of communications between youth and adults, and (d) opportunities for values clarification to help

with intelligent decisions, coping skills, and alternatives to drugs. These factors provide some of the basic elements needed for student guidance and curriculum development. Such considerations will aid students in the development of more effective ways of handling problems rather than seeking solutions through the risk-taking use of drugs.

4. The established goals of the program should be behaviorally centered and realistic in terms of achievement. Although factual, nonbiased information about drugs is necessary, such understandings by themselves usually do not have much effect on the life-styles of the young. The didactic, authoritative, teacher-centered, "scare" approaches to learning will have little if any impact on most students. Students need to be involved attitudinally and engaged actively in discussions, explorations, discoveries, and other activities that relate directly to the social context in which they are living if practices in the use and abuse of drugs are to be affected. The objectives must also focus on values clarification, development of self-concept and communication, decision-making, and coping skills experiences.

5. The school atmosphere should focus on the improvement of the quality of human interaction and human relatedness, especially between teachers and students. This approach has been referred to as the humanistic approach, or the humanistic emphasis. Schools, and especially teachers, need to be more concerned with pupils than with the content they teach. Efforts at improvement in communication is necessary. The drug problem is a human problem.

6. School activities must be related to and coordinated with those efforts taking place outside the school and should involve the participation of the community, including parents. The support of the community and its resources is most important for effective programs. Drysdale indicates this need in this statement: ". . . it is a partnership of State agencies that must be joined with a partnership of community agencies in each locality if we are to make a comprehensive and effective effort to combat the critical problem of youthful drug abuse."[7] By the same token, schools can encourage and motivate communities to develop and make available a variety of services that are useful to the young persons attending their institutions. The need for parental help must not be overlooked for effective results. A parent educational program could be one method of parental participation.

7. The formal educational program should be graded, sequential, and comprehensive in order to reach all students. It should begin in kindergarten, although it could start earlier in districts that have preschool programs. Many authorities believe the most effective educational program to be one that reaches children and youth at the earliest age that they start to be involved in the use of drugs and especially before they start experimenting with illegal drugs. The curriculum must also give consideration to the misuse and abuse of legal drugs. Primary prevention is thought to be of the greatest importance in reducing the drug problem.

8. Student involvement in the planning, management, and implementation of the drug program is essential. Although the manner and extent of pupil participation is not clear and is in need of identification, and although the degree of effectiveness of such involvement is not known, the action is logically and defensibly sound. Areas in which the use of young persons has been tried by schools include the following: determining student needs, conducting surveys, program planning, cross-age tutoring, peer counseling, ex-addict presentations, developing teaching materials, teacher and parent education, and evaluation.

9. Teachers, counselors, and other school personnel involved in the guidance of students with special drug problems must not only be academically competent and qualified, but must be able to communicate effectively with young persons.

These basic fundamentals clearly identify the importance of a multidimensional, multiphasic school program to implement the principles outlined that will meet the differential needs of students. Therefore, as a result of an exploration of activities now occurring in schools in many of the states, together with an extensive review of the literature and of suggestions by a variety of authorities in education, pharmacology, medicine, and other fields, and in the light of the varied experiences of the authors in the drug scene and in educational circles, a conceptual model of a school drug program has been developed. It is based on a philosophical approach to the school drug problem that includes education as a part of a broader program. The significance of this theoretical concept has been demonstrated by increasing implementation of segments in recent years. The total approach needs to be utilized in the nation's schools if effective drug education programs are to occur.

THE PROGRAM

The multiphasic differential school drug program model that has been designed includes the following four distinctive phases: (1) education, (2) services, (3) school atmosphere, or climate, and (4) coordination. These phases, however, cannot be developed without the consideration of certain administrative problems, which will be introduced in later chapters.

The following details outline the parts of the school drug program that will receive extensive coverage in the succeeding chapters.

I. Drug education
  A. Students
    1. Formal education
      a. Patterns of instructional organization
        (1) Direct teaching in health education
          (a) Drug education—cognitive, affective, action (practices, skills) goals
          (b) Mental health or affective education—values clarification, physical-emotional needs, self-concept, decision making—coping—risk-taking, communication
        (2) Correlated teaching
        (3) Alternative education
      b. Curriculum development—direct teaching
        (1) Scope and sequence
        (2) Curriculum guide—concept approach, objectives, content, methods, resources, evaluation
      c. Mini-courses—social, cultural, and recreational alternatives to drug abuse; peer counseling, cross-age tutoring, and others
    2. Informal education
      a. Counseling—one-to-one, small group interaction sessions
      b. Alternative activities to drug abuse
    3. Resource centers
    4. School and community resource personnel
  B. Parents
    1. Formal education
    2. Informal education

II. Drug services
  A. Identification of abuse drugs
  B. Identification of drug users and abusers
  C. Assistance for users and abusers
  D. Follow-up procedures
    1. Counseling and guidance
    2. Use of community resources
    3. Adjustment of school programs

III. School atmosphere
  A. Student alienation and unrest
  B. Physical and psychological needs of students
  C. Creating humaneness in schools

IV. Coordination of the program
  A. Administrative factors for program implementation
  B. Administration organization
    1. Leadership
    2. Advisory drug committee
  C. Policies and procedures
  D. Role of personnel
  E. Finance
  F. In-service preparation
  G. Evaluation

REFERENCES

1. American School Health Association: Teaching about drugs: a curriculum guide, K-12, ed. 2, Kent, Ohio, 1971, Association Press.
2. Barrins, P. C.: How to face up to drug abuse in your schools and your community, Am. Sch. Board J. **158:**17-20, 1970.
3. Bureau of Narcotics and Dangerous Drugs, United States Department of Justice: Guidelines for drug

abuse prevention education, Washington, D.C., 1970, Government Printing Office.

4. Cohen, S.: The drug dilemma: a partial solution. In Resource book for drug abuse education, Washington, D.C., 1969, National Clearinghouse for Mental Health Information.

5. Cornacchia, H. J.: Teaching in difficult areas in health, J. Sch. Health 41:193-196, 1971.

6. Demos, G. D., and Bennett, J. C., editors: Drug abuse and what we can do about it., Springfield, Ill., 1970, Charles C Thomas, Publisher.

7. Drysdale, E. J.: Youthful drug abuse: the problem and program, J. Drug Educ. 1:93-99, 1971.

8. Finlator, J.: The drug scene: the scope of the problem faced by the schools. In American School Health Association: Teaching about drugs: a curriculum guide, K-12, Kent, Ohio, 1970, Association Press.

9. Greenberg, J. S.: Drug abuse and the schools, J. Drug. Educ. 1:171-175, 1971.

10. Lewis, D. C.: How the schools can prevent drug abuse, N.A.S.S.P. Bull. 54:43-51, 1970.

11. Miller, T. J.: Drug abuse: schools find some answers, Sch. Manage. pp. 27-31, 1970.

12. National School Public Relations Association: Drug crisis: schools fight back with innovative programs, Washington, D.C., 1971, Association Pres..

13. Nowlis, H.: Drugs on the college campus, Garden City, N.Y., 1969, Anchor Books.

14. Ochberg, F. M.: Drug problems and the high school principal, N.A.S.S.P. Bull. 54:52-59, 1970.

15. Petrillo, R. F.: Comprehensive action model to combat drug abuse in high school, J. Sch. Psychol. 8:226-230, 1970.

16. Prettyman, R. L., and others: Drug abuse and the school scene, Sci. Teacher 37:45-47, 1970.

17. Report of the Ad Hoc Committee on Drug Abuse, Dallas, 1970, Superintendent of Schools, Dallas Independent School District.

18. Taylor, R. M., and Rackers, J.: How Missouri high school principals deal with student use of tobacco, alcohol, narcotics and drugs, Sch. and Country 56:7, 1970.

19. A teacher resource guide for drug use and abuse for Michigan schools, Lansing, 1970, Michigan State Department of Education.

20. U.S. Dept. of Health, Education, and Welfare, National Institute on Drug Abuse, Domestic Council on Drug Abuse Task Force: White Paper on Drug Abuse, September, 1975, Washington, D.C., 1975, U.S. Government Printing Office.

7
Drug education

Neither information nor education . . . has been given a fair test.

HELEN H. NOWLIS[67]

Every major group in the population . . . would require students to attend a program on the effects of drugs and alcohol . . .

Seventh Annual Gallup Poll[24]

. . . education and prevention should play a more important role in the national program than in the past.

White House Paper
on Drug Abuse
1975[85]

While many innovative, energetic programs are being designed in individual school systems, an overall concept of what school drug education is, or should be, is lacking.

Educational Research Service[17]

Drug education can hopefully reduce the amount of drug misuse and help students to make responsible decisions regarding their experimental and recreational drug use.

National Institute on Drug Abuse[62]

Drug education as an integral part of the preventive phase of a school drug program has been widely advocated by Yolles,[91] Langer,[45] Lewis,[49] Mikeal and Smith,[55] Kurzman,[44] the Seventh Annual Gallup Poll,[24] the National Institute of Drug Abuse,[62] and the White House Paper 1975.[85] These sources indicate that adequate programs available to children before they start using drugs could measurably reduce the drug problem.

The status of drug education programs today is perhaps best expressed by the National Commission on Marihuana and Drug Abuse when it concluded, "In the Commission's view, no drug education program in this country . . . has proven sufficiently

successful to warrant our recommending it."[17] Goodstadt said, ". . . there is almost a total lack of evidence indicating beneficial effects of drug education."[29] Nowlis remarked, ". . . within the past several years, education . . . has fallen into disrepute. It has been judged ineffective if not counterproductive in many instances. . . "[67] The Seventh Annual Gallup Poll reported, "The success of such required programs (drugs and alcohol) has been spotty in places where they have been tried."[24] The problem of quality programs is perhaps related to the comments made in the Educational Research Association Report that revealed, ". . . the present confusion over school drug education results from four factors: (1) definition, (2) goals,

(3) approaches, and (4) evaluation . . ."[17]

Yolles[91] indicates that educational efforts must be appropriate for specific population groups and should have the best educational and scientific bases available. The omission or lack of consideration of these points, in addition to the numerous fragmented and incomplete efforts that are under way in schools, are sufficient reasons to suspect the quality of many programs today.

The comments of the authorities indicate that school drug education programs are needed but may not be beneficial or preventive. They may not be turning youth off drugs or reducing their use; they may not be helping youth to identify alternatives to drugs, to establish values, or to aid in the development of decision-making, coping, and communication skills. Apparently better understanding by school personnel and new approaches are needed if education is to have any significant impact on young people. This chapter provides information that will be useful to administrators, teachers, and others not only in defining a complete approach to the situation but also in developing and conducting quality drug education programs. It will address itself to the criticisms about education introduced in Chapter 1 as well as to numerous other points. It will attempt to offer positive suggestions for the improvement of present educational offerings.

Essentially the material that follows considers both student and parent educational programs. Such complementary efforts are necessary for permanent and lasting results with young people. The student phase includes (1) formal education, patterns of instructional organization, curriculum, and minicourses, (2) informal education, (3) resource centers, and (4) role of personnel needed in the program—teachers, counselors, nurses, students, and the community. The parent phase will give consideration to both formal and informal education.

DRUG EDUCATION FOR STUDENTS

Instructional programs must give attention to the variety of student drug users— the nonusers, the experimenters, and the periodic, the compulsive, and the relapse users. To adequately meet these needs it is necessary to integrate the drug education program with all phases of the school curriculum. Whatever occurs within the school will have implications for drug education because the drug problem is a "people problem." In addition, both formal and informal drug education programs must be provided. The formal phase will more effectively reach the majority of young people who are nonusers and experimenters in the regular classroom setting. The informal phase, which usually occurs in various settings outside the classroom, is generally more appropriate for the periodic, compulsive, and relapse users of drugs. No program, however complete, can ever be designed to meet the needs of all students at all times. Nevertheless if the broad spectrum of educational offerings includes both formal and informal aspects and is integrated throughout the school program, the chances will be greatest not only of reaching but also of positively influencing many of the young people in school.

Student formal education

Numerous authorities agree that a comprehensive, sequential program of drug education should be provided in schools at all grade levels from K through 12. We need to reach students before they start using illegal drugs so that hopefully they will not want to begin. We need to help young people use all drugs wisely. This is the primary preventive approach. Many programs are now emerging that could achieve such a goal if they continue to be financially supported for a minimum of 3 to 5 years with qualified leadership. However, there are few model programs to direct schools, and there are only limited illustrative programs from which schools may seek guidance, although programs are becoming more numerous. Numerous curriculum guides have been developed, but many are narrow in their perspective. School personnel in need of help should find this chapter useful and practical. The material on curriculum should be of special assistance.

Where to put drug education in the curriculum is a frequent administrative problem. Should drug education be a separate, self-contained subject, or should it be a unit or a segment in another course or area? There does not seem to be any support for the separate subject status and the latter approach is the one most widely used. However, a further question can be asked, should drug education be a part of health education, science, social science, English, physical education, biology, chemistry, government, or some other subject, or should the organizational arrangement take some other form? It actually has relationships to all of these subject fields and might well be included in any or all of them. Would it perhaps be simpler to conduct one or two large assembly programs with all students in attendance and not be concerned about where to place drug education in the curriculum? These questions all relate to the patterns of instructional organization for drug education. How best to organize the instructional program to accommodate drug education is a significant question for administrators.

Patterns of instruction

No one organizational arrangement for drug education has been demonstrated to be the most effective in schools to date. Philosophically, it would be ideal to have a totally integrated instructional approach. Thus wherever formal education is offered, not only would the direct and correlated patterns exist, but they would be related to informal education and with all the other phases of the school drug program. Although efforts should be made to achieve such a goal, realistically it may be difficult to reach. The complexity of operating such a system, the limitations in funds, and other restrictions imposed on schools are the main obstacles inhibiting such a program.

Nationally, schools do not appear to be making efforts to move forward and provide the integrated arrangement. At this stage many schools are struggling merely to include formal education in their curriculum, which is evidenced by the sporadic, piece-meal, and crash programs that are emerging. Some administrators believe that a simple solution to drug education is to have an assembly with all students present, bring in a few speakers, and give students the facts. In other situations students participate in a special day- or week-long program in which the drug problem is emphasized. These approaches are questionable practices that have little impact on students. Quite often they act as substitutes for other, more appropriate educational arrangements.

The organizational patterns of formal drug education usually refer to the direct and correlated patterns of instruction. More recently a third category, called alternative education, has been added to this classification. The direct pattern includes drug education as part of a subject that usually deals with a variety of health problems and seeks changes in the health behavior of students; this occurs in health education. The correlated pattern means that instruction is correlated to other subjects in the curriculum that generally do not focus on health matters or practices, as in social studies or biology. In health education, attitudes and behaviors are oriented toward health and are people centered; in other curriculum areas the purposes are more likely to focus on cognitive objectives. Cognitive ends by themselves usually have little or no impact on healthful living.

*Alternative education** refers to an organizational approach that is more readily adaptable to the needs of particular students not usually found in conventional schools. This arrangement offers flexibility of curriculum, is more responsive to change, and generally has fewer rules and bureaucratic restraints. Some of the types that have emerged in the past 15 years include open school, schools-without-walls, learning centers, multicultural schools, and continuation schools. Additional information is found in Chapters 8 and 9.

In the secondary schools the direct and correlated patterns of instruction are easily

---

*National Institute on Drug Abuse: Alternatives, Washington, D.C., 1976, U.S. Government Printing Office.

distinguished. However, it is more complex at the elementary level. In elementary schools using the direct arrangement one might find drug education as a part of a subject area such as health education. Thus drug education would have status with other subjects such as language arts or social studies. The direct pattern could also refer to specific drug units that may be part of health education or entirely separated as distinct areas of instruction, provided time is allowed in the curriculum. The direct arrangement could also mean that the drug education program is related to social studies and science. In such instances drug education could be said to be co-related but often is said to be integrated into the curriculum. At the elementary level the words "correlated" and "integrated" are frequently used synonymously. Perhaps the distinction can be made that if elementary students are exposed to only one teacher daily, as in the self-contained classroom, a subject may be said to be integrated into the curriculum, whereas if students experience a variety of teachers daily in differing subject areas, a subject is said to be correlated into the curriculum.

Both the direct and the correlated patterns of instruction present problems and difficulties that need to be resolved in order to achieve the greatest degree of effectiveness. The correlated pattern is probably more complex and less likely to effect changes in the health behavior of students. The direct approach is believed to offer the best promise for providing the most effective drug education at both the elementary and secondary levels. Support for this position will be presented shortly.

The correlated organizational pattern of drug education is frequently used in schools today. Perhaps administrative ease is the primary reason for the selection of this arrangement. It is relatively simple to decide to put new content and new social problems or matters into already existing curriculum subjects, especially if no subject such as health education is offered.

Drug education may be correlated with numerous subject areas and can be approached through different methods to achieve various objectives. Examples of this correlation with the major subject areas might include the following:

Biology	Effects of drugs on the circulatory, respiratory, nervous, and other systems of the body; possible chromosomal and brain damage; other drug-induced organ damage
Chemistry	Chemical properties of alcohol, tobacco, and drugs; effects of smoking on chemical exchange of oxygen and carbon dioxide in the lungs; process of alcohol breakdown in the liver; percentage of alcohol in the blood
English	Preparation of essays, themes, poems, and speeches; reading and interpreting popular magazine articles, books, and pamphlets; analyzing themes of rock music
Driver education and safety	Effects of alcohol and drugs on accidents; cigarettes and fires
Government	Manufacturing, processing, distribution, sales, and taxes on the economics of the nation; role in the control of sale and distribution of drugs; prevention, rehabilitation, and treatment of addicts
History	Use of drugs by man throughout the ages; opium in Chinese settlements; morphine addiction of U.S. soldiers in the Civil War; the frontier and drugs; foreign, national, and state laws
Physical education	Drugs and their relationships to fitness and performance in athletics
Mathematics	A statistical information analysis of costs, profits, taxes, and other economic factors related to alcohol, tobacco, and drugs; percentages, graphs, budgets, and charts
Psychology	Motivational research in advertising; how to change attitudes and behaviors toward drugs; why people use drugs
Social studies	Incidence of drug use in society; foreign, national, state, and local laws; drugs in the culture and society; drugs and crime, poverty, and inequalities; student unrest and alienation

Teachers in all subject fields, in addition to cognitive learnings, can provide opportunities for student experiences in self-concept, problem solving, values clarification, as well as communication and decision-making skills development.

The following conditions should be operative if drug education is to be correlated into the curriculum:

1. Curriculum materials should be available that identify the specific content for each subject area with clearly stated goals to be achieved.
2. Teachers should be selected who are interested, or willing to become interested, in including drug information in their subject fields.
3. Provision is made for appropriate in-service preparation of teachers with supportive help from resource teachers when desired to maintain interest and obtain current information.
4. Responsible school personnel should be administratively assigned to (a) coordinate the correlation efforts, (b) help keep teachers up to date and interested, and (c) periodically evaluate the program.
5. It should be included as part of a broader, integrated, school drug program as outlined herein. It should be a segment of a formal and informal, comprehensive drug education program that also includes the direct approach.

The primary advantage of the correlated approach may be the fact that the drug problem needs a multidisciplinary educational attack. Drugs relate to people in all phases of life. If the topic is placed in any one area, such as science or social studies, the goal of a multidisciplinary program may not be achieved. If drug education is placed in several subject areas, problems of coordination immediately need to be resolved.

All too frequently when new content areas are proposed for school curricula, administrators are prone to use only the correlated approach because of the organizational ease of making it operational. It is a simple solution that quickly resolves the dilemma of where to place the topic in the school curriculum. Unfortunately when such action has occurred in the past, little or no consideration was given to the correlation problems previously identified. Neither was much if any thought given to the goals to be achieved or to the quality of the educational pro-

gram. Such action and lack of concern could well be the main difficulties with present drug education programs and the reason for their ineffectiveness.

Additional problems with the correlated approach support the need to consider a different way to present drug education in the curriculum. Frequently the objectives in these programs are not behavior or even health centered; some teachers may not wish to introduce other content into their crowded subject areas; no one may be available to coordinate the program. Therefore drug programs are dumped into the curriculum by administrative edict, and teachers are not always enthusiastically receptive. In addition, many teachers will not be interested or will not feel qualified to teach about drugs. Thus although the initial effort in launching a correlated program may meet with some success, it is doomed to failure or disappearance within a relatively short time because of the difficulties outlined. This will be especially true if no one periodically rejuvenates the program, motivates teachers, and occasionally assesses results. A few individual, dedicated teachers will continue their efforts, but when it becomes apparent that administrative support has waned, and when other matters of greater importance need attention, drug education will be pushed aside in order to take care of more pressing problems.

The logical, probably more natural, and perhaps most effective way of organizing the formal instructional program for drug education places this social health problem in a course or subject area that deals with all student health problems. Health education would be such a subject area. This pattern of instruction is the direct pattern because the content relates better with health problems, including venereal disease, communicable and chronic diseases, mental health, smoking, nutrition, and family health. Health education is gaining wide acceptance by students because it provides meaningful, relevant, and useful information.

The advantages of presenting drug education as part of health education include the following:

1. Curriculum materials in health education have been developed over the years and would continue to be developed with drugs included as one important area. A sequential, comprehensive drug program throughout the grades is more easily and more effectively achieved through an ongoing program of health education.

2. The concept approach to the teaching of health education, including drug education, identifies behaviorally centered objectives. This is the philosophical concept under which current health education curricula are developed and operated.

3. Mental health is an aspect of affective education and is generally included in the teaching of health education. Self-concept, decision-making, emotions understandings, and communication skills could be taught concurrently with a drug education unit.

4. The teachers of established health education programs in junior and senior high schools are interested, generally well qualified, and desire to add drug education to the health program. It is easier for these teachers to maintain this interest, to become knowledgeable, and to become familiar with current information.

5. Teachers of health education are usually concerned not only with the acquisition of information—cognitive domain—but also with the modification of attitudes and practices. Thus goals are more apt to be established accordingly.

6. Drug education as part of health education programs has been endorsed and promoted by at least 13 state departments of education, including California, Colorado, Delaware, Illinois, Maine, Maryland, Michigan, Nebraska, New Jersey, New York, Pennsylvania, Utah, and Washington. In a recent unpublished survey* of state drug education coordinators in the United States it was revealed that of 78% (30 states) of those states reporting, many, or all of them, followed this arrangement.

*Conducted by H. J. Cornacchia and D. E. Smith.

7. Drug education can more easily be evaluated and adapted to changing comditions and local community problems if it is included in health education.

The main problem with including drug education in health education is that vast numbers of schools do not yet include this subject in their curricula. Although many schools are adding this subject, many others are still in need of a health education program. Related to this problem is an auxiliary one. In a few schools where health education is provided, it is a weak and poorly taught area. These problems may be due to a variety of reasons, including insufficient administrative support and recognition of the subject; ineffective teaching, primarily due to poorly qualified and uninterested instructors; and the absence of a responsible administrative coordinator to oversee the program. These situations can be rather easily resolved.

If the fragmented, incomplete approach to drug education is to be modified to provide an instructional program with impact on young people, such a program must include a formal education component that incorporates both the direct and correlated instructional patterns outlined herein. However, if only one such arrangement is possible, we believe that the program more likely to be ongoing, continually improved, and effective in the lives of young persons will present drug education as a part of health education. Consideration must also be given to the inclusion of alternative education.

Curriculum

To provide continuity with a minimum of overlapping and duplication of content, a scope and sequence should be developed that indicates the nature of the drug content and the grade or grade levels at which this material is to be introduced in each school or school district. This local approach is necessary to develop a curriculum that is relevant to any given community. The student drug needs and interests survey (p. 157) and Tables 7-7 to 7-10 offer specific help in local scope and sequence preparation. An outline of the content may include:

Definitions
Historical aspects
Classification
   Legal and illegal
   Pharmacological—stimulants, depressants, narcotics, etc.
Physiological factors
   The nervous system
   Uses—medical, mood modifiers
   Effects
   Abuse potential—high-risk, low-risk
   Duration of action
   Method of administration
Psychological factors
   Physical and emotional needs
   Why people use, misuse, abuse
   Characteristics of potential drug abusers
   Alternatives to drugs
   Problem solving, coping, decision making
Sociological factors
   Patterns of use and abuse
   Misuse and abuse effects on home, family, school
   Factors affecting use and abuse—environment, business and economics, life styles, housing, employment, etc.
   Role of home, school, community
   Rehabilitation and treatment
   Laws
   Community resources
   Identification of abusers
Spiritual factors
   Values—self-concept
   Moral issues—effects on self, home, community
   Humanism—individual and community responsibility for abusers

Upon the completion of the scope and sequence material, a teacher's curriculum guide should be prepared for use at all grade levels where drug education is to be included. Such a guide may be developed locally, obtained from another school district, or adapted from state guidelines. The content should be locally relevant.

A curriculum guide could include the scope and sequence, consideration of the direct or correlated patterns of instruction, a statement of philosophy, and a variety of appropriate units prepared for the various grades. These units should include behav-

ioral objectives, content, teaching activities, teaching aids, and practical procedures for evaluation. Material in this book will aid in general preparation as well as helping teachers who wish to develop their own guides.

Concept approach.* The current philosophical ideal used in health education and applicable to drug education is the concept approach to curriculum. It emphasizes the learning of comprehensive ideas rather than mere factual information. Concepts are identified as ideas, generalizations, or conclusions that in simple form may be sensory perceptions of external objects or events (sight, smell, accident, eating) or in more complex form are high-level abstractions. (Drugs may result in health and safety problems for individuals.) Concepts cannot be taught directly but rather are the result of learning. What students learn, therefore, are not unrelated, isolated facts, but rather understandings and attitudes that enable them to form conclusions and make intelligent decisions about drugs. Thus the most effective teaching must be directed toward conceptual development.

The conceptual approach refers to the organization of various levels of abstractions, or generalizations, about drugs into a framework, or hierarchy, of concepts basic to the drug education curriculum. The essential categories of concepts that form the philosophical foundation for the drug education curriculum are the following: (1) definition of health applied to drug education; (2) values in the curriculum; (3) key concepts, the unifying threads of the curriculum; and (4) basic drug education concepts. These are the fundamental principles to be used in curriculum development and should receive major consideration by teachers in drug instruction programs.

Definition of health applied to drug education. Health has frequently been defined as a state of physical, mental, and social well-being and not merely the absence of disease or infirmity for effective living. Positive

*Adapted from Health education approach to curriculum design, School health education study, St. Paul, Minn., 1967, 3M Company.

health involves a multidimensional state of the organism that helps a person to function better or to adapt and adjust more easily to his society. This definition of health identifies man as a composite of interrelated segments that act independently or collectively to affect the individual's well-being. It correlates with the approach to the primary prevention concept that is advocated by the National Institute on Drug Abuse.

When applied to drug education, and more specifically to adequate and effective teaching, a fourth dimension, the spiritual phase, must be added to this definition in order to identify the interrelationships of the physical, social, and mental aspects in a more meaningful manner. In drug education programs to date the focus of attention has been on the physiological or pharmacological effects of drugs on the human body. This emphasis alone provides an important clue to the probable ineffectiveness of numerous programs. The need is for greater emphasis on the psychological, social, and spiritual aspects of the educational program. These phases have been limited or ignored in drug education programs. Greater attention to these aspects will provide more opportunities for the achievement of goals in the affective and action domains.

Fig. 7 is an isosceles triangle representing graphically the degrees of emphasis that the various dimensions of health as applied to drug education should receive in the instructional program. It should be noted that the physical phase is basic but is of lesser importance than the equally significant psychological and social aspects. However, the spiritual aspect is the core or the action director. This configuration emphasizes that an individual, as a result of values, moral principles, and physical and emotional needs, not only influences, or is influenced by, the social atmosphere in which that person lives but also helps to determine one's behavior.

Psychological or social factors bring about the physical health of the individual. If a person has an unfulfilled need and seeks an escape, the environment may provide the appropriate drug to change the mood or feelings or to reach the goal. By the same token the television commercial or the peer-group influence may help an individual find

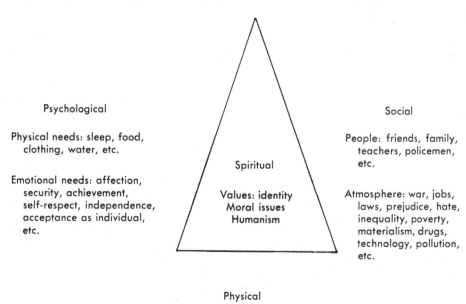

FIG. 7. Health dimension emphasis in drug education.

the drug to satisfy an emotional need. A person with good psychological or social health is perhaps more likely to enjoy good physical health. Such a person may be better able to adjust to society and have less desire to seek drugs that may affect his body. However, it is not necessarily true that a person with good physical health has good psychological or social health, or that a person with poor physical health has poor psychological or social health. The individual and his interrelationships with his environment basically control the status of the human organism. In arriving at decisions affecting one's physical body, the individual is guided by his values and moral principles, or by his lack of them, and by their application to other individuals.

The highest level of psychological health results from the individual's fulfillment of a variety of physical and emotional needs, which shape behavior. Failure to acquire adequate food, housing, and health together with lack of affection, achievement, self-respect, self-image, and coping and communication skills may affect one's physical health. Such omissions may be important causal factors in drug misuse and abuse.

Social health results from the interaction of individuals with their environment. This means not only influencing society but also being influenced by it. An individual is physically affected by many hazardous and harmful substances and materials—alcohol, tobacco, and drugs—that have been created, developed, or promoted. By the same token television encourages us to drink more beer and use more aspirin. The speed in our world and the rapid changes in technology may be creating personal anxieties that demand an escape from the world through drugs. If the drug abuse problem is to be reduced, greater concern and emphasis must be given to the psychological and social aspects of health in the drug education program.

Probably the most important influence on health, yet the one most frequently overlooked or omitted in teaching, is the spiritual aspect. The decisions individuals must make about health are dependent upon the values and moral codes by which these individuals live and their concerns for their fellowmen (the humanistic aspect). The emphasis on greed, avarice, prejudice, hate, destruction, inequality, and racism should be removed from the world and replaced with concern for people. It has been said quite frequently that the drug problem is a people problem. This concern for humanism must be brought into the drug education program. One way this can be achieved is by helping young persons to find their identities and to find meaningfulness in life. The achievement of spiritual health and the emphasis on moral issues and values can only occur if education focuses on the learner as a person. The teacher must realize and accept his role as not solely a specialist in subject matter but as an expert in knowing and understanding children. He must be able to communicate with students, to make learning relevant, to respect the dignity of individuals regardless of race, color, and creed, to give students a share of the power, and to allow the freedom to make choices but in so doing he should provide a variety of alternatives.

Values in the curriculum. Social turmoils with numerous dichotomies, confusing and conflicting occurrences, are creating difficulties in the establishment of values by children and young persons. Factors related to these difficulties include the following:

1. Family changes—mothers working and not home, broken homes
2. Influence of communication media—radio, TV, movies, publications
3. Technological innovations—cars, jets, computers, satellite communication
4. Less influence of church on growing child and on people in general
5. World events—violence and destruction, impoverished and hungry people, war
6. Value conflict of peace and war in society
7. Teacher emphasis on factual teaching only
8. Conflict of conformity and self-reliance, independency

9. Dichotomies of values—good and bad, moral and immoral, wealth and poverty

10. Affluence—emphasis on materialism, secularism

11. Existence of unemployment, hunger, inequality, prejudice

12. Conflict of authoritarianism and democracy

13. Pressures exerted for high academic performance—grades, courses

14. Dehumanization of schools

15. Extensive exciting stimuli that create a psychological numbness in students

As a result of these factors, a sizable number of young persons are questioning the values of society. These youth seem less secure and are searching for the ultimate meaning of life. They are asking such questions as: Who am I? What am I? Why am I here? What really matters? Thus a variety of different patterns of behavioral problems are appearing in schools among a sizable number of students. These problems include apathy (not being involved); inconsistent behaviors (flighty interests, uncertainty about choices, fluctuating achievements); drifting (no plans); drop-outs (dissent through negative action); overconformers (lack of purpose leading to band-wagon behavior); overdissenters (radical activists); and role-playing (cover for lack of clarity of direction). Other youths have never given thought or are uncertain about what they believe to be important in life.

Freud and the mental health movement indicated that the uncertainty about, or the lack of, values may be added to the explanations for children's behavior problems. Raths, and others[70] discovered that when children with certain behavioral problems were exposed to particular value experiences, these problems were often eased in intensity, or frequency, or both. Maslow,[52] Frankl,[21] and Keniston[43] further indicate that individuals need a sense of purpose and belief. People actively search for meaningfulness and identity in life as guides to good mental health. In addition, people need to acquire decision-making, coping, and communication skills.

There are indications that the use of drugs is closely related to the factors just identified. Young people are searching for ways to break out of the shell and the numbness in which society has placed them. Perhaps they are using drugs as one means of breaking through, of escaping. Youths are seeking immediate pleasure and satisfaction rather than deferring gratification and enjoyment. They are testing new, experimental values such as responsiveness, genuineness, spontaneity, and sensation in order to find meaningfulness in life. Although the vast majority of students do not seek meaning and experience primarily via psychoactive compounds, many are uncertain, unclear, and in need of help in understanding their purposes in life. Thus the need for learning about values and developing a value system becomes apparent.

No one clear, accepted definition of values exists; however, values manifest how a person decides to use his life. Values give direction to life and hence may be considered the determiners of behavior. Schools have been emphasizing intellectual values, but it is evident that facts alone are an insufficient basis for learning because they have relevance only in the context of human experience.

Values may be seen as goals that can be learned in the educational process. Such objectives have particular reference to the use, misuse, and abuse of drugs in the affective or attitudinal domain and in the experiential realm. Attitudes themselves have a multiplicity of understandings. Suffice it to say that attitudes refer to learned predispositions to action or behavior that may have varying effects on individuals. The degree and intensity of an attitude determine the potential and extent of the behavior or action. Table 7-1 presents a hierarchy of attitudes illustrating this concept.

There is no consensus regarding how to categorize values. Rucker et al.[77] offer the following list as a possible guideline:

1. Affection—congenial human relationships, love, friendship, and emotional security

TABLE 7-1. Hierarchy of attitudes*

	Attitude	Definitions	Behavioral manifestations
Overt action	1. Interest	Emotional responses to stimuli; feelings	1. Attention, awareness, appreciation by listening, talking, reading, writing, and other ways
	2. Opinion		2. Verbal or written expression
Internalization	3. Belief	Emotional acceptance of a concept, proposition, or doctrine; a preference; a decision about something; a conviction to or about something	3. Willingness to be identified with a proposition, or concept, self-expression with verbal, written, or performance action
	4. Value	A high, deep, and long-lasting degree of emotional acceptance and commitment to a concept, proposition, or doctrine; to cherish or prize; a faith; a potential goal	4. Pursues, seeks, and wants; takes action in satisfying ways through participation—convincing others, spending time, effort, and funds

*Modified from Rosser, J. M.: J. Sch. Health **41:**386-390, 1971.

2. Respect—use of individual talents, self-esteem assured
3. Skill—develop individual talents to potential limits
4. Enlightenment—respect for scholarship, seeking truths, student solves own problems; present both sides of issue
5. Power—student involvement in classroom decisions, democracy in action
6. Wealth—guide student to produce wealth in form of services and materials himself
7. Well-being—foster good physical and mental health for each student
8. Rectitude—student to develop moral responsibility and standards for own behavior; sharing of values

Another authority, Fraenkel,[20] indicates the diversity of values that exists in the following catalogue:

1. Intelligent use of forces of nature
2. Recognition of the worth and dignity of the individual
3. Use of intelligence to improve human living
4. Increasing effectiveness of the family as a basic social institution

5. Effective development of moral and spiritual values
6. Intelligent and responsible sharing of power in order to attain justice
7. Cooperative interest in peace and welfare
8. Widening and deepening the ability to live more richly
9. Recognition and understanding of world interdependence
10. Intelligent acceptance by individuals and groups of the responsibility for achieving democratic social action
11. Intelligent utilization of scarce resources to attain modest general well-being

Young persons learn values through exposure to a variety of meaningful experiences and through interaction with the environment. Therefore the sources of their attitudes are adults, peer culture, the family, the church, the communication media, the school, and friends and social groups who influence their decisions.

The school has a role to play as one source of value development but Simon states, "It is values, ultimately, which give a man the stars by which he steers his life; yet the schools are doing almost nothing to help young people make sense out of the clamoring and bewildering appeals rampant in these baffling times."[80] Thus old "shall nots" may be irrelevant today.

The teaching of values should be included in the school curriculum because the drug problem is a people problem; values can be significant aids in helping individuals with their search for meaning in life and with solving behavioral problems. One promising approach to value teaching is offered by Raths and others[70] who state that value-clarification involves a series of strategies or methods for helping students to learn values. Specific methods will be found later in this chapter and in the book by Raths and others.[70]

A value must meet these seven criteria:

Choosing	1.	Choosing freely—individual should not be coerced and should have freedom of selection.
	2.	Choosing from alternatives—a variety of alternatives must be provided.
	3.	Choosing thoughtfully—consideration should be given to the consequences of each alternative.
Prizing	4.	Prizing and cherishing—choice has a positive tone and is held in high esteem.
	5.	Affirming—when something is cherished it is publicly and verbally supported; doing something.
Action	6.	Acting upon choices—life is affected through reading, spending money, and budgeting time.
	7.	Repeating—persistency and endurance become a pattern of life.

Application of the criteria identified should make it obvious that most individuals will have few values. However, so-called value indicators, or potential values, may be evidenced in a variety of ways through such expressions as goals or purposes, aspirations, attitudes, interests, feelings, beliefs, activities, worries, and problems.

The inclusion of the values approach in the curriculum has been greatly expanded in schools throughout the United States. Many school districts now focus their drug education programs on this procedure. Such methods will hopefully guide students to alternative routes to the attainment of valid goals rather than the use of drugs. The values clarification method should help students realize that how one chooses to live one's life, how and where one hopes to seek experiences, and how one searches for meaning are important. Knowing that there are better and more lasting ways to experience the fullness, depth, and richness of life than through ingesting drugs should aid young persons in reaching their own decisions. Thus energies will be focused on the causes of drug misuse and abuse rather than the symptoms.

Whether the values clarification process eliminates or reduces drug abuse is not known today. Blum[6] says that when it is used with understandings about drugs, there is evidence of impact. However, Loggins[51] states that no one can tell whether the method works. A New York State Commission[72] claims it is difficult for students to clarify values when teachers themselves do not have clearly defined goals about drug misuse and abuse. They state that values are not learned by exposure to a 1-hour daily discussion.

Key concepts. In organizing the hierarchy of concepts basic to the drug education curriculum, certain key concepts are applicable to all individuals and therefore are essential understandings not only in curriculum development but more importantly in the instructional program. We have chosen three key concepts that serve as unifying threads and that should permeate the entire drug education curriculum.

1. Every person is a growing and developing organism born with certain hereditary factors. In the growth process each individual develops some characteristics common to all individuals, but shares certain traits with fewer individuals, and maintains other attributes that are distinctly his own. Although everyone usually has two arms, two legs, and two eyes, everyone does not have white skin or black skin; each person has his own features and his own personality that identify him in a unique way. With regard to the drug problem, students have different physical and psychological needs that must receive attention. Drug education programs in schools therefore must include consideration

of the diverse characteristics of students as well as the types and extent of drugs each individual uses or abuses. Byler's and Berlow's questions on pp. 157 and 160 provide indications of such needs.

2. The growing, developing organism, the individual, is constantly affected by and in turn affects certain biological, social, psychological, economic, cultural, and physical forces in the environment. Racism, prejudice, war, destruction, peer groups, the family, the school, and other social factors have varying degrees of impact on individuals. However, action can be taken to modify these environmental conditions. Applied to the drug field, television and newspapers continually try to influence people to use tobacco and alcohol. If all or many individuals suddenly decided to stop smoking cigarettes or drinking alcoholic beverages, such action could have considerable economic effect on the tobacco and alcohol industries.

3. People must make their own decisions about whether or not to use drugs. They must learn how to cope with such peer-group pressures in deciding whether or not to smoke, to drink alcoholic beverages, or to use marijuana. In the educational process, all the alternatives, both positive and negative, must be presented to students so that they will have the best opportunity for free and intelligent choices. The instructional program must be one of education and not indoctrination.

In summarizing, it can be stated that growing, developing young persons can be affected by the pressures of their peers to use drugs. In turn they can partially affect the social climate by not associating with such peer groups or by refusing to use the drugs. However, the decision to participate must be made by the students themselves and not by the teacher, the parent, or another adult. This concept is extremely important in the drug education program. Many teachers today are still using the "scare" approach or are imposing their own value systems on young people when teaching about drugs. Such approaches have not been successful, nor will they be.

Basic drug education concepts. The application of the definition of health to drug education together with knowledge of the drug use, misuse, and abuse problem in society and other material presented in this chapter lays the groundwork for the formulation of the basic concepts found in Table 7-2. These concepts are the foundation for the entire drug education curriculum. They are the main generalizations, or conclusions,

TABLE 7-2. Basic drug education concepts

Number	Concept	Application to definition of health
I	Drugs differ in kind and degree; they have multiple uses with a variety of effects on individuals.	Physical
II	Proper use of drugs may be beneficial to individuals, the family, and the community.	Physical
III	Improper use of drugs may result in health and safety problems to individuals, the family, and the community.	Physical
IV	Numerous factors and forces influence the availability as well as the use and misuse of legal and illegal drugs by individuals and the community.	Psychological-social
V	The individual, the family, and the community have interrelated and reciprocal responsibilities to help control the availability, to prevent the misuse and abuse, and to assist individuals who become misusers and abusers of drugs in society.	Social
VI	The use and misuse of drugs by individuals involve moral principles and issues, and are related to one's sense of values as well as to the humane and just treatment of all people in society.	Spiritual-philosophical

that should be learned in the educational program. Some schools and teachers may desire, or find it advisable, to develop sub-concepts for specific grade level groups or for individual grades. This is an acceptable practice and may enable such individuals to focus more easily on the concepts to be achieved.

Objectives. The fundamental concepts for drug education previously described serve as the bases for developing the objectives desired in the instructional program. Objectives are necessary, since they give direction to teaching and learning. They identify the *why* of teaching and form the basis for the evaluation to determine the effectiveness of the educational program. Objectives enable teachers and other school personnel to determine the quality of the instructional offering. The objectives should be concisely and clearly written so that they give clues to the teacher and are useful in the evaluation process.

When considering objectives, this statement from the White House Paper on Drug Abuse should be noted: "We should stop raising unrealistic expectations of total elimination of drug abuse from our society. . . . Prevention, education . . . will curtail their number, but will not eliminate drug use entirely . . . we probably always will have a drug problem of some proportion . . ."[85]

Goals, specifically identified as objectives later in this chapter, should stress behavioral changes and be written in behavioral terms. They should include purposes of a cognitive (understanding and knowledge), affective (attitude), and action (practice) nature. These behaviors should stress preventive drug education. Thus the formal educational program can aid in both primary and secondary prevention.

Many drug education programs have had little impact on young persons because school personnel have not been sure of their direction. They have not been realistic in the provision of attainable objectives. Goals have been inadequately defined. Purposes need to be written behaviorally, stated clearly and concisely, formulated for use in the evaluation procedures, and considered from the psychological, social, and spiritual emphases previously described. Application of these principles to the drug education goals at a variety of grade levels will be found later in this chapter.

The Task Force on Responsible Decisions About Alcohol[82] have outlined illustrative general objectives that are useful in any drug education curriculum.

1. Skills—evaluate risks (bodily harm, ethnic, social, financial); ability to communicate with peers, adults, and self; decision making (intelligent use of drugs); coping, problem solving (stress, emotions, relatives, friends); needs fulfillment (success, affection, self-esteem); values clarification (life goals).

2. Attitudes—responsibility for one's behavior; respect for the safety of others; issues awareness; empathy; personal moral integrity; breakdown of stereotyping; support for nondrinker; values clarification; positive self-image; disapprove peer group pressure.

Student drug needs and interests. To prepare objectives that are appropriate for local communities, whether predominantly low-income areas or suburbs, to make the instructional program meaningful, and to involve students in curriculum development, drug interests and needs should be identified. Insight and guidance as to the diversity and extent of objectives and guidelines for content can be determined from such data. A variety of procedures may be used to obtain this information but only two will be described herein. Teachers and school districts will want to conduct their own needs-interests survey for use in instructional programs. Byler[8] and Berlow[4] provide information for use in constructing survey instruments. The evaluation devices in Chapter 11 will also be helpful.

Byler[8] completed an extensive study of the health education needs and interests of over 5000 students in Connecticut. The excerpted data about drugs are presented in the question form the students used and are organized into grade level groupings around the following categories:

1. Classification of drugs

2. Physical and pharmacological effects of drugs
3. Psychological reasons why drugs are used
4. Social considerations
5. Spiritual values

STUDENT NEEDS AND INTERESTS*
GRADES K TO 2
Drugs

Physical. Are hospitals where they help us? Do dentists help you? Do they give shots so it will not hurt? Will it hurt to have my tonsils out?

GRADES 3 AND 4
Alcohol

Physical. What does alcohol have in it? If you drink wine or booze, will you get drunk? Could you die from too much alcohol? What would happen if I should drink some whiskey?

Psychological. Why do people drink so much? Do people drink things with alcohol because they like them?

Drugs

Physical. What is LSD? Is marijuana dangerous? How do they affect you? What does glue sniffing do to you? Why might people who take dope have a deformed child?

Psychological. Why do so many people take shots of marijuana, STP, LSD, "snow," and "speed?" Why do people smoke pot?

Social. Why do people make drugs when they know drugs can cause bad health and death? Why were these drugs invented and why are people bringing them to America?

Tobacco

Physical. Does smoking cause lung cancer? How many more smokers get heart attacks than nonsmokers? Will one cigarette a day hurt you? Twenty packs? Is smoking more of a hazard to young people than to older people? My father smokes a lot and he bought these pills. How could they help him stop smoking?

Psychological. Why do so many people smoke? Is it hard to give up smoking?

Social. Why do people continue to make cigarettes?

Mental health

Psychological and social. If you worry too much, will you become sick? My mother and father do not love each other anymore; which one shall I love? Why am I so lonely? Why do humans always fight with one another? Why do I not have any friends? Why do I hate my sister? My brother?

---

*Adapted from Byler, R.: Teach us what we want to know, New York, 1969, Mental Health Materials Center, Inc.

GRADES 5 AND 6
Drugs

Physical. What do drugs do to you? What are drugs and the differences between drugs and drugstores? How does it feel to get high on LSD? If a girl takes LSD and has a baby, will the baby be deformed?

Psychological. Why do people take drugs? Why can't people stop taking overdoses of drugs? Can anyone ever break the drug habit?

Social. How are different drugs made? How do people start taking "dopejuice"? My brother takes dope; what shall I do?

Spiritual. If we had a better sense of values would there be a need to take LSD?

Tobacco

Physical. What pleasures do people derive from smoking?

Psychological. Why do people want to smoke? Why do high school students want to smoke? Why do adults think they can't give up smoking?

Social. Why do they sell cigarettes?

Mental health

Psychological. Why do I act happy, sad, and angry? Why don't people like me? Why do I lose control of my temper? Why do I sometimes hate everybody? Why am I afraid of darkness, ghosts, etc.? Why are Negroes treated differently than white people? Why do my problems sometimes overcome me?

Social. What is a real friend? Why can I not get along with my brother? My sister? Why do people marry if they do not love each other? What are the different races of people?

Spiritual. Who am I? What is life? What makes me tick?

GRADES 7 AND 8
Alcohol

Physical. What is alcohol? How does alcohol get into the bloodstream? What emotional reaction is caused by drinking? Can alcohol cause brain damage to the unborn child if the mother drinks during pregnancy? What are the effects of alcohol on the body and mind?

Psychological. Why do people drink? Why do people become alcoholics?

Social. What is an alcoholic? Why is alcohol on the market? How can young people drink without parents knowing it when stores do not sell alcohol to people under 21 years of age?

Drugs

Physical. What are drugs? Are drugs habit forming? Could dope ever be properly used? Is dope a drug? Is it liquid? A cigar? A cigarette? What is a "trip"? What are the effects of marijuana and LSD on the body and brain? Does LSD affect the unborn child if the father uses it? If the mother uses it? Which medicines are good or bad? What do narcotics look like "so I can protect myself against pushers"?

Psychological. Why do people like to "trip-out" on drugs? Why do some teen-agers use drugs? Do hippies use drugs? How can a person stop using drugs?

Social. How many people use drugs? Which drugs are useful and which are not? How can we help people who use drugs? If someone offers you LSD should you tell your parents or someone older? Why do high school students sell marijuana? Why does the government not stop the sale of drugs? Why do newspapers make so much of drugs that young people want to try them?

Tobacco

Physical. Does smoking produce cancer? Does smoking affect the heart? Lungs? Brain? Does smoking stop tension?

Psychological. Why do people smoke? How can people stop smoking?

Social. Why are cigarettes made? Why do men in Vietnam receive free cigarettes if smoking is not good for people?

Mental health

Psychological. Why do people rob, murder, and commit suicide?

Social. Why do Negroes not have the right to live as whites do? Why do young persons drop out of school? What makes slums? How do you get rid of slums?

GRADE 9
Alcohol

Physical. How does alcohol make a person drunk? What are the effects of alcohol on the body and brain?

Psychological. Why do people drink? What causes alcoholism?

Drugs

Physical. Is there such a thing as a safe drug? Are drugs as harmful as people say?

Psychological. Why do people use drugs? How does a person become addicted?

Social. Should marijuana be made legal? What is the extent of the drug problem?

Tobacco

Physical. Is it certain that you can get cancer from smoking cigarettes? How dangerous is smoking? What substance in tobacco causes cancer?

Social. Why do stores continue to sell tobacco to youngsters?

Spiritual. Is it right or wrong for stores to sell tobacco to youngsters?

GRADE 10
Alcohol

Physical. What are the effects of drinking on health? What is the difference between sensible and unwise drinking? What are the results of excessive drinking? When under the influence, is a person able to make a decision to benefit himself?

Psychological. Is there harm in drinking if you are not an alcoholic?

Social. What are the dangers of drinking and driving? If alcohol is injurious, why is it so easy to buy?

Drugs

Physical. What are the dangers of taking drugs during pregnancy? What are the effects of drugs on offspring? Are drugs as enjoyable as they sound? How many times must you take drugs in order to get hooked?

Psychological. Are there any common factors in the background of drug addicts? Why should I not try drugs if everybody else does?

Social. Why are some drugs that are not habit forming made illegal?

Spiritual. What and who is God? How does he feel about love, sex, etc.? What is right? What is wrong? How are values established? How can I be more considerate, more helpful, and less critical? Why am I here?

Tobacco

Physical. What are the pleasures of smoking? What are the dangers to health?

Psychological. How can I achieve happiness?

Social. If cigarettes are dangerous, why are they easy to buy? How do you get along with people of your own age? How can we get along better with our parents?

GRADE 11
Alcohol

Physical. What are the real hazards of drinking? What are the effects of drinking on the body? On the mind? How does drinking affect athletic performance?

Psychological. Why are young persons drinking more hard liquor and less beer?

Social. Can teen-agers be taught to control social drinking and alcohol consumption?

Drugs

Physical. Who should you believe about drugs—the users, the experts, or the "slanting" press? What should teen-agers know about stimulants and drugs?

Psychological. Why do most teen-agers on drugs have a weary outlook, and why do they think it is "cool" to use drugs? How does a person become addicted? What are the psychological effects of drugs?

Social. What legal problems can drug users and pushers face?

GRADE 12
Alcohol

Psychological. If adults drink, why can't students?

Social. Why not lower the drinking age?

Drugs

Psychological. How can students be helped who have problems at home, school, and with friends and who want to get away from problems? How can students be helped to face reality?

Berlow,[4] a member of the staff of the School of Pharmacy, University of North Carolina, compiled a list of questions about drugs from discussion groups conducted by selected advanced pharmacy students in schools; it is reproduced in part here. Although they do not indicate grade levels, these questions can be utilized for teacher preparation, for developing tests for the student to give himself, for use in problem-solving experiences, for the preparation of survey inventories to determine local student interest, and in a variety of other ways. The questions focus on the following general areas: classification and nature of drugs, physical or pharmacological effects of drugs, psychological reasons why people take drugs, and social considerations.

A COLLECTION OF QUESTIONS ABOUT DRUGS*
WHY DO PEOPLE TAKE DRUGS?

Why do people think drugs are the solution to their problems?

Why do most people think that teen-agers will eventually resort to drugs? We are not all alike.

Why is it important to stay off drugs?

Do you become sexually aroused if you take LSD or marijuana?

Can the will power of a person keep him from using drugs?

Why do hippies mostly take drugs?

Why do people take drugs and say they did not?

Do you think the commercials on TV urge students and adults to try drugs?

If I myself believe that drugs are not harmful and I am all for drugs, do you think that I am wrong in feeling this way?

Is it a fact that many rock music groups use LSD to produce their music?

WHO TAKES DRUGS?

If you know a person who is taking drugs, should you associate with him? Will he try to slip you some?

How many people in the United States take drugs?

What was the percentage of drug use in Vietnam?

What percent of black people and what percent of white people are hooked on drugs?

Are drugs as prevalent in the other countries of the world as in the United States?

What are the ages of most people who take drugs?

---

*Excerpted from Berlow, L.: Kids 'n drugs, Chapel Hill, N.C., 1971, University of North Carolina, School of Pharmacy.

At what age do kids start taking drugs?

Suppose someone were to drug your food, how would you know?

WHERE DO DRUGS COME FROM?

How did drugs first come about?

Do the people who try to push drugs take them?

Where do the pushers get the drugs?

What plants do the different drugs come from?

How do drugs get in the country if they are against the law?

Can you spot a pusher?

WHAT CAN DRUGS DO TO ME?

Why do drugs kill a person?

Do drugs really change a person's personality?

How long would you have to stay on drugs before they completely destroyed your body?

Can smoking stunt your growth? Can it cause lung cancer?

What long-range effects on hormones, genes, mental and physical abilities come from the use of drugs?

If an expectant mother is physically dependent on heroin, will her baby be?

Is it true that some drugs damage the chromosomes?

How does a person look when he has been taking drugs?

Approximately how long does it take for drugs to enter the bloodstream?

What are the effects produced by pot, pep pills, LSD, and heroin?

If you take drugs will it affect your parents' and friends' emotions toward you?

If you were 15 years old and were caught with drugs, what would happen to you?

Can drugs cause any well-known diseases?

What effect does the drug have on the person when it wears off?

How dangerous can an afterflash be?

CAN I GET HOOKED ON DRUGS?

Do you think it is true that you use drugs once and you are hooked?

What do you do if you are hooked and scared to tell anybody but you want to get off drugs?

What do you do if someone in the family is on dope and you do not want to get them into trouble but you want to help them?

Could people get unhooked on drugs?

What drug is the hardest to stop taking?

How do you know when you are actually hooked?

Can speed or heroin become a day-to-day necessity after just injecting it for the first time? If not, how many times does it take to get hooked?

Why is it so hard to keep getting drugs after you are hooked?

What is the average age of a drug addict?

Can you become physically or psychologically dependent on legal amphetamines such as Vivarin or No-Doz?

Why does it make you go crazy if you stop taking
dope?

If you take drugs today, years from now will they
still be affecting you?

If you would just smoke one cigarette, would it harm
you? Also, would it lead to worse drugs?

CAN I GET INTO TROUBLE TAKING DRUGS?

Is it true that if you are caught with drugs you can
lose your right to vote?

What is the penalty for pushing heroin?

If you are caught while on probation where do you
go or what kind of sentence do you get?

If you know a person who shoots drugs and know
people who sell drugs, should you report them?

How many people use and are caught using drugs
each year?

Are drugs illegal in other countries?

If you are riding in a car with guys who are drinking
and are stopped, can the police do anything with
you if you are not drinking?

WHAT ABOUT . . . ?

Can you smell drugs?

If you are on two different drugs, what will happen?

What does THC mean?

What is the most popular kind of drug?

Does cough medicine hurt you besides making you
drunk?

How much do drugs cost?

What different kinds of drugs do truck drivers use to
stay awake on the job?

What is the difference between marijuana and LSD?

Can you take drugs without their becoming a habit?

Could water injected into the body have any effect on
a person?

How do parents find out that their child is taking
drugs?

Can you inject the blood from one person who was
high into another to get the same effect?

Which is the most dangerous drug among opiates,
sedatives, tranquilizers, cocaine, stimulants, hallucinogens, and marijuana?

When a person injects a drug could you take this
drug out the same way you put it in?

How many aspirin can you take to get high?

Which drugs have no medical uses?

Can a boy or girl my age take a drug and really not
know about it?

Is it possible that drugs can also be used as medicine?

Can an overdose of aspirin affect you?

How can coffee or tea act as drugs?

What is the difference between ups and downs?

MARIJUANA

Can marijuana kill you?

How does inhaling marijuana through the nose affect
the body?

If I take grass once can I stop?

How is marijuana sold? How much? What prices?

If there has been no proof of the harm of marijuana,
why is the penalty so harsh?

What would happen if you were caught in possession
of marijuana?

Is marijuana intoxicating?

Do you think that eventually marijuana will be or
should be legalized like alcohol?

If grass is growing in your backyard and you do not
know it can you be put in jail?

Can you have a bad trip on marijuana?

Why do people call marijuana mary jane, pot, grass,
etc.? What is the sticky substance on the marijuana plant?

Is the withdrawal process of marijuana severe?

Has it been proved that marijuana is habit forming,
and does it lead to harder drugs?

If you know where marijuana grows, should you tell
the cops?

Would a person get more effect from ground hash or
unground hash?

Which is worse, smoking grass or chewing it?

LSD

Can LSD cause chromosome damage?

How long do you have to stay on LSD before you
are addicted to it?

What would happen to someone if he got caught for
pushing LSD?

What part of the body does LSD affect?

What causes a bad trip?

If your brother is on LSD and you are locked in the
room with him, what can you do?

What is acid? What can it do to a person who takes it?

Is it true that an LSD trip can recur as much as a
year after taking LSD?

Can people put LSD on food and take it?

How many forms does LSD come in?

How long does it take for a drug to take effect and
how long does a trip last?

If a pregnant woman takes LSD only one time, can it
have any effects on the baby?

GLUE SNIFFING

Does sniffing glue harm your body?

Does glue sniffing cause drug abuse?

Can you be sent to prison for sniffing glue?

Is glue sniffing dangerous and does it lead to harder
drugs?

NARCOTICS

What illnesses need narcotics and drugs?

Can there be physical dependence with codeine?

If a doctor prescribed something with a narcotic in
it, could someone become addicted?

What cough syrups containing narcotics such as
codeine can be bought without a prescription?

What is the name of the dope that is taken by needle?

MORPHINE AND HEROIN

What would happen if you drank alcohol and took
heroin at the same time?

If a child were born to a heroin addict, would this child also be an addict?

How much of an overdose of heroin would it take to kill you?

How much heroin can you buy for $100?

Why do you have to inject heroin in a vein or under the skin?

Why do people take heroin?

Which is the most dangerous drug, LSD or heroin?

Can heroin kill you instantly?

What effects do heroin and morphine have on the body?

Are heroin and morphine used for medical purposes? Is this legal?

STIMULANTS

Do diet pills really work or is it in your mind?

Is cocaine a very deadly drug?

If you take an overdose of stimulants will it affect you later in life?

What are pep pills? Why are pep pills habit forming?

I know someone who takes an aspirin every night before going to bed. Is this good or bad?

DEPRESSANTS

Are tranquilizers dangerous if you become addicted to them?

What are yellow jackets?

What are some necessary precautions to take in the use of sleeping pills?

How many sleeping pills does it take to kill somebody?

Do you think young people should take sleeping pills?

Can you get hooked on sleeping pills? How?

AND WHAT ABOUT ALCOHOL?

What is the best treatment for alcoholism?

Is it true that the day after you drink alcohol you have a headache and a hangover?

What happens when alcohol and drugs mix?

What effects can cough syrup with alcohol in it have on your mind and your body?

I am an alcoholic. What should I do?

Can a small amount of alcohol hurt the body?

I know a person who drinks beer and liquor, and he is always complaining about seeing a devil in the middle of the road while driving. Would this be a sign that he is an alcoholic?

HOW CAN PEOPLE ON DRUGS GET HELP?

What could you do if a friend admitted to you that he or she was taking drugs?

Can drug addicts be cured?

How do you stop someone from taking drugs when you know it is dangerous? How do you get through to him?

What are the chances for an addict to be treated successfully?

Is it possible for addicts to get help without being turned in?

Drug education objectives. One of the major problems in drug education programs is the lack of clearly defined, reasonably achieved, and adequately covered drug education objectives. In the numerous curriculum guides and other resource materials we reviewed, there were many diverse approaches. Therefore, in an attempt to bring consistency and clarity to this matter, the broad perspective of objectives identified in Tables 7-3 to 7-6 have been assembled in grade level groupings. They should provide guidance and assistance to teachers and curriculum directors. These objectives have been prepared using the basic philosophical concepts previously outlined.

In addition to the cognitive, affective, and action domain classification of goals, further clarity is attempted by identification of those goals that may not be observable in the classroom or that may have delayed achievement in the action domain. Any attempt to evaluate the accomplishment of such nonobservable and delayed purposes may be difficult, if not impossible.

Drug education content. The degree of emphasis to be placed on the physiological, psychological, sociological, and spiritual aspects of drugs at the various grade levels is not known at this time. Such factors as the community, the level of sophistication of the students, and the teacher's knowledge of drugs must be given consideration. However, it is believed that at the primary grades the major emphasis should be on the physiological or pharmacological aspects, with some minimal reference to the other areas. In the middle grades there will probably be the need for an increase in the psychological and sociological phases, with some introduction of the spiritual side. At the junior and senior high school levels the focus should be on the psychological, sociological, and spiritual aspects, with limited concern for the physiological. This philosophical approach will need exploration and experimentation in the instructional program.

The content of drug education to be pre-

TABLE 7-3. Drug education objectives, grades K to 2*

Domain	Objectives for students†	Basic concepts‡
Cognitive	1. Identifies drugs commonly used	I
	2. Illustrates ways common drugs are used by individuals	I
	3. Lists beneficial effects of drugs	II
	4. Identifies substances that can be harmful or misused	III
	5. Lists responsible people who can help when medicines are needed	II, III
	6. Explains why medicines should be taken under supervision of parent as prescribed or recommended by a physician or dentist	IV
	7. States conditions under which individuals show lack of responsibility when using medicine	V
	8. Cites ways in which individual shows respect for drugs	V
Affective	9. Is aware of differences between alcohol and other drugs and of their usage by individuals	I, IV
	10. Displays interest in learning about the beneficial as well as harmful effects of drugs	II, III
	11. Desires to use drugs in useful and responsible ways	IV, V
	12. Shows interest in discovering people who can help when medicines are needed	V
Action (nonobservable or delayed)	13. Uses only substances that aid in proper growth and development	II
	14. Takes medicines and drugs only under responsible supervision	III
	15. Refuses to accept substances from strangers	III, IV, V
	16. Limits or refrains from use of drugs, except medicines prescribed and recommended, until grown-up	III, V

*Adapted from California State Department of Education: Framework for health instruction in California public schools, K-12, Sacramento, Calif., 1970, State Printing Office; and Health education: a conceptual approach to curriculum design, School health education study, St. Paul, Minn., 1967, 3M Company.
†Consideration should be given to the inclusion of such mental health aspects as emotions (fear, joy, anger, hate), self-concept, and decision making.
‡Roman numerals refer to basic concepts in Table 7-2.

sented was developed from the objectives already discussed. Tables 7-7 to 7-10 are not meant to be all-inclusive but rather illustrative in nature. Additional material may be necessary to achieve the established goals, particularly in such mental health areas as emotions, risk-taking, communication skills, problem-solving, coping, decision-making, tolerance, responsibility, and peer pressure.

Methods of teaching

The teaching techniques selected for the formal program should help achieve the established behavior goals. Although the process for modifying behavior, especially drug misuse and abuse behavior, is not known, a variety of guidelines and principles of learning exist that teachers in drug education programs will find useful.

Guidelines. Some important guidelines are as follows:

1. Know your students and the community in which they live. Try to become familiar with their values, culture, and ethnic backgrounds. Attempt to understand their feelings about life, the world, the school, and other psychological and social matters. Be familiar with community attitudes toward drug use, including that of alcohol.

Text continued on p. 176.

TABLE 7-4. Drug education objectives, grades 3 to 6*

Domain	Objectives for students†	Basic concepts‡
Cognitive	1. Identifies varieties of drugs used by individuals	I
	2. Lists reasons for drugs in society	III
	3. Explains medical uses of commonly used drugs	II
	4. Explains physiological effects of some of the commonly used drugs	I
	5. Lists reasons persons react differently to chemicals contained in drugs	I
	6. Cites examples of misuse and abuse of drugs	III, IV
	7. Identifies difficulties or possible problems from misuse and abuse of drugs	III
	8. Explains why misuse and abuse of drugs may start early in life	IV
	9. Lists ways society tries to protect individuals from abuse of drugs	IV
	10. Identifies ways to protect self against misuse and abuse of drugs	III, IV
	11. Starts to analyze information about drugs on television, in newspapers and magazines	IV, V
Affective	12. Displays interest in learning about varieties of drugs and their effects on the body	I, II, III
	13. Asks questions about problems involved with misuse or abuse of drugs	III, V
	14. Seeks further information about community efforts to help people who misuse and abuse drugs	V
	15. Discusses ways to protect self against misuse and abuse of drugs	V, VI
	16. Expresses desire to use drugs responsibly and usefully	II, VI
Action (nonobservable or delayed)	17. Uses only substances that aid in proper growth and development	II
	18. Takes medicines and drugs only under responsible supervision	III
	19. Limits or refrains from use of drugs, except medicines prescribed or recommended, until grown-up	III
	20. Refuses to use illegal drugs	III, IV
	21. Starts to develop own practices and habit patterns to protect self against abuse of drugs	III, V

*Adapted from California State Department of Education: Framework for health instruction in California public schools, K-12, Sacramento, Calif., 1970, State Printing Office; and Health education: a conceptual approach to curriculum design, School health education study, St. Paul, Minn., 1967, 3M Company.
†Include emotions, decision-making, and coping and communication skills.
‡Roman numerals refer to basic concepts in Table 7-2.

TABLE 7-5. Drug education objectives, grades 7 to 9*

Domain	Objectives for students†	Basic concepts‡
Cognitive	1. Recalls varieties of drugs used by people	I
	2. Describes how medicines can be used to benefit individual	II
	3. Lists variety of individual and social factors that influence misuse and abuse of drugs	IV
	4. Interprets role of business and advertising in sale of drugs	IV, V
	5. Identifies differing effects of variety of drugs on the body	I, IV
	6. Compares benefits of smoking, drinking, and using drugs with possible detrimental effects	II, III
	7. Identifies reasons why people do and do not use, misuse, and abuse drugs	IV
	8. Illustrates ways to cope with social and emotional pressures of life other than through use of drugs	IV, V
	9. States procedures used by community to control availability and sale and use of drugs	V
	10. Discusses need for development of a value system	VI
	11. Recalls signs and symptoms of drug misusers and abusers	
Affective	12. Is attentive to information presented on varieties of drugs used by people, their benefits, their hazards, and their differing physiological effects	I, II, III
	13. Shows interest in comparisons of benefits and detrimental effects of alcohol, tobacco, and drugs on individuals and society	II, III
	14. Gives opinions regarding role of business and advertising in sale and availability of drugs	II, III, V
	15. Asks questions about alternatives to drug use	IV, V
	16. Displays interest in developing a value system	VI
	17. Is aware and discusses long-term results from frequent and regular misuse and abuse of drugs	IV, V
Action (observable)	18. Makes judgments about drugs and drug users after reviewing all aspects of problem	IV, V, VI
	19. Seeks to discover one's own identity and purposes in life	VI
	20. Participates in a school education-information program	V
	21. Seeks help from school personnel if having a drug problem	IV, V
Action (nonobservable or delayed)	22. Refrains from regular use of drugs that may lead to dependency, disease, or disability	III, IV, V, VI
	23. Avoids use of drugs that may affect ability to think clearly and react normally	III, IV, V, VI
	24. Refuses to use illegal drugs	III, IV, V, VI

*Adapted from California State Department of Education: Framework for health instruction in California public schools, K-12, Sacramento, Calif., 1970, State Printing Office; and Health education: a conceptual approach to curriculum design, School health education study, St. Paul, Minn., 1967, 3M Company.
†Include values clarification, communications skills, development, coping skills (tension, stress, peer pressure), and risk-taking.
‡Roman numerals refer to basic concepts in Table 7-2.

TABLE 7-6. Drug education objectives, grades 10 to 12*

Domain	Objectives for students†	Basic concepts‡
Cognitive	1. Analyzes nature and content of prescription and nonprescription as well as legal and illegal drugs	I
	2. Reviews physiological effects of alcohol, tobacco, and drugs	I
	3. Compares beneficial and harmful effects of drugs on the body	II, III
	4. Interprets reasons why people use, misuse, and abuse drugs	IV
	5. Identifies various alternatives to use, misuse, and abuse of drugs	IV, V
	6. Identifies predisposing characteristics of potential drug abusers	IV, V
	7. Compares patterns of drug use and abuse in children, youth, and adults in religious, racial, and social situations	IV, V
	8. Summarizes nature and extent of legal and illegal drug use and abuse in children, youth, and adults	IV, V
	9. Lists individual and social problems that result from misuse and abuse of alcohol, tobacco, and drugs	III, IV, V
	10. Identifies society's contributions to use, misuse, and abuse of drugs	IV, V
	11. Suggests ways individual, family, and society can reduce use, misuse, and abuse of alcohol, tobacco, and drugs	III, IV, V
	12. Identifies social situation or conditions when individuals may be apt to use, misuse, or abuse drugs with suggested ways to avoid or to handle such occasions	IV, V
	13. Analyzes effects of laws on use, misuse, and abuse of legal and illegal drugs	IV, V
	14. Lists resources available in school and community where individuals or families with drug problems may obtain help	V
	15. Discusses rightness and wrongness of use, misuse, and abuse of drugs by individuals and their relations to right of individuals to make their own decisions	VI
	16. Recalls historical use of drugs by man	I
	17. Identifies procedures to help drug abusers in emergencies and crisis	I, III

*Adapted from California State Department of Education: Framework for health instruction in California public schools, K-12, Sacramento, Calif., 1970, State Printing Office; and Health education: a conceptual approach to curriculum design, School health education study, St. Paul, Minn., 1967, 3M Company.
†Include values clarification, needs fulfillment, responsibility, empathy, and coping and communication skills.
‡Roman numerals refer to basic concepts in Table 7-2.

Table 7-6. Drug education objectives, grades 10 to 12—cont'd

Domain	Objectives for students	Basic concepts
Affective	18. Asks questions about nature, content, and physiological and beneficial and harmful effects of drugs and other related matters	I, II, III
	19. Gives opinions about reasons persons use drugs	IV
	20. Talks about problems of use, misuse, and abuse of drugs	III, IV
	21. Displays interest in wanting society to resolve the drug problem	V
	22. Expresses desire to help individuals and society solve the problem of drugs	IV, V, VI
	23. Reacts to laws and law enforcement aspects of the drug problem	V
	24. Is interested in developing an individual value system	VI
	25. Is concerned with fair and just treatment of all individuals in schools and in community	VI
Action (observable and nonobservable)	26. Makes judgments about drugs and drug users after reviewing all aspects of the problem	VI
	27. Seeks to discover one's own identity and purposes in life	VI
	28. Attempts to develop an individual value system appropriate to one's potential, interests, and abilities	VI
	29. Voluntarily participates in activities and agencies or organizations attempting to rehabilitate drug abusers	V
	30. Helps organize or participate in school or community educational-information programs for students and others to aid those in need of help or with drug problems	V
	31. Shows tolerance and respect for others' views and opinions	VI
	32. Seeks help if he has a drug problem	V, VI
	33. Is able to provide guidance and help to individuals in crisis situations	V
	34. Seeks alternative behaviors to drug use and abuse	IV, V
Action (nonobservable or delayed)	35. Refuses to use illegal drugs	IV, V
	36. Refrains from use of drugs in situations that may be unsafe or hazardous to health	III, V
	37. Avoids use of drugs that may reduce ability to think clearly and act normally	III, IV
	38. Refrains from use of drugs that may lead to dependency or habit-formation	III, IV, V

TABLE 7-7. Drug education content, grades K to 2

Question-answer application of concepts and objectives	Objectives*
What are drugs? Substances, other than food, that affect body structure and function	1

In what form are the commonly used drugs taken?
   Medicines (prescription and over-the-counter):
     Pills—aspirin; injections—penicillin; liquid—cough medicine; capsule—anti-histamine; ointment—zinc oxide or menthol
   Others:
     Liquids—whiskey, beer, wine, coffee, tea, gasoline, kerosene, airplane glue; smoking—cigarettes, cigars, pipes
	1, 2, 9

What are the beneficial effects of medicines?
   Prevent infection
   Relieve pain
   Control coughs
   Ease upset stomach
	3, 10, 11

What substances can be harmful if misused?
   Cola drinks
   Coffee and tea
   Alcohol, beer, wine
   Medicines—aspirin, vitamins, diet pills, antibiotics, and antihistamines
   Glue
	4, 10, 13

Who are the responsible people who can help when medicines are needed? Parents, nurses, doctors, dentists, pharmacists	5, 6, 14

Why should medicines be taken under a parent's or responsible person's supervision?
   To ensure correct drug for illness
   To ensure proper dosage
   To ensure proper frequency of use
	6, 11, 14

What are the conditions under which a person may take a wrong medicine?
   Not reading the label
   Taking in the dark
   Accepting substances from strangers
   Using another person's medicine
   Taking more than the prescribed dose
   Taking medicine from an unlabeled bottle
	7, 11, 13, 14

How may a person show respect for drugs?
   Use only when necessary
   Take only in recommended amounts and at recommended times
   Take only under supervision
   Do not accept substances from strangers
	8, 11, 15, 16

*Numbers refer to behavioral objectives found in Table 7-4.

TABLE 7-8. Drug education content, grades 3 to 6

Question-answer application of concepts and objectives	Objectives*
What are the various types of drugs used by people?	1, 10, 13
General classifications: stimulants, depressants, hallucinogens, psychedelic tran- quilizers, and narcotics	
Legal: prescription and nonprescription (over-the-counter); alcohol, tobacco, coffee, tea, cola drinks, aspirin, vitamins, laxatives, cough depressants, diet control items, oral antiseptics	
Illegal: marijuana, heroin, LSD	
Why are drugs needed by man?	2, 3, 10, 12
To control disease	
Relieve pain and suffering	
Escape from reality	
Relaxation and relief from tension	
What are the medical uses of some of the commonly used drugs?	1, 2, 3, 12, 17, 18
Alcohol—antiseptic, diet stimulant	
Tobacco—emetic (nicotine)	
Marijuana—none	
Amphetamines—control appetite, relieve mild depression, weight control	
Barbiturates—relieve high blood pressure, epilepsy, hyperthyroidism, sleep	
Narcotics (morphine)—pain relief, euphoria	
Tranquilizers—relieve anxiety and tension	
Hallucinogens—possible treatment in mental and emotional illness and alcoholism	
What are the effects of some of the commonly used drugs on the body?	1, 4, 10, 13
Stimulants—relieve fatigue, alertness, activeness	
Depressants—relaxation, sleep, tension escape	
Sedative-hypnotics—euphoria, relaxation, anxiety reduction, sense alteration	
Hallucinogens—distortion of senses, consciousness expansion, exhilaration	
Narcotics—euphoria, escape, pain relief	
Tranquilizers—anxiety and tension reductions	
Inhalants—get "high," intoxication	
Why do people react differently to drugs?	1, 2, 5, 10, 12, 13, 19
Body size	
Rate of metabolism	
Dosage or amount taken	
Amount of time elapsed while taking drug	
Sensitivity	

*Numbers refer to behavioral objectives found in Table 7-5.

Continued.

TABLE 7-8. Drug education content, grades 3 to 6—cont'd

Question-answer application of concepts and objectives	Objectives
What are illustrative ways drugs can be misused or abused? 　Use medicines prescribed for someone else 　Take more than the recommended or prescribed amount 　Do not follow prescribed or recommended time table 　Use nonprescription drugs unwisely 　Take drugs for kicks	2, 3, 4, 6, 10, 12, 13, 19, 20
What problems may arise when drugs are misused or abused? 　May become physiologically or psychologically dependent 　May cause organic damage 　May cause death 　May develop drug-reaction sensitivity 　May lose incentive for school, work, play, appearance, friends	4, 5, 6, 7, 10, 12, 13, 19
Why does the misuse and abuse of drugs possibly start early in life? 　Curiosity 　Imitating adult use of drugs 　Using accidentally 　Peer influence 　Acting on a dare 　Experimentation 　Boredom	8, 12, 13, 19, 20
What does the community do to help protect individuals from the abuse of drugs? 　Federal, state, and local laws control sale and distribution of legal and illegal drugs 　Law enforcement agencies implement laws 　Establishes courts to penalize breakers of the laws 　Provides rehabilitation and treatment services 　Provides educational programs	4, 6, 7, 9, 11, 13, 14, 20
What can an individual do to protect himself against the abuse of drugs? 　Develop a healthy body 　Follow the suggestions outlined herein 　Learn to get along with all persons and to treat all persons equally 　Decide upon values and goals in life and seek to achieve them 　Know sources of help should you need it 　Seek alternatives through play, sports, camping, fishing, hobbies, work 　Learn to make intelligent decisions 　Critically analyze information on television, in newspapers, and in magazines	10, 11, 13, 15, 16, 19, 20, 21

TABLE 7-9. Drug education content, grades 7 to 9

Question-answer application of concepts and objectives	Objectives*
What are drugs? Substances, other than food, that affect body structure and function	1
What are the common varieties of drugs used by people? Stimulants Depressants Sedative-hypnotics Hallucinogens Inhalants Narcotics	1, 2, 12
What are ways that drugs can be beneficial to people? Prevent infection Prevent premature deaths Prevent epidemics Weight control Decrease infant and maternity mortality rates Ease pain and suffering Aid in surgery Sleep and relaxation Control of chronic diseases and disorders—heart, cancer, diabetes, epilepsy	2, 12
What are the individual and social factors that may influence the misuse of drugs? Self-medication Attempts to escape reality Discovery of new drugs Activity of criminal element Ease of transportation of drugs Advertising Ineffective law enforcement Inadequate law enforcement Widespread use of drugs Ease of obtaining and purchasing drugs Business profit motive Excess leisure time Nonrelevant school programs Discrimination and inequality in schooling, housing, jobs	3, 13
What are the effects of drugs on the body? Effects from tobacco: 　Immediate—cardiovascular stimulation; mucous membrane, minor drying effect and irritation with acute use, subsequent production of secretions with chronic use; may improve short-term human performance; blood chemistry, chronic use may cause some impairment of interchange of O_2, CO, and CO_2 　Long-range—heart disease, lung cancer, emphysema, other circulatory disorders Effects from alcohol: 　Immediate—intoxication; reaction time slowed; sense organs, disinhibition and relaxation at low dosages and dulling effect at high dosages; blood chemistry, alcohol in blood supply affects bodily functions; neuromuscular coordination may be impaired 　Long-range—alcoholism, liver malfunction, brain damage	5, 12, 16, 22, 23

*Numbers refer to behavioral objectives found in Table 7-6.

Continued.

TABLE 7-9. Drug education content, grades 7 to 9—cont'd

Question-answer application of concepts and objectives	Objectives

Effects from other stimulants, depressants, or hallucinogens:
   Immediate—stimulation or depression of nervous or circulatory system, hallucinations, distortion of senses, death caused by overdose
   Long-range—dependence, chromosomal change, mental disorder, shortening of life expectancy
 Synergistic effects (result of combination of drugs): Death, masked symptoms	

What are some of the beneficial and detrimental effects of the use and misuse of drugs?
   Benefits: relaxation, stimulation, acceptance by peer group, social value, sign of adulthood, satisfies curiosity, possible pleasure, escape from reality
   Detriments: organic effects, possibility of death, economic cost high, possible loss of inhibitions, danger of dependency, loss of friends, loved ones, and job
	6, 11, 12, 16, 22, 23, 24

What are the reasons why people do, or do not, use or misuse drugs?
   Do's: stay awake, sleep and relaxation, ease pain, feel different, escape from reality, rebellion, curiosity, pleasure, group acceptance, social need
   Don't's: fear of dependency, feel secure and emotionally mature, have success experiences, accepted as individuals without bias and prejudice, have equality of opportunities, have viable alternatives to drug use, enjoy school, have friends among teenagers and adults
	7, 15, 18, 23

What are some of the viable alternatives to the use of drugs?
   Establish realistic goals
   Seek success in school
   Remain in school
   Develop and participate in leisure time activities—hiking, camping, fishing, art, music, drama, writing, sports, travel, reading, helping others
   Make intelligent decisions
   Acquire appropriate social relationships
   Develop a value system
   Participate in activities to help change injustices, inequities, and the like
	8, 13, 15, 16, 20, 22, 24

What does the community do to protect against the abuse of drugs?
   Establishes laws and law enforcement agencies
   Provides educational programs
   Establishes public and private agencies and organizations authorized to implement laws, to control business and advertising, and other things
   Provides rehabilitation and treatment services
	4, 5, 9, 18, 21, 22, 23, 24

Why should an individual develop a value system?
   To identify his purpose in life
   To determine realistic goals in life
   To decide ways to achieve goals
   To assess his potential, abilities, and skills
   To develop independence, security, acceptance as an individual, recognition, status, and peace with the world
	10, 16, 19, 21, 22, 24

What can the teenager do to help solve the drug problem?
   Learn facts about drugs
   Use necessary drugs carefully
   Avoid unnecessary drug use
   Resist peer pressure to experiment
   Help others learn about drugs
   Develop wide interests
   Recognize early signs of personal inadequacy in dealing with problems and seek help
	6, 7, 12, 14, 16, 18, 19, 21, 22, 24

TABLE 7-10. Drug education content, grades 10 to 12

Question-answer application of concepts and objectives	Objectives*
What is the nature and content of drugs? (See Chapter 4)	1

Legal
  a. Prescription:
    Stimulants—amphetamines (Benzedrine, Methedrine)
    Sedative-hypnotics—barbiturates (Nembutal, Seconal)
    Narcotic—morphine
  b. Nonprescription (over-the-counter): sleeping aids, cough depressants, nasal decongestants, alcohol
Illegal
  a. Stimulants—cocaine (also prescribed as local anesthetic for mucous membranes)
  b. Sedative-hypnotic—marijuana
  c. Narcotic—heroin
  d. Psychedelics—LSD

What are the physiological effects of drugs on the body? (Refer to Table 7-9)	2, 3, 17
What are the beneficial and harmful effects of drugs on the body? (Refer to Table 7-9)	13, 19, 25, 34, 35, 36
What are the reasons why people use and abuse drugs? (Refer to Table 7-9)	4, 6, 11, 18, 26, 34
What are the alternatives to the use and abuse of drugs? (Refer to Table 7-9)	5, 25, 31, 34

What are the characteristics of potential drug misusers and abusers?   4, 6, 19, 22
  Little tolerance for frustration
  Difficulty in coping with stress
  Tensions and conflict in family situation
  Alienation with community and family
  High levels of energy and poor impulse control

What are the patterns of drug use and abuse found in society?   7, 17
  Types: nonusers, experimenters, periodic, compulsive, and relapse users; also social, ritualistic-religious, and instrumental—for valid medical reasons

What is the nature and extent of drug use and abuse?   8
  Children and youth:
    Alcohol, 60% to 90%
    Tobacco, 40% to 60%
    Marijuana, 6% to 40%
    Amphetamines, 5% to 15%
    Barbiturates, 2% to 15%
    Solvents, 2% to 12%
    Heroin, 1% to 3%
  Adults:
    7 million experimenters, 5 million moderate, and 3 million chronic users of illegal drugs
  Prescription and nonprescription drugs—used daily but most individuals in some form; 202 million prescriptions in 1970 for stimulants, sedatives, tranquilizers, and antidepressants; billions of dollars spent yearly on alcohol, tobacco, cough syrups, laxatives

---

*Numbers refer to behavioral objectives found in Table 7-7.

Continued.

TABLE 7-10. Drug education content, grades 10 to 12—cont'd

Question-answer application of concepts and objectives	Objectives

What are the individual and social problems that result from the misuse of drugs?
   Crime
   Accidents
   Prostitution
   Suicides
   Deaths from overdose
   Dependency necessitating rehabilitation and treatment services
   Work absenteeism
   Cost of rehabilitation and treatment services
   Personal and family relations problems
   Loss of job
	9

What are the hazards from the use of drugs in driving an automobile and in sports? Accidents, poor performance, organic damage	3, 11, 34, 35
What are the social factors that contribute to drug misuse? Stress brought on by personal and adult pressures, technological change, Vietnam war, discrimination, inequality and lack of consideration for humaneness, need for success in school and elsewhere, emphasis on materialism, dichotomy of principles and practice regarding morals, and others (Also refer to Table 7-9)	10

What can be done to reduce the misuse of drugs?
   Individuals:
     Learn about drugs
     Make intelligent decisions about use of unnecessary drugs
     Resist peer pressures to experiment and use
     Develop a variety of interests and behaviors that foster emotional maturity
     Accept responsibilities
     Establish attainable goals
     Extend help to others
     Seek help if abusing drugs
	11, 14, 17, 19, 20, 21, 30, 31, 32, 37

What can be done to reduce the misuse of drugs?
   Community:
     Support community efforts to control drugs and rehabilitate users
     Support law enforcement
     Establish reasonable laws
     Educate public
	14, 16, 20, 22, 25

TABLE 7-10. Drug education content, grades 10 to 12—cont'd

Question-answer application of concepts and objectives	Objectives
What social situations may cause individuals to misuse drugs and how might they be handled?	12, 20, 32, 34, 35
Situations: invitation to party; social meeting with unknown people; peer group pressures; friends who encourage experimentation; excessive free time and nothing to do; few, if any, friends and family members; failure at school; loss of job opportunity; availability of drugs at school or elsewhere, etc.	
Possible actions: eat food before attending party; be selective in choice of friends; be able to refuse drugs graciously and stand firm in decisions; weigh carefully all the alternatives; try to increase circle of friends—try to be friendly; have varied interests including recreational; ask for help when unsuccessful at school; try to get along with others	
What effects do laws have on the use and misuse of drugs?	13, 20, 22, 32
Some drugs legal and easy to get	
Controls the age of purchaser of alcohol and tobacco	
Prevents the availability of illegal drugs	
Some may be too harsh on penalties and make mere possession of marijuana a felony	
Help to deter use and misuse of illegal drugs	
May cause large expenditures of funds for enforcement and prosecution of offenders	
Should all drugs be legalized?	13, 20, 22, 32
Yes:	
Reduces crime	
Reduces cost of law enforcement and prosecution	
Reduces number of teenage criminals	
Right of individual to make own decisions	
No:	
Easy availability of dependent drugs may create greater health hazards and deaths and other problems	
Business and social groups might apply greater pressures to experiment	
People should learn to solve problems without chemicals	
What community resources are available to help people with drug problems?	14, 17, 21, 28, 29, 30, 34
School counselor, nurse, physicians, psychiatrists, clergy, and others; free clinics, "drop-in" centers, short- and long-term rehabilitation and treatment modalities —hospitals, Synanon, Gateway House, Reality House	
How should one go about developing a value system?	15, 23, 24, 30, 31, 33
Determine who you are and why you are here	
Decide what you would like to do or to be	
Set reasonable, attainable goals	
Seek help from counselors, friends, teachers, clergy, parents, and others	

2. Present the positive as well as the negative side of the drug abuse problem, including the dichotomies that exist between these two extremes. Some drugs for some people, and other drugs for many people, are beneficial, pleasant, and useful.

3. Be well informed about drugs, including the broad spectrum of concepts presented herein. Try to build trust in your students through truth.

Untruths, exaggeration, sensationalism and moralizing kill the effectiveness of drug education. If 20% of the students in a classroom of 50 have used a drug, there are at least ten students carefully measuring the teacher's word against empirical knowledge. At least 30 students will know the ten users and be briefed by them. With 40 of the audience of 50 in a good position to judge the accuracy of the teacher's statements about a drug he has never tried, any discrepancies will be quickly noted and used to breach distrust of the total situation.*

4. Present a variety of alternatives to behavior for decision making. To be able to make intelligent, rational decisions, all viewpoints and all sides of the picture must be presented openly, clearly, and with the opportunity for freedom of expression.

5. Utilize the community in your educational program in a variety of ways, including the following: field trips, discussions with ex-addicts, and interviews with and presentations by experts and parents.

6. Keep the lines of communication with students open regardless of attitudes and feelings that may arise. Avoid student stereotypes because of appearance, language, or other factors. Prevent personal, critical, and moral judgments from ending discussions. Explore opportunities to increase and improve communication. Be a good listener.

7. Involve students through critical thinking, discussion, problem solving, analysis, development of responsibility, and in other ways. Opportunities for self-direction should be provided, encouraged, and supported.

Principles of learning.[12] Motivation is essential to learning and depends on the following factors:

*Guidelines for drug abuse prevention, Washington, D.C., 1970, Bureau of Narcotics and Dangerous Drugs, U.S. Department of Justice.

1. The individual's readiness to learn is related to the meaningfulness of the material presented. The drug needs and interests introduced earlier will be helpful in selecting goals and content.

2. The experiences and environment to which individuals are exposed affect learning. Many of the teaching techniques provided in this chapter as well as consideration of the environmental factors (Chapter 8) will be invaluable.

3. Guidance is necessary for the most effective learning. Although learning takes place within the student, teachers should select experiences, create the atmosphere in the classroom, and extend opportunities for individualized, self-directed learning. The amount of help needed and provided should differ with the individual student.

4. Learning is a self-active process. Students must talk, interact, do, and be actively involved in numerous aspects of the drug problem. This may necessitate going outside the classroom and even outside the school for the greatest learning to occur.

5. Much learning is soon forgotten and only a fraction is ultimately remembered. Thus the stress on attitudes, practices, behavior, and on the conceptual approach to drug education becomes imperative. The generalizations, conclusions, and attitudes about drugs will be more likely to remain than will the informational details.

6. The ability to solve problems, to reason, and to think reflectively involves training and must be learned. All the factors previously mentioned are related to this one. If helping students with drug problems is to be effective, the experiences must be meaningful, must be relevant, must involve students, and must provide the direction and guidance of teachers and other school personnel.

Teaching techniques. The teaching techniques supplied here are practical applications of the guidelines and principles of learning already introduced. These techniques have been grouped into four categories for easy reference: alcohol, drugs, tobacco, and psychic-social-spiritual.

Text continued on p. 202.

ALCOHOL

	GRADES*
Advertisements	
Students bring ads to class for analysis.	J,S
Bulletin board	
Students illustrate some commercial or medical uses of alcohol.	I,J
Students post a variety of ads with analysis statement.	I,J
Buzz group	
Why do people drink alcoholic beverages?	J,S
Why do young people experiment with alcoholic beverages?	J
Chart	
Students construct a chart illustrating level of alcohol in blood, number of drinks consumed, and effect on the body.	S
Debate	
Drinking alcoholic beverages is a hazardous practice.	J,S
To drink or not to drink.	
Decision making—coping	
You are at a friend's house whose parents have gone out for the evening. You are watching TV and have already consumed a can of beer each. You are about to open a second when your friend's parents unexpectedly walk in and see you. How would you feel? What would you do?	J,S
Betsy's father is said to be an alcoholic. One of her classmates says, "I heard your father is an alcoholic. Is it true?" How should Betsy deal with this? Should such a question be asked? Why? How can Betsy be helped?	J,S
Demonstration	
Place a small (3-inch) goldfish in a solution of ½ ounce of alcohol in ¾ pint of water (the amount in a 12-ounce bottle of beer). In almost 20 minutes the fish will be "under the influence" (floating to the surface). When the effect of the alcohol can be seen, remove the fish and place him in fresh water to revive him.	I
Discussion	
Effects on the body.	I,J,S
Explain: "Action of alcohol starts at the highest brain centers and works progressively to the lowest brain centers as the blood level increases."	J,S
Medical, industrial, social, religious uses.	I,J,S
Compare nutritive values of foods and alcoholic beverages—wine, whiskey, beer.	J,S
Auto accidents and drinking alcoholic beverages.	S
Safe and unsafe alcohol.	J,S
Should I drink alcoholic beverages?	I,J,S
Why do teenagers start to drink?	J,S
Why do adults drink alcoholic beverages?	I,J,S
Why do some teenagers not drink?	J,S

*Letters refer to suggested grade level for which the activity is appropriate. P = primary, I = intermediate, J = junior high school, and S = senior high school.

Continued.

ALCOHOL—cont'd

	GRADES
At what age should one be permitted to drink?	J,S
Effect of advertising media on teenage drinking.	S
Why do hangovers occur?	S
Differing attitudes toward drinking in your community.	J,S
Nature, types, and methods of production of alcoholic beverages.	I,J,S
Oxidizing rate of alcohol in the body.	J,S
Personality characteristics of alcoholics.	J,S
Predisposing factors to alcoholism.	J,S
Laws relating to alcohol use.	J,S
Extent of and attitudes toward alcoholism in society.	S
Differing effects of alcohol on individuals.	I,J,S
The economics of alcohol and industry.	S
Rehabilitation and treatment services in the community.	S
Effects of problem drinking on families.	J,S
Ways to alleviate drinking problems in the home.	J,S
Types of drinkers: social, occasional, problem.	J,S

Exhibit

Display beer, whiskey, and wine glasses with caption: "Each contains same   J,S
amount of alcohol?" Why are they different sizes?

Field trip

Visit Alcoholics Anonymous or an alcoholic treatment center or clinic.   J,S

Interview

Policeman regarding auto accidents and alcohol. Physician or psychiatrist   J,S
regarding methods of treatment of alcoholics. Counselor regarding
problems relating to alcoholics and the family, alcoholism in industry,
etc.

Newspaper

Prepare a special edition of the high school newspaper that contains nu-   S
merous articles prepared by students about alcohol abuse and misuse
with helpful hints for coping with its use.

Opinionnaire

Prepare an opinionnaire and use as a motivating device to discuss drinking,   J,S
drunkenness, and alcoholism as follows:

	AGREE	DISAGREE	DON'T KNOW
A user of alcohol is one who:			
1. Takes one drink before dinner always.	_____	_____	_____
2. Takes one drink after dinner always.	_____	_____	_____
3. Takes one or two drinks periodically.	_____	_____	_____
4. Takes alcohol at a religious ceremony.	_____	_____	_____
A misuser of alcohol is one who:			
1. Gets drunk occasionally.	_____	_____	_____
2. Always gets drunk at socials where alcohol is served.	_____	_____	_____

ALCOHOL—cont'd

3. Takes a drink before or after dinner. _____ _____ _____
4. Gets drunk after 2 to 3 drinks. _____ _____ _____
5. Takes alcohol at a religious cere- _____ _____ _____
   mony.

An abuser of alcohol is one who:

1. Is addicted. _____ _____ _____
2. Gets drunk only on weekends. _____ _____ _____
3. Gets drunk after 2 to 3 drinks. _____ _____ _____

Pretest

Prepare pretest about alcohol and its effect on body systems. (Chapter 11)   J,S

Problem solving

You know three people: one drinks excessively, one drinks moderately,   J,S
one abstains. Compare their personal traits, ambitions, appearance,
popularity, and other appropriate characteristics.

Problem solving

What suggestions would you have for a student who has one or more par-   J,S
ents with a drinking problem?

Have students complete the following, attempting to establish guidelines   S
for the use of alcoholic beverages by their sons and daughters. After
completion divide students into small groups to read each other's papers
and report results to class. Teacher conducts discussion.

DRINKING SITUATIONS	YES/NO	WHEN	AMOUNT	TYPE	WHY
Drink at home	_____	_____	_____	_____	_____
Drink outside home	_____	_____	_____	_____	_____
Drive when drinking	_____	_____	_____	_____	_____
Serve liquor to friends	_____	_____	_____	_____	_____

Question box

Have designated place in class where students may place questions.   I,J,S

Reports

Cultural and religious uses of alcohol throughout history.   J,S
Effectiveness of Alateen and Alanon programs.   J,S
Relation of alcohol to nutritional problems.   J,S
Golin's "Robber of Five Million Brains" in *Journal of American Medical As-*   S
sociation (**167:**1496, 1958).
State alcohol use and control laws.   J,S
Tests to determine intoxication: alcoholometer, Breath Alyzer, drunkom-   S
eter, blood tests, etc.
Alcoholism and home and family relations.   S
Differentiation between drinking, drunkenness, and alcoholism.   S
Role of Alcoholics Anonymous in the rehabilitation of alcoholics.   S
Effects of alcohol on the body.   I,J,S
Government and private agencies involved in problem of alcoholism.   J,S
Extent of alcohol use in the United States.   S

Continued.

	GRADES
Research	
Ingredients, manufacturing techniques, and alcoholic content of beer, wine, whiskey, vodka, gin, and rum.	J,S
The economic factors of alcohol in society.	S,
Why some people drink alcoholic beverages and others do not.	J,S
Uses of alcohol in food, medicine, beverages, cosmetics, and other products.	J,S
Various state legal standards defining intoxication as a percentage of alcohol in blood.	J,S
Alcohol and its effects on the brain.	J,S
Comparison of effects of alcohol with those of other drugs.	J,S
Resource person	
Invite a member of Alcoholics Anonymous to speak to the class.	S
Invite a social worker or family guidance counselor to discuss alcoholism and home and family problems.	S
Policeman to demonstrate alcohol intoxication tests used.	J,S
Pharmacologist to discuss effects on body.	J,S
Role play	
Saying "No" when offered an alcoholic beverage.	J,S
Pressures to consume alcoholic beverages by peer group in social situation.	J,S
Survey	
Students identify types and amounts of alcoholic bevarages consumed by classmates.	S
Student attitudes about use of alcoholic beverages.	S
Tape recording	
"Man-in-the-street" interview as to attitudes toward use of alcohol.	J,S
Interview ex-alcoholic about his attitude and reaction to use of alcoholic beverages.	J,S
Interview physician, pharmacologist, guidance counselor, and others about any aspect of alcohol and alcoholism.	J,S
Collect TV and radio commercials for class analysis.	J,S
Values clarification	
What is your opinion of the following? Why? What would you do?	J,S

1. A person buys a beer in a grocery store to give to her friend who is under age.
2. Person who comes to school stone drunk.
3. A student who reports to a counselor of his involvement in alcohol and counselor reports to his parents.
4. Father who drinks a couple of beers each evening to be sociable and yells when he hears his 15-year-old son has been drinking at a party.
5. A star athlete who drinks alcoholic beverages frequently and to excess at times.
6. A wino who asks you for money.
7. Your father and mother who become the life of the party when drunk.
8. A drunken driver who kills your best friend.
9. A classmate drinking beer on school grounds.
10. A parent who permits teenagers to drink alcoholic beverages at home.

DRUGS

Action group

    GRADES*

Students participate in community and school action groups designed to resolve drug problem.   S

Advertisements

Students study radio and TV ads on drugs and prepare reports on product name and type, program seen with, time of day, length of commercial, appeal used, and group appeal directed toward.   S

Collect ads for discussion, analysis, evaluation, preparation of scrapbook and displays, and reports.   I,J,S

Collect ads from different magazines and newspapers over a period of months. Categorize by magazine, type of drug, frequency of appearance, space allocation, and analysis of information provided.   S

Brainstorming

Ways students can contribute to drug control in the school and community.   J,S
Values held by students and significance in own lives.   J,S

Bulletin board

Students post current newspaper and magazine articles as well as appropriate pictures and ads. Might be titled "The Chemical Cop-Out" or "The Choice is Yours." May be organized around specific drugs, music, law enforcement, research, and the like. Use to stimulate class discussion.   I,J,S

Students prepare reports (also useful for school newspaper) titled "To Smoke or Not to Smoke"; "Pot's a Put-On"; "Are We a Drug-Taking Society?"; "Watch Out for Con Men"; "To Drink or Not to Drink"; "How to Say No"; etc.   J,S

Buzz group

Discuss these questions on how to make your own decisions about drug use: I
  1. Me, drugs, and my future.   J,S
  2. Should marijuana be legalized?   J,S
  3. Is marijuana no worse than alcohol or tobacco?   J,S
  4. Do marijuana and LSD always make you happy and like other people?   J,S
  5. Is there a drug problem at school? In the community?   J,S
  6. Is there influence from the university students on the drug problems at high school?   S
  7. What factors contribute to drug abuse?   J,S
  8. What should you do if you learn your classmates are using illegal drugs?   J,S
  9. What needs to be done to resolve the drug problem at school? In the community?   J,S

Cartoons

Have talented students prepare cartoons on various aspects of drug use in society: medical use, religious use, abuse, etc.   I,J,S

*Letters refer to suggested grade level for which the activity is appropriate. P = primary, I = intermediate, J = junior high school, and S = senior high school.

Continued.

DRUGS—cont'd

GRADES

Chart

A committee of students could be assigned to research a variety of drugs   I,J,S
and cooperatively prepare a chart for classroom or school display that
contains broad classifications and specific drug names, form, dosage,
source, legal or illegal, effects on body, and others. Younger students
may wish to limit this this to common household medicines.

Debate

Questions for debate include:

1. Is the antiestablishment feeling of some young people a factor in the   S
teen-age drug abuse problem?
2. Should narcotic or drug addicts be treated as criminals or as sick   S
people?
3. Should marijuana be legalized?   J,S
4. To smoke or not to smoke.   J,S
5. To drink or not to drink.   J,S
6. To use or not to use drugs.   J,S
7. Should the British system of legally providing narcotics to addicts be   S
adopted in the United States?
8. Does the U.S. government have the right and the duty to control the   J,S
availability and use of drugs?
9. Have "rock music" and "rock music festivals" contributed to the   J,S
greater use of drugs by young people?

Demonstration

Burn some Lipton tea leaves. Odor similar to the burning of marijuana.   J,S
Administer tranquilizers or barbiturates and amphetamine drugs to Daph-   J,S
nia (minute freshwater crustaceans) to observe effects.
Pharmacologist at local medical center may be willing to illustrate effects   J,S
of certain drugs on small animals.

Discussion

Read warning labels on containers and discuss meaning of the skull and   P,I
crossbones sign.
The family medicine cabinet.   P,I
Medicines: Why take them? How do they help? How much do you take?   P,I
Who decides when and what to take? Why? Why is prescription needed
for some and not others?
What are drugs? Medicines? Why are they available?   P,I
What to do if you feel sick or dizzy after taking a drug or medicine with or   P
without supervision.
What to do if no responsible person is available and an emergency exists.   P,I
Difference between tattling and responsible reporting if stranger offers   P,I
candy; if older child dares someone to use a drug; if you think some-
one is abusing drugs.
Ways to help someone in need.   P,I
Who do you discuss a serious problem with? (See *That's What Friends Are*   P,I
For by Sylvia Van Chief and Florence Heidi.)
What made you feel sad or glad at times? (See *The Sorely Trying Day* by   P,I
Russel and Lillian Hoben.)

DRUGS—cont'd

	GRADES
Keeping confidences. (See *A Friend Is Someone Who Likes You* by Joan Anglund.)	P
Meaning of use, misuse, abuse, addiction, physical and psychological dependence, habituation, and tolerance.	I,J
Categories and types of drugs, including coffee, tea, and cola drinks.	I,J,S
Effect of drugs on the body, including habit-forming aspect.	P,I,J
Why do people take drugs? What are the alternatives?	P,I,J,S
Differences between over-the-counter and prescription drugs.	I,J,S
Drugs and allergies, infections, and malnutrition.	I,J,S
First aid procedures for poisoning or for overdose of drugs.	I,J,S
Peer pressure and drug use; "taking a dare."	I,J,S
Laws and penalties regarding illegal drugs.	I,J,S
Impact of advertising on sale and use of drugs.	I,J
Dangers of self-medication.	J,S
Ways to relieve worry, tension, and frustration.	I,J,S
The drug-oriented society and patterns of drug use.	J,S
Ways to solve a problem with drugs; ways to solve any problem.	J,S
Drugs and autos, athletes, studying, housewives.	J,S
Psychological and sociological effects of drugs.	J,S
All drugs may be dangerous to ingest.	P,I,J,S
Why do some people not use drugs?	I,J,S
Hazards of potentiation with, for example, alcohol and barbiturates.	J,S
Economics of drugs.	J,S
Government control of use and sale of drugs. Relate to freedom and independence.	J,S
Attitudes of people toward addicts, drug abusers, hippies, etc.	J,S
Community resources available for drug abusers.	J,S
Marijuana is the new social drug.	S
Influence of propaganda and motivational research control on individual's decisions.	S
Personalities of drug abusers.	J,S
Methods of rehabilitation and treatment of drug abusers.	S
History of drugs.	J,S
Drugs and social problems: war, crime, poverty, racism, inequalities, etc.	S
Potential drug abusers: risk personalities, risk behaviors, risk environments.	J,S
Legalization of marijuana.	J,S
Physical and psychological needs of people.	J,S
Improving interpersonal relations.	I,J,S
Student alienation and unrest.	S
Values and their meaning in life.	I,J,S
Is it right or wrong to use, misuse, and abuse drugs?	J,S
Role of the school, home, church, community, and individual in drug problem.	J,S
Dramatization	
Characters illustrate sadness, depression, happiness, joy, fear, anger, and other emotions. Students discuss ways to help.	P
Making an emergency telephone call.	P
Ways to ask for help when in need.	P

Continued.

DRUGS—cont'd

GRADES

Student urged to take a dare. Discuss consequence. Have students prepare several different endings and discuss.

P

Teacher reads story to pupils, then they act out the parts. Choose different children to play each episode. Pantomime may be used without props. Such simple objects as a toy telephone, bottle, or spoon may be used.

P

Story:

Dennis has a little sister named Prue. One day Prue got sick. Mother took her temperature. Then Mother went to phone the doctor.

The Doctor came to see Prue. He said Prue must have some medicine. He wrote out a prescription.

Dennis went with his father to the drug store to have the prescription filled. His father gave the prescription to the pharmacist. The pharmacist read the prescription. Then he mixed the medicine in a dish and poured it into a bottle.

"This medicine is meant for Prue," the druggist said. "It is not good for anyone else. It might even make another child sick." "I will not touch it," Dennis promised. "You must never touch any medicine, even if it was mixed especially for you, unless Mother or Father are with you," the druggist said. Then the druggist put a label on the bottle to tell just how much medicine Prue should take and when she should take it.

When Dennis and his father reached home, Mother looked at the bottle of medicine very carefully before she opened it. "I must be careful to give Prue just the amount it says on the label," Mother said. "Will you get me a clean teaspoon, Dennis?"

Dennis gave his mother a clean teaspoon. She measured the medicine and gave it to Prue. Prue made a face but she swallowed it because she knew it would maker her well.

Mother looked at the clock. "The label says I should give Prue some more medicine in 1 hour. It is 2 o'clock now." She held up two fingers. "When will it be time to give Prue her medicine again?" Dennis held up three fingers. "At 3 o'clock," he said. "I will watch the clock and tell you. May I put the medicine away?" "No," said Mother. "It is good of you to offer but children should *never* touch medicine. I will put it in the medicine cabinet where it belongs and lock it up until we need it again." And she did.

At 3 o'clock Dennis called Mother and she took the medicine out of the cabinet and gave Prue another spoonful. Just then the telephone rang. Mother heard the phone but did not pay any attention to it. Instead, she put the medicine in the cabinet and locked it up before answering. "It is most important to put the medicine away before answering the phone," she said. "Dennis, would you answer the phone for me?" Dennis answered the phone, saying, "Mother will come in a minute; she is putting the medicine away."

As soon as Prue was well, Mother took her medicine and poured what was left of it into the toilet. Then she flushed the bowl, washed the bottle carefully, and put it in the trash can. "Why did you do that?" asked Dennis. "There was some left. I could have used it if I got sick." "Oh, no," said Mother. "You will have your own medicine if you are sick. It is not safe for one person to take another person's medicine." Then she hugged Dennis. "But we hope you will never be sick," she said. Dennis hoped so, too.

DRUGS—cont'd

	GRADES
Drawings	
Students make drawings and pictures of beneficial effects of medicine and substances that can be harmful if misused.	P
Students prepare illustrations of how specific mood-modifying substances affect people physically, socially, and psychologically.	I
Exhibit	
Display labels and containers of over-the-counter drugs and others for student examination and discussion.	P,I
Display a variety of pamphlets, books, and other items in class, in the library, or elsewhere for review.	J,S
Students participate in a classroom or school "Drug Fair." A variety of displays are prepared: bulletin boards, charts, posters, pamphlets, books, films, filmstrips, reports, oral presentations, a question corner. Parents, the community, and teachers may be invited.	I,J
Field trip	
Visit local jail to discuss drug law violations with officials and see interior.	I,J,S
Attend court in session on illegal drug case.	J,S
Tour community rehabilitation and treatment agencies such as Teen Challenge, Synanon, Damien House.	J,S
Visit the street drug scene to meet and talk with drug users and abusers.	J,S
Interview	
Pharmacist to discuss common nonprescription drugs.	I
Addicts and ex-addicts about their involvement, attitudes, feelings.	J,S
Physician or pharmacologist about the use and effects of drugs.	I,J,S
Police to discover what happens when a drug abuser is arrested, especially a minor.	J,S
Friends and neighbors about attitudes toward drug use and abuse.	J,S
Judge regarding his views on the drug problem.	J,S
Magazine and newspaper articles	
Collect articles for scrapbook, current information reports and summaries, class presentations, motivation.	I,J,S
Map	
Prepare world map indicating the sources, distribution, processing, and marketing of legal and illegal drugs.	J,S
Mural	
Students make a mural depicting all the people responsible for controlling drugs and tracing the route of a drug from producer to consumer.	P,I
Music	
Expose students to various types of music depicting people's moods—rock music, ballads, classical, and country—and relate the music to drug scene. When words to songs are available, lyrics could be analyzed.	I,J,S

Continued.

DRUGS—cont'd

Opinionnaire

Place a check in the appropriate space on the right.

GRADES: J,S

	AGREE	DISAGREE	DON'T KNOW
A drug user is one who uses drugs:			
1. Once and stops.	____	____	____
2. Ten times and stops.	____	____	____
3. More than ten times and stops.	____	____	____
4. Once a week but not every week.	____	____	____
5. Occasionally and can stop when so desires.	____	____	____
A drug misuser is one who uses a drug:			
1. Once every week and stops after several weeks.	____	____	____
2. Ten times and stops.	____	____	____
3. Daily for several months and stops.	____	____	____
4. Takes overdose, almost dies, and stops.	____	____	____
A drug abuser is one who uses a drug:			
1. Once every week.	____	____	____
2. Once every day.	____	____	____
3. Several times most days.	____	____	____
4. All the time and must steal to sustain the habit.	____	____	____
5. Because he is addicted.	____	____	____
6. And can buy whatever drugs needed.	____	____	____

Panel discussion

Topics for consideration include:

	GRADES
1. Are we a drug-oriented society?	J,S
2. What can a teenager do to help solve the drug problem in school? In the community?	J,S
3. What drug laws need changing?	J,S
4. How can young people achieve emotional maturity?	J,S
5. What are the alternatives to drug use and abuse?	J,S
6. How can a drug abuser get help in school? In the community?	J,S

Parent involvement

Invite parents to a presentation on drugs given by a physician, pharmacologist, or other qualified person.	I,J,S
Conduct a program with a variety of speakers covering a broad spectrum of drug topics.	I,J,S
Arrange for sessions of student-parent discussions about drugs. Have specialists on hand to assist.	J,S
Students prepare programs for parents followed by question and answer period.	I,J,S

Peer group

Students prepare program on drugs for presentation to other classes.	I,J
Students conduct survey among students, "What can we do about the school drug problem?"	J,S

DRUGS—cont'd

	GRADES

Establish a volunteer speakers bureau comprising teams of two to four speakers to visit fifth, sixth, seventh, or eighth grade classes in nearby schools to discuss drugs.   J,S

Posters

Students prepare posters to be used in school anti-drug abuse program.   J,S

Pretest

Prepare pretest (also use as posttest) to discover student knowledge, attitudes, and practices regarding drugs. (See Chapter 11 for illustrative questions.)   I,J,S

Problem solving

Students respond to these statements by checking on the right: J,S

	AGREE	DISAGREE	DON'T KNOW
1. It is my life and I can do with it as I please.	_____	_____	_____
2. My responsibility is to myself and no one else.	_____	_____	_____
3. If you experiment with drugs, that is your problem, not mine.	_____	_____	_____
4. If you have a pain or a problem just pop in a pill; it is the shortest trip to joy.	_____	_____	_____

Pupils respond orally to these questions: P
1. Who can help you if you misuse a medicine?
2. What should you do?
3. Whom should you tell?
4. Whom should you call?
5. If you found a box of pills or an open bottle of medicine at home what would you do? Why?
6. If a friend offered you something to eat or drink and you were not sure what it was, what would you do? Why?

If you discovered that your brother, sister, or friend was experimenting with drugs, what would you do?   J,S

What are the consequences of being discovered at a party where illegal drugs are being used or in a car where they are found? What effect might this discovery have on your life? What could you do to prevent this occurrence?   J,S

Project

Organize students into teams to prepare a special edition of the school newspaper about drugs. Students should work on topics or sections of their choice. Some talented young people may do the art work; others may be organizers; most should have research and writing responsibilities.   J,S

Continued.

DRUGS—cont'd

	GRADES
Publicity campaign	
Conduct a school-wide, student-run drug use information campaign using the school newspaper, student-made signs, materials, displays, assemblies, films, and outside speakers or resource persons.	J,S
Puppets	
Students use prepared puppets or make them out of paper bags and other materials to depict dramatically a variety of situations for discussion, such as something I could not have, loss of a pet dog, dislike of a neighbor.	P
Questions	
Students bring to class written questions about drugs that they have prepared or others have asked them to have answered. Time is set aside for a question and answer session.	I,J,S
A question box for anonymous questions or concerns is provided.	J,S
Students raise questions about drugs and list them on the chalkboard. Assignments are made individually or by group to research the answers and make reports to class.	J,S
Reports—oral or written	
The nature of community resources available and the services they provide.	J,S
The effects of drugs on the body.	I,J,S
Students select drugs to research and prepare material on medical use, effects, dosage, form sold, hazards, and other information.	J,S
Health problems related to drug abuse—malnutrition, VD, infectious diseases, etc.	J,S
Legal responsibility of the school in regard to drugs.	J,S
Drug laws pertaining to minors.	J,S
Having the courage of my convictions.	J,S
The importance of maintaining freedom of choice.	J,S
How students can help in the school drug program.	J,S
Legal, financial, physiological, psychological, and familial problems of the narcotic addict.	J,S
Driving and drugs.	S
Cost and problems of maintaining a heroin habit.	S
Where would I like to be 10 years from now and what would I be doing?	J,S
Addicted mothers and their unborn children.	J,S
The American vs. the British system of dealing with narcotic addicts.	J,S
Comparison of various types of drug withdrawal symptoms.	J,S
Several case histories of drug abusers.	S
Describe a friend with a well-balanced personality and give reasons why so well-adjusted.	S
My philosophy of life.	S
How to say "No" to drugs.	J,S
The school drug problem.	J,S
Precautions to follow when using drugs.	J,S
Physical, psychological, and social aspects of drugs.	J,S
Why students use drugs.	J,S
How can parents help students with drug problems? Or how could they have helped to prevent the problem?	J,S
How I feel about using drugs.	J,S
Alternatives to drug use.	I,J,S

DRUGS—cont'd

	GRADES
Peer pressure and drug abuse.	J,S
Prescription and nonprescription drugs.	J,S
The law and drugs.	S
My school and its likes and dislikes.	S
My friends and their likes and dislikes.	S
My family and its effect on my life.	S
What are my values in life? What attitudes have the greatest meaning and influence on my life?	S
Is there rightness and wrongness in this world?	S
Who am I? Why am I here? Where am I going?	S
The story of drug abusers such as Judy Garland, Janis Joplin, Jimi Hendrix, Bill Stern.	S
What makes me sad, happy, angry?	I,J

Research

	GRADES
Role of the World Health Organization in drug control.	J,S
Federal and state drug laws.	J,S
Historical development of drugs.	J,S
Current information about various drugs.	J,S
Illegal heroin and marijuana traffic and efforts to control it.	J,S
Cultural and religious use of drugs.	J,S
Properties of marijuana, including strength, varying strength, effects on body, and other current information.	J,S
Functions and responsibilities of government agencies involved in the standardization, purity, and safety of drugs.	J,S
Route of legal drugs to illegal markets.	S
International control of illegal drugs.	S
Current status of methadone in treatment of addicts.	J,S
Addiction in pregnant women and resultant fetal problems.	S
Services rendered by community rehabilitation and treatment centers for youth and how adequate they are.	S
Tests to determine whether a person is under the influence of drugs (nalline, urinalysis, chromatography).	S
Personality characteristics of drug abusers.	S
Treatment modalities for addicts.	S

Resource and information center

	GRADES
Students conduct programs for peers, parents, and others, with pamphlets, information, speakers, and rapping. May also have hot-line if school funds available.	J,S
Students obtain books, pamphlets, and other materials for use in classroom	I,J,S

Resource person

	GRADES
A variety of community and school personnel may be invited to meet with students and discuss numerous topics. Some of these individuals are pharmacists, pharmacologists, physicians, psychologists, psychiatrists, policemen, attorneys, district attorneys, judges, probation officers, narcotic squad officers, treatment center representatives, counselors, drug abusers, and ex-addicts.	I,J,S

Continued.

DRUGS—cont'd

Role play   GRADES

These situations can be dramatized:
1. A parent giving medicine to a sick child.   P
2. Mother takes sick child to doctor who prescribes medicine later ob-   P
   tained at drug store. Mother takes child home and gives exact
   amount.
3. Adolescent who feels his problems can only be resolved by escaping   I,J
   through drugs.
4. Refusal to accept the offer of a marijuana cigarette.   I,J
5. Different moods or emotions of people with discussion of meaning   P,I
   and action to take—anger, happiness, anxiety, fear, etc.
6. A friend offers his friend a pill that he has been taking in an attempt   P,I
   to help the second person who is complaining of a minor ailment.
   The friend refuses the pill and indicates the possible problems in
   accepting medicine from unauthorized individuals.
7. Teenager is caught with illegal drugs in his possession.   J,S
8. Student admits to parents he is using drugs.   J,S
9. Clergyman speaks to teenage drug abuser about youth's involvement   J,S
   in drugs.
10. A girl is at a party and a "joint" is passed around.   J,S
11. A man is employed and has a good position but is dependent on   S
    heroin. His employer discovers the problem.

School newspaper

Provide column in each publication for questions to be answered by stu-   J,S
dent researchers.
Periodic articles on drugs written by students should be included.   J,S
An entire edition might be devoted to a variety of articles on drugs as part   J,S
of an antidrug campaign or drug education week.

School program

Organize school into a a series of committees to control and prevent the   S
spread of drug abuse. Students should be actively involved in the planning and execution of the program. A plan of action that would not be
solely educational could evolve and include parent and community participation.

Scrapbook

Students collect newspaper and magazine articles, advertisements, pic-   I
tures, and other appropriate materials and organize in a useful manner.
Could become part of school or classroom resource and information
center or be taken home for parent reference.

Self-test

Ask students to verbally identify the person responsible for: P
1. Making safe drugs.
2. Writing prescriptions.
3. Choosing drugs to be used.
4. Filling prescriptions correctly.
5. Choosing over-the-counter drugs.
6. Reading labels and following directions.

DRUGS—cont'd

7. Keeping drugs in a safe place.
8. Helping younger children.
9. Taking drugs only under supervision.

Show and tell

Students describe experiences with medicines and identify what they con-   P
sider to be ways to act responsibly.

Show pictures of medicines taken in the home such as aspirin, laxatives,   P
and cough syrups. Have students respond to these questions:
1. How should they be taken?
2. Who should give them?
3. Where should drugs be stored at home?

Cut out pictures of people representing different emotions—fear, pain,   P,I
anger, joy, hate. Place them on the bulletin board with possible caption: "These people feel," or "How do you think these people feel?"
Have children view pictures and explain why the people in the pictures
acted as they did.

Songs

Students analyze and discuss the lyrics of popular songs that refer to drugs.   J,S

Story

Teacher prepares unfinished story wherein students can supply answers to   P
appropriate questions in regard to proper use of medicines. For example, Jane's mother was given a prescription to get some medicine
_____ .

Questions:
1. Who would give her the prescription? Why?
2. Where would she take it? Why?
3. What would be on the label? Why?

Teacher may read this story or duplicate it so that students may read it.   P
Afterward, children may complete it with verbal conclusions or write an
ending.

Grandma Periwinckle has not been feeling too well lately. She went to
see her doctor. He wrote a prescription which she took to the pharmacist at the drug store. She went back to the pharmacy a few hours later
and picked up the pills. She read the label, which said, "Take two every
four hours." Also printed on the label was "CAUTION: KEEP OUT OF
REACH OF CHILDREN." Grandma Periwinckle put the pills in her purse
and went home. Just as she arrived at the door, her little grandson,
Jeffrey, came around the corner with his mother. Grandma Periwinckle
went into the bedroom where she took off her coat and put it, along
with her purse, on the bed. She then returned to the living room to talk
to Jeffrey's mother. Usually Grandma Periwinckle is very careful to
keep all her medicines and household products on high shelves because, even though she has no small children of her own, Jeffrey and
his friends visit her quite often. She always warns the children never
to put anything into their mouths without asking first. But this time she
forgot that purses containing medicines should also be put out of
children's reach. As she was talking in the living room, little Jeffrey

Continued.

GRADES

walked into the bedroom and emptied her purse. Along with her cosmetics, her change, and her handerkerchief, he found the bottle of pills.
Tell what happened then.

Survey

Conduct anonymous, open-ended survey of students regarding their experiences in the use of drugs—types, frequency, reasons.   I,J,S

Students prepare survey form to be used in class or schoolwide to determine incidence and type of drug abuse in school.   I,J,S

Teacher asks students to identify interests and concerns in drugs. Use to determine content of material to be presented to students.   I,J,S

Students identify substances in home medicine cabinets that can be classified as drugs.   I

Students survey adults for reasons why they use such drugs as alcohol, tobacco, and aspirin.   I,J

Students prepare in class a list of benefits of marijuana as revealed by drug abusers. They then research the topic and compare findings.   J,S

Prepare survey form with yes or no answers to these questions. Do you: J,S
    1. Drink coffee every morning?
    2. Take more than three aspirin a week?
    3. Participate in extracurricular activities?
    4. Participate in sports?
    5. Enjoy dancing?
    6. Use sleeping pills often?
    7. Drink milk every day?
    8. Eat hamburgers frequently?
    9. Use stay-awake pills?
   10. Use pep pills?
   11. Take diet pills?
   12. Have regular physical examinations?
   13. Drink alcoholic beverages?
   14. Use cold remedies frequently?
   15. Feel sick often?
   16. Like school?
   17. Have hobbies?

Visit local pharmacies seeking answers to these questions: J,S
    1. What drugs are in greatest demand? What are they used for?
    2. Do any of the nonprescription drugs contain dependency-producing substances?

Survey drug section of a shopping center and list the various medicines available.   J,S

Survey the community resources where individuals with drug problems are helped.   J,S

Survey the social and recreational activities available to teen-agers in the school, church, and community.   S

Tape recording

Interview a physician for answers to questions raised in class about drugs   I,J
Radio and TV ads for class discussion.   J,S

Volunteer student services

Students volunteer to spend time helping at the various rehabilitation and treatment centers in the community. Later they report their experiences to the class for discussion.   S

TOBACCO

	GRADES*
Advertisements	
Bring newspaper and magazine ads to class for analysis regarding accuracy and further research.	I,J,S
Tape radio commercials and discuss in class.	J,S
Students prepare reports analyzing ads in terms of appeal and factual aspects, misleading or deceptive.	J,S
Brainstorming	
Students raise relevant questions about tobacco and health; these are placed on blackboard. Individuals or groups conduct research and report findings in class.	I,J,S
Buzz group	
Discuss such questions as: Should you smoke? Why do people smoke? Do people learn to smoke in groups or alone? Why do some people not smoke? Are school smoking regulations necessary? Why is it difficult to stop smoking?	J,S
Cartoon and picture collecting	
Collect cartoon characters or pictures of people who are smoking from newspapers and magazines. Remove captions. Have students place their own captions under each cartoon or picture. (Student attitudes toward smoking may be revealed.)	I,J
Chart	
Students prepare chart or charts illustrating death rates, life-expectancy rates, incidence of lung cancer, heart disease, and respiratory problems of heavy smokers, moderate smokers, and nonsmokers.	J,S
Debate	
To smoke or not to smoke. Are school smoking regulations necessary? Should cigarette advertising be banned? Is cigarette advertising deceptive and misleading?	J,S
Demonstration	
Use a smoking machine (American Cancer Society) to demonstrate the residue found in cigarettes and discuss implications.	I,J,S
Take pulse rates before and after smoking a cigarette and discuss reasons for difference.	J,S
Diagram	
Diagram and describe on chalkboard the effect of tobacco smoke on respiratory system.	J,S
Discussion	
Effects of smoking on the circulatory, respiratory, and digestive systems, on athletic performance, and on other areas.	I,J,S

*Letters refer to suggested grade level for which the activity is appropriate. P = primary, I = intermediate, J = junior high school, and S = senior high school.

Continued.

TOBACCO—cont'd

	GRADES
Advantages and disadvantages of smoking.	I,J,S
Why young people begin to smoke.	I,J
Effect of smoking on others at social functions, in public places, and in other situations.	J,S
Effectiveness of cigarette filters.	J,S
Relationships between use of alcohol, tobacco, and drugs.	J,S
Difficulty in breaking smoking habit.	I,J,S
Cultural and sociological influences on the attitudes and habits of smokers.	J,S
Use of tobacco by society.	J,S
Laws relating to tobacco.	J,S
Effect of antismoking campaign.	I,J,S

Dramatization

A 10-year-old child is encouraged by his friends to smoke a cigarette.	I
Prepare skits or puppet shows satirizing smoking ads.	I

Exhibit

Models of cancerous and noncancerous lung tissue (American Cancer Society).	J,J,S
Microscopic lung tissue from smoker, nonsmoker, and exsmoker. (See pathologist at local hospital.)	I,J,S
Charts, graphs, and other statistics (American Cancer Society).	J,S
Variety of filters in cigarettes.	J,S

Field trip

Visit local health department, hospital, and voluntary health agencies to discuss smoking and health.	J,S

Forum

Students conduct discussions, debates, and programs in classrooms, assemblies, and other places; letters to the editor, pro and con column in newspaper.	J,S

Health fair

Students plan and conduct variety of activities, including health agency exhibits, student-prepared exhibits, presentations, films, filmstrips, and pamphlet distribution.	J,S

Notebook

Include a collection of ads with student analysis resulting from research.	J,J
Current newspaper and magazine articles with brief summaries.	I,J

Parents' day

Parents attend classroom or school display of student activities such as fact gathering, experiments, contacts with health agencies, survey results, conclusions, and summary of individual work.	I,J

Parodies

Develop parodies, satires, and singing commercials on cigarette ad slogans such as "Why filter springtime?" and "Don't smoke. The life you save may be your own."	J,S

TOBACCO—cont'd

	GRADES
Posters	
Effects of tobacco on the body.	I,J
For school, home, or community antismoking campaign.	J,S
Pretest	
Conduct a pretest on tobacco and health.	I,J,S
Problem solving	
Conduct research on a problem using following procedure: (1) collect data, (2) analyze data, and (3) draw conclusion.	I,J,S
Publicity campaign	
Prepare posters, buttons, and newspaper articles to discourage smoking.	I,J,S
Reports—individual or group	
Examine materials received from agency contacted and report to class.	I,J
Reasons for decision to smoke or not to smoke.	I,J,S
In-depth study of advertising based on motivational research.	J,S
Analysis of current newspaper and magazine articles.	I,J,S
Development of a safe cigarette.	J,S
Effects of tobacco on body.	I,J,S
Laws against sale to minors.	J,S
Economic cost of smoking one package of cigarettes a day for a week, a month, a year, a lifetime.	I,J,S
Resource person	
Invite nurse, physician, representative from voluntary health agency, and others to discuss smoking and health.	I,J
Invite members of local withdrawal clinic to speak.	S
Role play	
How to refuse a cigarette offered.	J,S
A home situation where teenager announces that he has started smoking.	J,S
Disciplinary action of principal against three students caught smoking at school.	J,S
A group of students discussing whether or not to smoke.	I,J
Survey	
Extent of student smoking.	J,S
Extent of parent smoking.	I,J
Why students or adults started smoking.	I,J
Attitudes of students, parents, coaches, and other people toward smoking.	I,J
People who have tried to stop smoking and the results.	J,S
Most popular brand of cigarettes sold in a few stores.	J,S

"What kind of smoker are you?"*

	ALWAYS	FREQUENTLY	OCCASIONALLY	SELDOM	NEVER
A. I smoke cigarettes in order to keep myself from slowing down.	5	4	3	2	1
B. Handling a cigarette is part of the enjoyment of smoking it.	5	4	3	2	1
C. Smoking cigarettes is pleasant and relaxing.	5	4	3	2	1
D. I light up a cigarette when I feel angry about something.	5	4	3	2	1
E. When I have run out of cigarettes I feel it almost unbearable until I can get them.	5	4	3	2	1
F. I smoke cigarettes automatically without even being aware of it.	5	4	3	2	1
G. I smoke cigarettes to stimulate me, to perk me up.	5	4	3	2	1
H. Part of the enjoyment of smoking a cigarette comes from the steps I take to light up.	5	4	3	2	1
I. I find cigarettes pleasurable.	5	4	3	2	1
J. When I feel uncomfortable or upset about something, I light up a cigarette.	5	4	3	2	1
K. I am very much aware of the fact when I am not smoking a cigarette.	5	4	3	2	1
L. I light up a cigarette without realizing I still have one burning in an ashtray.	5	4	3	2	1
M. I smoke cigarettes to give me a lift.	5	4	3	2	1
N. When I smoke a cigarette, part of the enjoyment is watching the smoke as I exhale it.	5	4	3	2	1
O. I want a cigarette most when I am comfortable and relaxed.	5	4	3	2	1
P. When I feel depressed or want to take my mind off cares and worries I smoke cigarettes.	5	4	3	2	1
Q. I get a gnawing hunger for a cigarette when I haven't smoked for a while.	5	4	3	2	1
R. I've found a cigarette in my mouth and didn't remember putting it there.	5	4	3	2	1

How to score:

Enter the numbers you have circled in the spaces below over the appropriate letters. Then total the scores on each line to get your totals. For example, the sum of your scores on lines A, G & M gives you your score on stimulation. Lines B, H and N give the score on handling, etc.

Scores can vary from 3 to 15. Any score 11 and above is High. Any score 7 and below is Low.

_____ + _____ + _____ = Stimulation
    A   G   M

_____ + _____ + _____ = Handling
    B   H   N

_____ + _____ + _____ = Pleasurable relaxation
    C   I   O

_____ + _____ + _____ = Tension reduction
    D   J   P

_____ + _____ + _____ = Psychological addiction (craving)
    E   K   Q

_____ + _____ + _____ = Habit
    F   L   R

Write

Request materials from voluntary health agencies about smoking and health.   I,J

*Reprinted with permission from The Journal of the Addiction Research Foundation of Ontario.

PSYCHIC-SOCIAL-SPIRITUAL*

GRADES†

Attitude questionnaire

Complete short answers to: I,J

1. Happiness is _____ .

2. Sadness is _____ .

3. I am fearful of _____ .

4. I am angry when _____ .
Conduct discussion when completed.

Have students complete open-ended questions such as: J,S

1. If I could go any place in the world on an all-expense paid vacation,

   I would go to _____ .

2. If I could be any person in the world, I would be _____ .

3. If I could make one change in the school program it would be _____

   _____ .

4. I believe the three most important things in life are _____ ,

   _____ , and _____ .
Have discussion of choices after completion.

Brainstorming

Students prepare list of problems they consider important and develop   I,J
plans to resolve them.

Bulletin board

Students prepare a display of pictures that expose a variety of emotions   I,J
such as anger, fear, love, and happiness. Title might be "Emotions We
Live With."

Students display pictures, advertisements, and cut-outs to help make decisions about drugs with captions and selections such as:

DRINK	DON'T DRINK	SMOKE	DON'T SMOKE	USE DRUGS	ABUSE DRUGS
☐	☐	☐	☐	☐	☐

Buzz group

Involve students in answering these questions: J,S
1. What is reality?
2. How do you make your own decisions to be a good leader and a sensible follower?
3. Does having the courage of one's convictions mean one is stubborn?
4. Does "everybody's doing it" mean everyone should do it?

Chart/posters

Illustrate in writing, pictures, or drawings ways to handle upset feelings,   I,J
anger, hate, and other emotions.

*Also refer to pp. 226-227.
†Letters refer to suggested grade level for which the activity is appropriate. P = primary, I = intermediate,
J = junior high school, and S = senior high school.

Continued.

GRADES

Checklist

Students prepare a checklist of personal or family values and discuss bases for them. — S

Communication

At the start of a new class divide the students into groups of two for a limited discussion, then place them all into larger groups of six to eight students with each individual being responsible for introducing the partner, based on impressions formed. — J,S

Construction

Have students make life-size outline of self on butcher paper. Have them color as desired, cut out with scissors, and display around the room. Students may need to help one another to make the outlines (a way to get to "know myself"). — P,I

Debate

How do value systems affect behavior patterns of individuals? Cover positive and negative aspects relating to persistence in completing a job, cheating, and premarital pregnancy. — S

Decision making-coping

Identify a problem that you have and discuss the steps you would take to try to solve it. — J,S

If you had a problem about being angry at your brother/sister, mother/father, or friend, who could you go to for help? Who should you go to when you have a problem? — P,I

Have students tell or prepare a list of the things about which decisions can be made at home, in school, at play, about food, and the like. Also, have have them prepare a second list about decisions they are unable to make. Hold a discussion. — P,I

View and discuss the Inside/Out Series,* thirty films for 8 to 10-year-olds that deal with social, emotional, and physical problems. — I

View and discuss the Self, Inc. Series,* fifteen films, for 11 to 13-year-olds to help them cope with emotional, physical, and social problems. — J

Discussion

What causes quarrels? How can they be prevented?	P,I
Ways feelings were hurt and how hurt was overcome.	P,I
Emotional needs and how they can be satisfied.	J,S
Constructive and destructive criticism.	J,S
Hate and inherent dangers.	P,I,J
Wholesome outlets for anger.	P,I,J
"He or she has no personality."	J,S
Causes of conflicts and frustrations and how to handle.	J,S
Who besides our family can help us—doctors, teachers, nurses, policemen, friends?	P,I
How can we make friends? Why are friends necessary?	P,I,J
Should you discuss problems with your parents?	P,I,J

*Agency for Instructional Television, Box A, Bloomington, Indiana 47401; or check audiovisual center of local school district.

	GRADES
How negative moods and feelings (anger, jealousy, rage, fear, worry, etc.) can produce anxiety and stress. What can be done?	P,I,J
Why is it frequently difficult to do what is right? What factors influence decision making?	I,J,S
How illness, lack of rest, and lack of food can affect feelings and cause irritability.	I,J
How anxiety affects learning and doing what we enjoy.	I,J
How talking with someone may help with problems.	P,I,J
Prepare list of what "turns kids on" and "turns kids off." Then prepare list of human needs—physical, social, etc.—and compare to determine relationships.	I,J
Prepare list of values and spend time determining if they are values or merely interests. Draw conclusions.	I,J
Meaning of "growing up."	I,J
Fears—of earthquakes, illness, war—and reasons why they develop.	I,J,S
Control of emotions.	P,I,J
Process to follow in making decisions (relate to drugs).	I,J,S
What are desirable and undesirable factors of belonging to a clique or gang?	J,S
Do parents, teachers, and other adults belong to cliques or groups?	J,S
Why do people join a clique or group? Are dress, behavior, appearance, and attitudes related to acceptance in the group?	J,S
Several races and cultures of people in society.	I,J,S
Cultural deprivation.	S

Drawings

Express feelings and emotions in drawings, paintings, clay modeling, and other self-expressive activities.	P,I

Exhibit

Prepare display of materials of different faiths, races, and countries and discuss.	I,J

Problem solving

Children prepare short, anonymous paragraphs of realistic problem situations to be read or dramatized in class with follow-up discussion in problem-solving techniques.	I,J

Reports—individual or group

When I wanted something I could not have.	I
"Me as I see myself" or "Me as I would like to be."	I,J
How brothers, sisters, or friends react to emotional situations.	I
Committee prepares list of recreational and social opportunities in school and neighborhood and discusses in class.	J,S
Characteristics necessary to get along with others.	I,J
Committees analyze propaganda methods and motivational researchers' ways to try to influence people—alcohol and tobacco industries and others.	S

Research

Students investigate how emotions affect the endocrine, digestive, respiratory, and circulatory systems.	I,J

Continued.

PSYCHIC-SOCIAL-SPIRITUAL—cont'd

	GRADES
Resource person	
Advertising agency representative to describe techniques used to sell products.	S
Psychologist or psychiatrist from local treatment center to discuss relationship between emotional stability and drug dependence.	J,S
Nurse to discuss emotions and the body functions.	I
Counselors, clergy, social workers, and others to discuss how they can help students.	J,S
Role play	
Feelings of difference in terms of race, religion, cultural customs, ethnic origin, and others followed by discussion.	I,J,S
Negative emotional behavior.	I,J
How to make new friends.	P,J
How to help an unhappy person or one with hurt feelings.	P,J
How to say "No" if someone offers you a marijuana cigarette.	J,S
How to say "No."	I,J
Approached by a stranger and offered a ride home.	P
Someone you do not know offers you some candy.	P
Self-image-concept	
Have each student rate himself/herself on a scale from 1 to 10, with 10 being the highest score.	P

As you are now ————

As others see you ————

As you want to be ————

How can you get to where you want to be?

Discovering ourselves.* Children look at themselves in mirrors to discover special things that make each one unique. Teacher leads discussion of growth and development characteristics and relate to preventive health behavior including drugs.

Drawing ourselves. Children prepare portraits of themselves on large pieces of paper using crayons or water color paints. Teachers can follow activity by asking students how they feel about their work? Why are people different? Others?   P

DUSO (Developing Understanding of Self and Others). This is a prepackaged, self-contained, set of materials that includes puppets, posters, tapes, records, role playing instructions, and cards with discussion questions. The purpose is to help children better understand their own social and emotional behavior and that of their friends.†

Magic circle.‡ This is a procedure to help children better understand themselves and others, increase self-confidence, and improve social skills. Small groups of students sit in a circle and students raise hands when   P,I

*Adapted from Mobley, B.: I'm glad that I am me, Olympia, 1973, Washington State Dept. of Education.
†See Dinkmeyer, D.: Developing understanding of self and others manual, Circle Pines, Minnesota, 1970, American Guidance Service, Inc.
‡Adapted from Lotecka, L.: We all get a chance to talk: the circle approach to affective/social education, McKeesport, Penn., 1974, MYCODA, Inc.

PSYCHIC-SOCIAL-SPIRITUAL—cont'd

GRADES

they wish to speak about favorite possessions, something that bugs me, something I do well, I did something I liked, communication without words, and others. Teacher thanks students for contributions and may ask simple question or two.

Semantic-Differential§   J,S

	1	2	3	4	5	6	7	
Active	___	___	___	___	___	___	___	Passive
Strong	___	___	___	___	___	___	___	Weak
Healthy	___	___	___	___	___	___	___	Sick
Clean	___	___	___	___	___	___	___	Dirty
Predictable	___	___	___	___	___	___	___	Unpredictable
Honest	___	___	___	___	___	___	___	Dishonest
"Cool"	___	___	___	___	___	___	___	"Square"
Good	___	___	___	___	___	___	___	Bad
Fast	___	___	___	___	___	___	___	Slow
Smart	___	___	___	___	___	___	___	Stupid

Rate each of the following individuals, using a scale of 1 to 7 for each set of contrasting adjectives identified to represent *your* opinions of these people:
  Myself
  A drug education teacher
  A marijuana smoker
  An alcoholic
  A drug addict

Story

Introduce group of pictures representing anger, sadness, hate, love, and joy and develop stories relating to why each emotion is expressed.   P,I

Obtain books containing stories about emotions for students to read and discuss.   I

Share stories and poems that create different moods.   I

Value analysis

Ask students series of questions and after responses ask "Why?"   J,S
  1. What aspect of health do you value most?
  2. If you had to give up one of your senses, which one would it be?
  3. If you had 6 months to live, what would you do?
  4. What do you like about yourself?
  5. If you could make one telephone call anywhere in the world, who would you call?

§Adapted from Simpson, M. L., and Koenig, F. W.: The use of the semantic differential technique in drug education research, J. Drug Education **5**:251-259, 1975.

Continued.

PSYCHIC-SOCIAL-SPIRITUAL—cont'd

GRADES

Value challenges*

Teacher consistently and regularly raises value issues with students by in- J,S
troducing provocative, controversial statements found in newspapers,
magazines, books, and on radio, or TV. These should be duplicated for
student reading and accompanied by a series of teacher questions that
might include: What is your reaction to the statement? Would you be
proud of this action? Does it make you want to change your life?

Value questionnaire*

Prepare a series of questions for student response and discussion pur- J,S
poses. Illustrative questions might include the following:
1. What do you most like to do with your free time?
2. What adult qualities do you admire?
3. Where will you be and what will you be doing in 10 years?
4. What injustices exist in the community?
5. How do you feel about money and material possessions?
6. Will you marry outside your race or religion?

Value report card*

Students anonymously turn in 4 × 6 value cards on which they describe J,S
things they care about deeply or value highly. One card is turned in each
week and contains one value. Some cards are read and discussed in class
periodically.

Value time diary*

Students maintain a time diary for 1 week—a daily chart divided into ½ J,S
hour time blocks. Actual uses of time are listed. These should be personal and not viewed by teachers or others. An attempt is made to help
students locate those things they most like to do, to discover wasted
time, to identify inconsistencies, and to focus on the difference between what one says and what one does. After tabulation by students
and clarification of activities, efforts are made individually to determine
what students really value.

*Adapted from Simon, S. B.: Promoting the search for values, Sch. Health Rev. **2:**21-24, 1971. Also review
Raths, L. E., and others: Values and teaching, Columbus, Ohio, 1966, Charles E. Merrill Publishing Co.; and
Simon, S. B., and others: Values clarification; a handbook of practical strategies for teachers and students,
Amherst, Mass., 1972, Values Associates.

Inventory of risk-taking behaviors and rewards. Distribute copies of the inventory shown in Fig. 8 to all students. Have them complete this and use it as a basis for discussion. The inventory may also be collected at the end of class if it is completed anonymously. Results could be tabulated and findings reported to the class for use in further discussions.

Drug education resource materials

Printed materials such as textbooks, pamphlets, and leaflets and visual items, including films, filmstrips, cassettes, transparencies, and posters, are teaching aids, or resource materials, that are helpful in drug education programs. They have a multiplicity of uses and frequently can provide direct experiences obtainable in no other way. They

| Type of Risk | Degree of Risk | | Degree of Reward |
	To Individual Lowest Highest 1 2 3 4 5	To Society Lowest Highest 1 2 3 4 5	To Individual Lowest Highest 1 2 3 4 5
Smoking cigarettes			
Lack of affection			
Drinking beer			
Use of "pep" pills			
Marriage			
Stealing			
Drinking alcohol and driving			
Lack of success experiences			
Smoking cigars			
Drinking wine			
Lack of identity			
Use of heroin			
Sexual intercourse			
Use of marijuana			
Smoking pipes			
Drinking whiskey			
Use of sleeping pills			
Inequality of opportunity			
Abortion			
Use of coffee, tea, cola			
Self-medication			
Use other's prescription drugs			
Pushing drugs			
Lack of job			
Fighting			
Arguing with friends, with parents			
Sniffing glue			
Inadequate housing			
Use of contraceptives			
Cheating or lying			
Use of aspirin			
Destruction of property			
Mainlining drugs			
Racial, ethnic prejudice			

List your three most important risks. Why are they risks? What are the rewards?

FIG. 8. Risk-taking behaviors and rewards inventory. Students insert most appropriate number (1 to 5) in columns and spaces. (Adapted from Carney, R. E.: Risk-taking behavior questionnaire. In Report on feasibility of using risk-taking attitudes as a basis for programs to control and predict drug abuse, Coronado Unified School District, California, 1970.)

are often referred to as the tools of education.

Literally thousands of items (many of which are not well prepared) are available; the problem is one of selection. Hammond[32] stated that of the 800 posters, charts, giveaways, pamphlets, and other items received by the National Coordinating Council on Drug Education, perhaps only thirty could be recommended. Therefore any materials for the instructional program should be carefully screened as to appropriateness and suitability. Chapter 11 includes several instruments for the evaluation of resource materials.

These basic resources should receive consideration when seeking drug education materials and information: (1) National Clearinghouse for Alcohol Information, (2) National Clearinghouse for Drug Information, (3) National Clearinghouse for Smoking and Health, and (4) National Coordinating Council on Drug Education. (Addresses can be found on pp. 215, 216.)

The Clearinghouses are agencies supported by the federal government and operate as central sources for the collection and dissemination of information, as well as coordinating organizations, agencies, and programs throughout the country. Their major activities include the distribution of information materials, the answering of mail and phone inquiries, the referral of specialized requests to appropriate government and private sources, the publication of source reference materials, and the operation of up-to-date and computerized information storage and retrieval systems. They have developed immense files of resource materials, including bibliographies, program descriptions, published guidelines, and technical data. Some of the other services provided by these agencies are: (1) prepare and distribute publications, (2) conduct literature and program searches, developing printouts of magazine article abstracts or inventories of federal supported programs, (3) maintain libraries of books, reports, journals, texts, and the like, and (4) produce newsletters and magazines.

The National Coordinating Council on Drug Education is the largest private organization in the field of drug abuse prevention and education. More than 130 groups of professional, law enforcement, government, youth, and service organizations and corporations are included as members who provide support. Its goal is to promote and develop effective drug abuse prevention materials and programs. Its staff of consultants has provided such services as editing, evaluation, training, workshops, and public speaking to communities, drug abuse councils, school districts, law enforcement agencies, service organizations, media, and industry. The Council has prepared the following nominally priced materials, available on request:

Drug Abuse Films, ed. 3—an evaluative report on over 220 films and audiovisuals
Annotated Drug and Alcohol Bibliographies—twenty-four categories such as Sports, Industry, and Altered States of Consciousness in a single reference
Common Sense Lives Here, ed. 2—a step-by-step guide to community drug abuse organization
National Drug Reporter—a biweekly newsletter on the latest developments in drug abuse education, prevention, treatment, and enforcement

The references that follow include sources of drug materials, including books, curriculum guides, films and filmstrips, library sources, newsletters, professional journals, textbooks, and other materials usable in the instructional program. It is recommended that local and state resources also be identified and located when seeking instructional materials. It should be noted that the cost and availability of items listed by agencies and organizations may, on occasion, change rather rapidly.

The wide variety of available references in the drug field makes it impossible to provide a comprehensive list of books. It is suggested that individuals seeking additional information will find a detailed list of volumes in *Annotated Drug and Alcohol Bibliographies*, 1975 (89 pp., $4.00), which can be ordered from the National Coordinating Council on Drug Education, 1346 Connecticut Avenue, N.W., Washington, D.C. 20036.

The following selected books should provide an appropriate introduction to the drug scene.

BOOKS

Aberle, D. P.: The peyote religion among the Navajo, Chicago, 1966, Aldine-Atherton, Inc.

Answers to the most frequently asked questions about drug abuse, Chevy Chase, Md., 1970, National Clearinghouse for Drug Abuse Information.

Bloomquist, E. R.: Marijuana—the second trip (revised), Beverly Hills, Calif., 1971, Glencoe Press.

Blum, R. H., and others: Drug education: results and recommendations, Lexington, Mass., 1976, Lexington Books.

Blum, R. H., and others: Horatio Alger's children, San Francisco, 1972, Jossey-Bass, Inc., Publishers.

Blum, R. H.: Drugs I: society and drugs. Drugs II: students and drugs, San Francisco, 1969, Jossey-Bass, Inc., Publishers.

Blum, R. H., and others: The utopiates: the use and users of LSD-25, Chicago, 1964, Aldine-Atherton, Inc.

Brecher, E. M.: Licit and illicit drugs, Boston, 1972, Little, Brown and Company.

Brown, D.: The milder hallucinogens: nutmeg, morning glory seeds and marijuana, London, 1965, Westmount Press.

Cahalan, D., and others: American drinking practices, New Brunswick, N.J., 1969, Rutgers Center for Alcohol Studies.

Cain, A. H.: Young people and drugs, New York, 1969, The John Day Co., Inc.

Center for the Study of Social Behavior, Research Triangle Institute: A national study of adolescent drinking behavior, attitudes, and correlates, Washington, D.C., 1975, National Institute of Alcohol Abuse and Alcoholism.

Cohen, A. Y.: Alternatives to drug abuse: steps toward prevention, Rockville, Md., 1973, National Institute of Drug Abuse.

Cohen, S.: The beyond within: the LSD story, New York, 1967, Atheneum Publishers.

Cornacchia, H. J.: Consumer health, St. Louis, 1976, The C. V. Mosby Co.

Diehl, H. J.: Tobacco and your health: the smoking controversy, New York, 1969, McGraw-Hill Book Co.

Fiddle, S.: Portraits from a shooting gallery: life styles from the drug addict world, New York, 1967, Harper & Row, Publishers.

Fort, J.: Alcohol: our biggest drug problem, New York, 1973, McGraw-Hill Book Co.

Fort, J.: The pleasure seekers: the drug crisis, youth and society, New York, 1969, Grove Press, Inc.

Fort, J., and Cory, C. T.: American drugstore: A(alcohol) to V(valium), Boston, 1976, Little, Brown and Co.

Kalant, H., and Kalant, O.: Drugs, society and personal choice, Toronto, Canada, 1971, Addiction Research Foundation.

Kaplan, J.: Marijuana—the new prohibition, Cleveland, 1970, World Publishing Co.

Kron, Y. J., and Brown, E. M.: Mainline to nowhere: the making of a heroin addict, Cleveland, 1967, Meridian Books.

Lieberman, F., P. Caroff, and Gottesfeld, M.: Before addiction, New York, 1973, Human Sciences Press.

Lingeman, R. R.: Drugs from A to Z: a dictionary, New York, 1969, McGraw-Hill Book Co.

Marijuana: a signal of misunderstanding, First Report of the National Commission on Marijuana and Drug Abuse, Washington, D.C., 1972, U.S. Government Printing Office.

Marin, P., and Cohen, A.: Understanding drug use: an adult's guide to drugs and the young, New York, 1970, Harper & Row, Publishers.

McCarthy, R. G.: Exploring alcohol questions (revised), New Brunswick, N.J., 1970, Rutgers Center for Alcohol Studies.

McCurdy, R. M.: Smoking, lung cancer and you, New York, 1973, British Book Center.

Milgram, G. G.: The teenager and smoking, New York, 1972, Rosen Press.

National Institute on Alcohol Abuse and Alcoholism: Facts about alcohol and alcoholism, Washington, D.C., 1974, U.S. Superintendent of Documents.

National Institute on Drug Abuse: Marihuana and health. In Perspective, Summary and Comments on the Fifth Annual Report to the U.S. Congress from the Secretary of Health, Education and Welfare, Washington, D.C., 1975, U.S. Government Printing Office.

National Institute on Drug Abuse: White Paper on Drug Abuse, September, 1975, Washington, D.C., 1975, U.S. Government Printing Office.

National Institute on Alcohol Abuse and Alcoholism: Alcohol and Health: Second Report to the U.S. Congress, Washington, D.C., 1974, U.S. Government Printing Office.

Nowlis, H. H.: Drugs on the college campus, New York, 1969, Anchor Books.

O'Donnell, J. A., and others: Young men and drugs: a nation wide survey, Springfield, Va., 1976, National Technical Information Service.

Rachel, J. V., and others: A national study of adolescent drinking behavior, attitudes and correlates: final report, Washington, D.C., 1975, Center for the Study of Social Behavior for the National Institute on Alcohol Abuse and Alcoholism.

Raths, L. E., and others: Values and teaching, Columbus, Ohio, 1966, Charles E. Merrill.

Ray, O. S.: Drugs, society, and human behavior, St. Louis, 1972, The C. V. Mosby Co.

Resource book for drug abuse education, ed. 2, Chevy Chase, Md., 1972, National Clearinghouse for Drug Abuse Information.

Roszak, T.: Making of a counter culture, New York, 1969, Doubleday & Co., Inc.

Rublowsky, J.: The stoned age: a history of drugs in America, New York, 1974, G. P. Putnam's Sons.

Simmons, J. L., and Winograd, B.: It's happening: a portrait of the youth scene today, Santa Barbara, Calif., 1966, Marc-Laird Publications.

Slotkin, J. S.: The peyote religion, New York, 1956, The Free Press.

Smart, R. G.: The new drinkers: teenage use and abuse

of alcohol, Toronto, Canada, 1976, Addiction Research Council.

Smith, D. E., editor: The new social drug: cultural, medical and legal perspectives on marijuana, Englewood Cliffs, N.J., 1970, Prentice-Hall, Inc.

Smith, D. E., and Gay, G. R.: It's so good, don't even try it once: heroin in perspective, Englewood Cliffs, N.J., 1972, Prentice-Hall, Inc.

Smith, D. E., and Wesson, D. R.: Uppers and downers, Englewood Cliffs, N.J., 1974, Prentice-Hall, Inc.

U.S. Department of Health, Education and Welfare, Public Health Service: The health consequences of smoking, a report to the Surgeon General, Washington, D.C., 1971, U.S. Government Printing Office.

Wesson, D. R., and Smith, D. E.: Barbiturates: their use, misuse and abuse, New York, 1976, Human Sciences Press.

Yablonsky, L.: Synanon: the tunnel back, Baltimore, 1969, Penguin Books, Inc.

Yablonsky, L.: The hippie trip, New York, 1968, Pegasus.

CURRICULUM GUIDES

Numerous drug education curriculum guides have been prepared and are available from state departments of education and local school districts. If such references are desired, it is recommended that state directors of drug education be contacted for information and assistance.

FILMS, FILMSTRIPS, AND OTHER AUDIOVISUAL MATERIALS

The materials identified in this section represent those recommended by a variety of reliable references (pp. 204, 206, 215, 216). *The Drug Abuse Films Directory*, ed. 3, published by the National Coordinating Council of Drug Education (NCCDE), was the primary publication used in compiling the films list. It is important to understand that the NCCDE in 1972 selected only 16% of the more than several hundred AV materials evaluated. Most of these have been listed here.

The following resources are worthy of consideration in order to keep up to date with new items that become available. In addition to annotated bibliographies being available, these agencies publish newsletters that are either free or nominally priced.

Mental Health Materials Center
419 Park Ave., South
New York, N.Y. 10016

Extension Media Center
University of California
2223 Fulton St.
Berkeley, Calif. 94720

Films
Alcohol

*Alcohol—How Much Is Too Much?** Aims Instructional Media Services, Inc., P.O. Box 1010, Hollywood, CA 90028, 11 min., color, sd., grades 5-9, 1973 (Miles, ARF).

Problem Drinking: A Call To Action Association Instructional Materials, 866 Third Ave., N.Y., NY 10022, 20 min., junior high, 1970 (Miles).

What's It Going To Get You, Peppy? Youth Film Distribution Center, 4 West 16th St., N.Y., NY 10011, 9 min., b/w, junior high, 1970 (Miles).

Alcoholism: A Model Of Drug Dependency CRM Educational Films, Del Mar, CA 92014, 19 min., senior high, 1972 (Miles).

A Short History Denver Alcohol Safety Action Program, 1845 Sherman St., Denver, CO 80203, 6½ min., senior high, 1971 (Miles. ARF).

Ninety-Nine Bottles Of Beer Hollywood Film Enterprises, 6060 Sunset Blvd., Hollywood, CA 90028, 23 min., sd., color, junior-senior high, 1973 (ARF) Experiences and feelings of young people and alcohol.

Trigger Films Addiction Research Foundation, 33 Russell St., Toronto, Canada, M5S 2S1, 2-5 min, senior high, 1973 (ARF). To increase awareness of consequences of alcohol abuse and alcoholism.

Community-Treatment-Rehabilitation

Community As The Doctor Dick Ham Productions, 352 Waverly St., Palo Alto, CA 94301, 29 min., color, sd., org. community programs, 1971 (NCCDE).
Describes the process of organizing a comprehensive drug program. Discusses issues of community cooperation, law enforcement, parents, political leaders, and fund raising.

Help Concept Films, 1155 15th St., N.W., Washington, DC 20005, 25½ min., sd., color, junior and senior high, 1970 (NCCDE).
Scenes filmed at a hot-line order crisis center.

H + 2: Concerning Two Heroin Addicts Stephen Bosustow Productions, 1649 Eleventh St., Santa Monica, CA 90404, 22 min., sd., color, parole officers, judges, social workers, etc., 1971 (NCCDE).
Describes the frustrations and failures of two heroin addicts who undergo rehabilitation and are released

---

*The letters or names identified in the parentheses at the end of each item were recommended in these sources: (Miles) = Miles, S. A., editor: Learning about alcohol, Washington, D.C., 1974, AAHPER; (ARF) = Addiction Research Foundation; (NCCDE) = National Coordinating Council in Drug Education; (Schapps) = Schapps, E., and others: Balancing head and heart, sensible ideas for the prevention of drug and alcohol abuses; Book 3: Implementation and resources, Lafayette, Calif., 1976, Prevention Materials Institute Press.

from jail to face the pressures and responsibilities of community life.

Not The Giant Nor The Dwarf NBC Education Enterprises, 30 Rockefeller Plaza, N.Y., NY 10020, 57 min., sd., color, senior high, 1971 (NCCDE). View of Gateway House, a therapeutic community in Chicago.

We Have An Addict In The House Doubleday Multimedia, 1371 Reynolds Ave., Santa Ana, CA 92705, 30 min. sd., color, 1972, (NCCDE).
Through a cross-interview technique and the portrayal of rehabilitation encounter sessions, this film explores the concerns of the drug user, his parents, and his friends.

What Did You Take? Knightsbridge Productions, Inc., 155 East 38th St., N.Y., NY 10016, 35 min., sd., color, health professionals, 1971 (NCCDE).
This film depicts the treatment of actual patients brought into the emergency room of Beth Israel Hospital for treatment of heroin, barbiturate, amphetamine, and LSD abuse.

Communication-Coping-Decision Making

Almost Everyone Does Wombat Productions, 77 Tarrytown Rd., White Plains, NY 10607, 14 min., sd., color, intermediate and junior high, 1970 (NCCDE, ARF).
Film emphasizes that all people have feelings, both good and bad, and focuses on how people learn to deal with their feelings by drinking a martini, smoking cigarettes, talking to a neighbor, and taking a pill to relax.

I Think Wombat Productions, 77 Tarrytown Rd., White Plains, NY 10607, 19 min., sd., color, primary, intermediate and junior high, 1970 (NCCDE, ARF).
The film reviews some of the influences which determine a young child's attitudes and behavior. These influences include advertising, expectations of parents, school, friends, and self.

Brian At Seventeen National Institute of Mental Health, Abuse Film Collection, National Audiovisual Center (GSA), Washington, DC 20409, 30 min., sd., b/w, teachers, school administrators, counselors, parents, 1971 (NCCDE, ARF).
This film enters the world of a high school senior and looks at his life in and out of school, exploring his relationships with teachers, administrative personnel, friends, and family.

Is It Always Right To Be Right? Stephen Bosustow Productions, 1649 Eleventh St., Santa Monica, CA 90404, 8 min., sd., color, general audience, 1970 (NCCDE).
Our world is depicted in an animated cartoon, in which age, race, and vocation create factions which impair communication. The gulf is breached when people admit that they may have been wrong.

For Adults Only Professional Arts, Inc., P.O. Box 8484, Universal City, CA 91608, 28 min., sd., color, middle class adults, 1970 (NCCDE).
Dr. Allan Cohen discusses drug-related situations, which often lead to communications breakdowns between adults and their children

Flip City: The Psychotropics And You Carleton Productions Ltd., 1500 Merivale Rd., Ottawa, Ontario, Canada, 44 min., sd., color, junior, senior, high, college, adult, 1971 (NCCDE).
This documentary takes a broad look at drug issues as revealed by comments from high school and college students, a "street" clinic director, college faculty, a judge, a doctor, and a law enforcement officer.

Disappointment: A Day That Didn't Happen Guidance Associates, 757 3rd Ave., New York, NY 10017, sd., color, junior and senior high, 1973 (Schapps).
The film depicts a young girl waiting for her favorite uncle who has just returned after a long absence. Anticipation mounts as the day wears on. Finally the uncle calls to say he will be unable to come, and the girl breaks into tears.

The Divided Man: Commitment Or Compromise? Stephen Bosustow Productions, 1649 Eleventh St., Santa Monica, CA 90404, 1973 (Schapps).
An animated film depicting the inner struggles of a person making a living with a decision.

Greenhouse Arthur Barr Productions, Inc., P.O. Box 7-C, Pasadena, CA 91104, sd., color, all ages, 1973 (Schapps).
Depicts a boy caught vandalizing a greenhouse by the old man who owns it. Boy agrees to work off his debt and grows to love the greenhouse.

Inside/Out National Instructional Television Center, Box A, Bloomington, IN 47401, sd., color, intermediate, 1973 (Schapps).
A series of thirty films designed to help children understand and cope with their emotions.

The Many American Film Series Learning Corporation of America, 711 5th Ave., New York, NY 10022, sd., color, intermediate (Schapps).
Six films about children of different ethnic backgrounds, depicting conflicts of lifestyles and values.

General drugs

Us Churchill Films, 662 N. Robertson Blvd., Los Angeles, CA 90069, 28 min., sd., color, general, 1972 (NCCDE).
The film begins with shots of slums, waste, pollution, student unrest, and war, and then shifts back and forth to particular and contradictory situations in which people are using drugs.

What Do Drugs Do? National Institute of Mental Health, Drug Abuse Film Collection, National Audiovisual Center, Washington, DC 20409, 12 min., sd., color, elementary, 1972 (NCCDE).
A film designed to inform elementary school students of the good and bad action of drugs and chemicals on the body, the risks associated with drugs, and the dangers of drug abuse.

Marijuana

Weed Encyclopaedia Britannica Educational Corp., 425 N. Michigan Ave., Chicago, IL 60611, 24 min., color, sd., junior and senior high, college, adult, 1971 (NCCDE).
The film covers some legal, historic, and sociological aspects of marijuana use. Reviews what is currently known about physical effects of marijuana use and discusses current research efforts.

Narcotics

Darkness, Darkness Haight-Ashbury Films, 701 Irving St., San Francisco, CA 94122, 37 min., sd., color, senior high, adults, 1970 (NCCDE).
The film listens to a dozen middle-class whites whose lives have been touched by heroin.

Scag Encyclopaedia Britannica Educational Corp., 425 N. Michigan Ave., Chicago, IL 60611, 21 min., color, sd., intermediate, junior and senior high, 1971 (NCCDE).
The film presents a comprehensive picture of the heroin problem in an accurate, objective manner.

School atmosphere

Films For Success In Schools (Glasser on Schools, The Reality of Success, School Without Failure, A Success-Oriented Classroom) Media Five Film Distributors, 1011 North Cole Ave., Hollywood, CA 90038, sd., color, education professionals, 1970, 1971 (Schapps).
A series of five films on the concepts and methods of William Glasser's Reality Therapy and his Schools Without Failure Progam.

Human Relations Media Five Film Distributors, 1011 North Cole Ave., Hollywood, CA 90038, color, sd., educational professionals (Schapps).
A set of three films with the titles: Why Human Relations? The Humanity of Teaching. Starting Tomorrow.

School Discipline Media Five Film Distributors, 1011 North Cole Ave., Hollywood CA 90038, color, sd., education professionals and parents (Schapps).
A set of three films: *What is Discipline, Anyway?; The Who, What, and Why of Authority: Minority Report.*

Self-concept—values

Grooving Benchmark Films, Inc., 145 Scarborough Rd., Briarcliff Manor, NY 10510, 31 min., sd., color, teacher's manual, intermediate, junior and senior high, 1970 (NCCDE).
A teenage group is filmed over a period of several days during confrontations and discussions regarding drug use. The drug users, nonusers, and ex-users talk about the reasons for trying various drugs and some experiences with drugs.

A Nice Kid Like You Extension Media Center, University of California, 2223 Fulton St., Berkeley, CA 94720, 38 min., sd., b/w, college, parents, teachers, professionals, 1969 (NCCDE).

Students from two unidentified eastern colleges reveal their feelings about drugs, sex, parents, the educational system, and American society.

Up Front Aims Instructional Media Services, Inc., P.O. Box 1010, Hollywood, CA 90028, 28 min., sd., color, teenager and above, 1971 (NCCDE).
Roy Evans portrays himself as a counselor and technical advisor as he raps with teenagers, young adults, and parents. A former user himself, he guides the discussion away from generalizations about drugs and evokes introspective conversations about the reasons which lead to drug use.

Self Awareness Film Modules On Drug Abuse Film Modules Distribution, 496 Deer Park Ave., Babylon, NY 11702, 17-21 min., sd., color, junior and senior high, 1972 (NCCDE).
The three film modules on fear, humiliation and anger, and compassion, describe the many experiences young people have lived through.

Stimulants

Speedscene: The Problem Of Amphetamine Abuse BFA Educational Media, 2211 Michigan Ave., Santa Monica, CA 90404, 17 min., sd., color, junior and senior high, 1969 (NCCDE).
Interviews with speed users interspersed with statements from medical authorities present evidence against the use of amphetamines for other than medicinal purposes.

Stimulants-depressants

Glass Houses See-Saw Films, P.O. Box 262, Palo Alto, CA 94302; Haight Ashbury Films, 701 Irving St., San Francisco, CA 94122, 22 min., sd., color, senior high, college, adult, 1972 (NCCDE).
This film records thirteen extemporaneous comments from blacks, whites, Chicanos, young, old, rich, and poor about their personal experiences with barbiturates and amphetamines.

Filmstrips
Self-concept

Adolescent Conflicts: Dealing With Anger Guidance Associates, 757 3rd Ave., New York, NY 10017, sd. with record or cassette, senior high, 1974 (Schapps).
A driving examiner who treats Sue unfairly causes her to vent her anger in a variety of ways—rage and retaliation, self-denigration, displacing her anger.

Communication: Person-To-Person Scholastic Book Services, 904 Sylvan Ave., Englewood Cliffs, NJ 07632, sd. record, posters, student logbooks, teachers' guide, junior high (Schapps).
The filmstrip demonstrates ways to communicate, common student communication problems, and ways of overcoming them.

Dare To Be Different. Guidance Associates, 757 3rd Ave., New York, NY 10017, sd. with record or cassette, discussion guide, senior high, 1969 (Schapps).
Makes use of interviews to explore the concepts of individualism and conformity.

Do We Live Or Exist? Guidance Associates, 757 3rd Ave., New York, NY 10017, sd., by record or cassette, discussion guide, senior high, 1971 (Schapps). This filmstrip reviews poverty, ecology, education, alienation, and love and hate, with students making personal comments on each.

Personal Commitment: Where Do You Stand? Guidance Associates, 757 3rd Ave., New York, NY 10017, sd. by record or cassette, discussion guide, senior high, 1971 (Schapps).
The filmstrip explores the nature of commitments to self, family, friends, and social groups and issues.

Your Personality: The You Others Know Guidance Associates, 757 3rd Ave., New York, NY 10017, sd. by record or cassette, discussion guide, senior high, 1969 (Schapps).
Teenagers discuss their own and others' likes and dislikes about themselves, and make distinctions between personality and character, self-image and its effects on personality, and self-awareness.

Teenage Rebellion: Challenge To Authority Guidance Associates, 757 3rd Ave., New York, NY 10017, 1971 (Schapps).
Rebellious behaviors are examined and means of gaining peer respect are illustrated, from sincere attempts at basic social change to rebellion.

First Things: Values Guidance Associates, 757 3rd Ave., New York, NY 10017, sd., with record or cassette, discussion guide, primary and intermediate, 1972 (Schapps).
These filmstrips use conflict situations to explore such concepts as truth, promises, fairness, rules, and property rights.

Reflections Of Myself Guidance Associates, 757 3rd Ave., New York, NY 10017, sd. with record or cassette, senior high, 1972 (Schapps).
A review of such common adolescent concerns as discovering identity, dealing with uncertain situations, romance, and relationships with peers, friends, and adults.

Values In Action Winston Press, 25 Groveland Terrace, Minneapolis, MN 55403, sd. with record, teachers' guide, intermediate (Schapps).
Ten filmstrips that present conflict situations that involve decision-making.

Adolescent Experience: Developing Values Guidance Associates, 757 3rd Ave., New York, NY 10017, sd. with record or cassette, discussion guide, senior high, 1973 (Schapps).
Discussions of the following experiences: fear of punishment, interactions with peer groups, religion, school, parental example, reaction to parents, development of personal convictions.

School atmosphere

The Effective Teacher: Drug Education Guidance Associates, 757 3rd Ave., New York, NY 10017, sd., with records or cassettes, 13-17 min., college, adult, teacher training, counselors, school administrators, parents, 1970 (NCCDE).
Four filmstrips; The drug problem in Perspective, Drugs and the Classroom, Curriculum Approaches to Drug Education, Classroom Dynamics in Drug Education.

General drugs

Let's Talk About Drugs Multi-Media Productions, Inc., P.O. Box 5097, Stanford, CA 94305, 38 min. in two parts, color, sd. with records, teacher's guide, 9 and 10-year-olds, 1970 (NCCDE).
Discusses these questions: What is a drug? Why are drugs different from other things taken into the body? What kinds of drugs are there? Why do people take drugs? What do drugs do?

Drugs: Friend Or Foe? Marsh Film Enterprises, Inc., P.O. Box 8082, Shawnee Mission, KA 66208, 15 min., color, sd. by record or cassette, teachers' guide, kdg.-3rd grade, 1970 (NCCDE).
R. E. Davis, M.D., leads a spontaneous discussion about drugs with a group of elementary children designed to create an awareness of the benefits of rational drug use and a knowledge of the dangers of drug misuse.

Marijuana

Marijuana: What Can You Believe? Guidance Associates, 757 3rd Ave., New York, NY 10017, 32 min. in two parts, color, sd., by record or cassette, discussion guide, senior high, college, adults, 1969 (NCCDE).
David Smith, M.D., defines marijuana use and discusses its effects in part I. Part II relates some of the experiences of five teenagers with marijuana and other drugs.

Depressants

Drug Information Series–Sedatives Guidance Associates, 757 3rd Ave., New York, NY 10017, 14 min., color with record or cassette, discussion guide, junior and senior high, college, adult, 1970 (NCCDE).
The information presented regarding sedatives includes alcohol, barbiturates, and marijuana.

Stimulants

Drug Information Series–Stimulants Guidance Associates, 757 3rd Ave., New York, NY 10017, 11 min., sd., with record or cassette, discussion guide, junior and senior high, college, adult, 1970 (NCCDE).
Covers the broad range of stimulants used daily: caffeine, nicotine, cocaine, amphetamine, and methamphetamine ("speed"). Concentrates on life-style of the chronic speed user.

Hallucinogens

Drug Information Series–Psychedelics Guidance Associates, 757 3rd Ave., New York, NY 10017, 12 min., sd. with record or cassette, discussion guide, senior high, college, adults, 1970 (NCCDE).
Names types of psychedelics; young couple relates experiences with use; physicians discusss perceptual and mood changes.

Narcotics

Drug Information Series–Narcotics Guidance Associates, 757 3rd Ave., New York, NY 10017, 15 min., color, sd. by record or cassette, discussion guide, junior and senior high, 1970 (NCCDE).

The filmstrip identifies drugs in the narcotic family: opium, morphine, codeine, and heroin, and the synthetic narcotics. It focuses on life-styles of the heroin addict.

Tobacco

Contact local chapters of the American Cancer Society and the American Lung Association for the latest and most popular films.

Transparency

School Health Education Study: Use Of Substances That Modify Mood And Behavior 3M Company, Box 3100, 3M Center, St. Paul, MN 55101, twenty visuals with teaching-learning guide and teacher-student resources. Level III contains five sets each of the visuals, K-12 (Level III = junior high), 1968 (NCCDE).

Focus on behavioral decisions of young adolescents, relating particularly to tobacco and alcohol.

Slide Tape

Any Drug Education Program That Talks Only About Drugs, Is At Best–A Waste Do It Now Foundation, P.O. Box 5115, Phoenix, AZ 85010, 45 min., color, two screen presentation, adults, 1971 (revised fall, 1972).

The slide presentation covers a short history of drugs, a doctor talking about drug use and abuse, discussion among young people, and conversations with parents and teachers.

NEWSLETTERS

Addiction And Drug Abuse Report (monthly)
Grafton Publications, Inc.
667 Madison Ave.
New York, NY 10021
Cost: $22 yearly

Catalyst (quarterly)
North Conway Institute
8 Newbury St.
Boston, MA 02116
Cost: Free on request

Drugs And Drug Abuse Education Newsletter (monthly)
Scope Publications, Inc.
474 National Press Building
Washington, DC 20004
Cost: $33 yearly

Drug Survival News (bi-monthly)
Do It Now Foundation
Institute For Chemical Survival
P.O. Box 5115
Phoenix, AZ 85010
Cost: $2.50 yearly

Grassroots (monthly binder service)
Stash, Inc.
118 South Bedford St.
Madison, WI 53703
Cost: $115 yearly
(Includes Capsules, Directory of Drug Information, and Treatment Organizations)

Mental Health Materials Center (monthly)
419 Park Avenue South
New York, NY 10016
Cost: $12.00 yearly

National Drug Reporter (monthly)
National Coordinating Council on Drug Education
1526 18th St., N.W.
Washington, DC 20036
Cost: $21 yearly

Newsletter (monthly)
The National Council on Drug Abuse
8 South Michigan Avenue
Suite 310
Chicago, IL 60603
Cost: $38 yearly

NIAAA Information & Feature Service (monthly)
National Clearinghouse for Alcohol Information
Department of Health, Education & Welfare
P.O. Box 2345
Rockville, MD 20852
Cost: Free on request

Pyramid (periodic)
39 Quail Court
Suite 201
Walnut Creek, CA 94596
Cost: Free on request

Stash Capsules (monthly)
Stash, Inc.
118 South Bedford
Madison, WI 53703
Cost: $8 yearly

Smoking And Health Bulletin (periodic)
National Clearinghouse for Smoking and Health
Bureau of Health Education
Center for Disease Control
Atlanta, GA 30333
Cost: Free on request

Smoking And Health Newsletter (periodic)
National Interagency Council on Smoking and Health
419 Park Ave. South
Room 1301
New York, NY 10016
Cost: Free on request

Street Drug Survival (quarterly)
Do It Now Foundation
National Media Center
P.O. Box 5115
Phoenix, AZ 85010
Cost: $1 yearly

The Journal (monthly)
Addiction Research Foundation
33 Russell St.
Toronto, Canada M5S 2S1
Cost: $16 yearly

U.S. Journal Of Drug and Alcohol Dependence
   (monthly)
U.S. Journal
7541 Biscayne Blvd.
Miami, FL 33138
Cost: $20 yearly

PROFESSIONAL JOURNALS

Addictions (quarterly)
Addiction Research Foundation
33 Russell St.
Toronto, Canada M5S 2S1
Cost: $10 yearly

Alcohol Health And Research World (quarterly)
National Institute on Alcohol Abuse and Alcoholism
Superintendent of Documents
Government Printing Office
Washington, DC 20402
Cost: $6.40 yearly

Bulletin On Narcotics (quarterly)
Division of Narcotic Drugs
Geneva, Switzerland (also New York)
United Nations Sales Section
Cost: $10 yearly

Community Mental Health Journal (monthly)
Behavioral Publications, Inc.
2852 Broadway, Morningside Heights,
New York, NY 10025
Cost: $25 yearly

Drug Dependence (quarterly)
National Clearinghouse for Mental Health Information
Westwood Towers
5401 Westbard Ave.
Washington, DC 20016
Cost: Free on request

Drug Enforcement (quarterly)
U.S. Department of Justice
Drug Enforcement Administration
1405 I St.
Washington, DC 20533
Cost: Free on request

Drug Forum (quarterly)
Baywood Publishing Company
43 Central Drive
Farmingdale, NY 11735
Cost: $35 yearly

Drugs In Health Care (quarterly)
(The Journal of the Drug Use Process)
American Society of Hospital Pharmacists
Research and Education Foundation, Inc.

4630 Montgomery Ave.
Washington, DC 20014
Cost: $15 yearly

International Journal of Addictions (quarterly)
Marcel Dekker, Inc.
270 Madison Ave.
New York, NY 10002
Cost: $45 yearly

International Journal Of Drug And Alcohol Depen-
   dence (bimonthly)
(research and intervention activities)
Elsevier Sequoia SA
P.O. Box 851
CH-1001 Lausanne 1, Switzerland
Cost: $21 yearly

Journal Of Drug Education (quarterly)
Baywood Publishing Company
43 Central Drive
Farmingdale, NY 11735
Cost: $35 yearly

Journal Of Drug Issues (quarterly)
P.O. Box 4021
Tallahassee, FL 32303
Cost: $25 yearly

Journal Of Psychedelic Drugs (quarterly)
Stash, Inc.
118 S. Bedford St.
Madison, WI 53703
Cost: $20 yearly

Journal Of Studies On Alcohol (monthly)
Center of Alcohol Studies
Rutgers University
New Brunswick, NJ 08093
Cost: $25 yearly (individuals)

Listen: A Journal of Better Living (monthly)
Pacific Press Publishing Association
1350 Villa St.
Mountain View, CA 94040
Cost: $6.50 yearly

Psychology Today (monthly)
Communications Research Machines, Inc.
Carmel Valley Rd.
Del Mar, CA 92014
Cost: $15 yearly

The Alcohol Digest (monthly)
2 Research Court
Rockville, MD 20760
Cost: $75 yearly

TEXTBOOKS

   Schools can obtain textbooks from the following
sources:

Allyn & Bacon, Inc.
Grades 4 to 8: What you should know about drugs,
   Donald A. Read, 1970

Grades 6 to 12: Drugs and people, Donald A. Read, 1972

Associated Press
Grades 7 to 12: You and Your Alcoholic Parent, Hornik, 1973

American Education Publications
Grades 7 to 12: Know about drugs: A guide for students, 1969

Barron's Educational Series Inc.
Junior high: You, Pearl Roam, 1964

Behavioral Publications, Inc.
Preschool-primary: Things I hate; The boy with a problem; Don't worry dear; I have feelings; other texts

Book-Lab
Grades 6 to 10: Let's talk about drugs, C. Collins, and others, 1973.

Children's
Grade 5 and up: Yerians, rainbows and jelly beans: a look at drugs

John Day
High school: Young people and drinking: The use and abuse of beverage alcohol, A. H. Cain, 1970.

Fearon Publishers
Grades 4 to 8: About drugs, Haskell L. Bowen and Les Landin, 1971
Grades 7 to 12: Going places with your personality, Charles Kahn and Robert Tong, 1971

Fell
Grades 9 and up: How to kick the habit: a guide to drug withdrawal, new edition, C. and S. Clifton, 1972

Ginn and Company
Grades 7 to 12: Youth and the drug problem, Henry T. Van Dyke, 1975

Harcourt Brace Jovanovich, Inc.
Grades 4 to 6: What you should know about drugs, C. W. Gorodetsky and S. T. Christian, 1970
Grades 6 to 8: Drugs and people, C. W. Gorodetsky and S. T. Christian, 1968

J. B. Lippincott Company
Grades 4 to 6: The good drug and the bad drug, John S. Marr, 1970

John Knox Press
Grades 8 to 11: Youth and alcoholic beverages, John S. Lyles, 1967

Laidlaw Brothers
Grades 4 to 8: Basic concepts of tobacco and smoking, R. H. Needle, 1970
Grades 7 to 8: Basic Concepts of Drugs: Their Use And Abuse, B. D. Summer, R. H. Needle, and A. E. Hill, 1972

Julian Messner
Grades 4 to 6: Alcohol and you, E. E. Lee and E. Israel, 1975; Drugs and you, A. Madison, 1971; Smoking and you, A. Madison, 1975
Junior and senior high: Alcohol—proof of what? E. E. Lee, 1976

Macmillan
Grades 7 and up: Heroin was my best friend, J. Berry, 1974

McGraw-Hill Book Company
Grades 7 to 8: The drug dilemma, S. Cohen; Tobacco & your health, H. S. Diehl
Grades 8 to 12: Know about drugs, M. O. Hyde, 1971; Mind drugs, M. O. Hyde, 1968

National Education Association
High school: people do drink and drive: a guide to personal decisions, 1973

Oxford Book Company
Grade 8: Drugs and you, Hal W. Chauncey and Laurence A. Kirkpatrick, 1970

Pendulum Press
Grades 6 to 10: Narcotics and drug abuse, new edition, E. S. Williams

Pergamon
Grades 7 and up: Drugs for young people, ed. 2, K. Leech and B. Jordan, 1974

Pflaum/Standard, Publisher
Dimensions in Personality Series, Walter J. Limbacher, series editor
Level K-1: Let's begin
Level 1: Now I'm ready
Level 2: I can do it
Level 3: What about me
Level 4: Here I am, 1970
Level 5: I'm not alone, 1970
Level 6: Becoming myself, 1970
Junior high: Search for meaning
Senior high: Search for values

P-H
Grades 10 to 12: Drug scene: help or hangup, W. L. Way, 1970

Ramapo House
Elementary: The play is yours: you and drugs, L. S. Finkel and R. Drawitz, 1973; It's really up to you: you and smoking, D. Gess, 1973; It's really up to you: you and alcohol, G. Patterson, 1973
Junior high: It's your decision: you and narcotics, R. Berg, 1973; It's your decision: you and smoking, J. Curran, 1973; It's your decision: you and alcohol, J. Patterson, 1973
Senior high: You and narcotics: choose for yourself, G. Shevlin, 1973; You and smoking: choose for yourself, R. Spillane, 1973; You and alcohol: choose for yourself, M. Ames, 1973

Reader's Digest Services, Inc.
Junior & senior high: Coping with our changing world; Adventures in understanding; Drugs, drinking, driving, smoking and you; Ways to personal power; Love, morals, and marriage; Sex and sexuality, 1975

Rosen Press, Inc.
Grades 9 and up: Teenager and alcohol, A. Ayers and G. B. Millgram, 1970

Scholastic Book Services
Grade 1: What you must know about drugs, Harvey R. Greenberg, 1970
Grades 8 to 12: The wets and drys: Drinking—what are the risks, M. P. Acker, 1974

Science Research Associates, Inc.
Grades 6 to 8: What you should know about smoking and drinking, W. W. Bauer and D. D. Dukelow, 1971
Grades 7 to 8: Facts about narcotics and other dangerous drugs, V. H. Vogel and V. E. Vogel, 1971; Facts about smoking and health, E. J. Salber, 1968

Scott, Foresman and Company
Grades 4 to 8: About you and smoking, N. W. Houser, and others, 1971
Grades 6 to 8: Drugs: facts on their use and abuse, N. W. Houser, and others, 1971

Stash Press
Senior high: Our chemical culture: drug use and misuse, M. J. Summers, and others, 1975

Steck-Vaughn Company
The Human Value Series
Grade 1: About me
Grade 2: About you and me
Grade 3: About values
Grade 4: Seeking values
Grade 5: Sharing values
Grade 6: Thinking with values

U.S. Government Printing Office
Senior high: Thinking about drinking, revised, 1972

William Morrow
Grades 4 to 6: Medicine, H. S. Zim, 1974
Grades 6 and up: To smoke or not to smoke, Terry Luther and D. Horn, 1969

SELECTED SOURCES OF OTHER DRUG EDUCATION MATERIALS*
Commercial

Allstate Insurance Company
Allstate Plaza
Northbrook, IL 60062
(drinking-driving phamplets)

American Guidance Services, Inc.
Publisher's Bldg.

*Fee may be charged for some items. Also refer to pp. 226-227.

Circle Pines, MN 55014
(coping series booklets; multimedia program, developing understanding of self and others)

Channing L. Bete Co., Inc.
45 Federal St.
Greenfield, MA 01301
(booklets)

Creative Visuals Guidance Dept.
Box 1911 G
Big Spring, TE 79720
(junior and senior high tapes)

DCA Educational Products, Inc.
424 Valley Road
Warrington, PA 18976
(transparencies)

Denoyer-Geppart, Times Mirror
5235 Ravenswood Ave.
Chicago, IL 60640
(filmstrips, transparencies, annotated catalogue)

Distilled Spirits Council of the United States, Inc.
Education Service
1300 Pennsylvania Ave.
Washington, DC 20004
(reprints)

Educational Development Corporation
4900 South Lewis Ave.
Tulsa, OK 74145
(drug I.D. kit; flip charts; etc.)

Eli Lilly and Company
Indianapolis, IN 46206
(drug abuse information kit)

Encyclopedia Brittanica
Educational Corporation, Dept. 10A
425 North Michigan Ave.
Chicago, IL 60611
(positive self-concept materials for teachers)

Eye Gate House
146-01 Archer Ave.
Jamaica, NY 11435
(filmstrips, cassettes, records, transparencies)

Guidance Associates
757 3rd Ave.
New York, NY 10017
(filmstrips, films, drugs and values)

Imagination, Inc.
1821 University Ave.
St. Paul, MN 55104
(posters, stickers, leaflets)

Schloat Productions
150 White Plains Road
Tarrytown, NY 10591
(films, filmstrips, records, casettes)

Marsh Film Enterprises, Inc.
P.O. Box 8082
Shawnee Mission, KA 66208
(filmstrips, records, casettes, teachers' guide)

Media Five Film Distributors
1011 North Cole Av.
Hollywood, CA 90038
(reality therapy, schools without failure, etc.)

Medical Economics, Inc.
Book Division
Box 149
Westwood, NJ 07675
(drug I.D. guide, books)

Methods and Materials Press
6 South Derby Rd.
Springfield, NJ 07081
(socio-guidrama playlets, decision-making)

Agency for Instruction Television
Box A
Bloomington, IN 47401
(videotapes, films)

Professional Arts, Inc.
P.O. Box 8003
Stanford, CA 94305
(films)

Progressive Playthings, Inc.
Pennant Educational Materials Division
P.O. Box 20633
San Diego, CA 92120
(value games, books, instruments)

REACT, Inc.
Dept. J
1008 N. Randolf St.
Arlington, VA 22203
(audio cassettes, audio tapes, and program guides on
    alcoholism)

Reader's Digest Services, Inc.
Education Division
Pleasantville, NY 10570
(life values series for junior and senior high)

Stanford Press
Educational Development Corporation
Palo Alto, CA 94305
(self-enhancing education materials)

Scholastic Book Services
904 Sylvan Av.
Englewood Cliffs, NJ 07632
(filmstrips)

Science Research Associates, Inc.
259 E. Erie St.
Chicago, IL 60611
(filmstrips, records, cassettes, pamphlets)

Sigma Information, Inc.
240 Grand Av.
Leonia, NJ 07601
(cassettes on drugs)

Society for Visual Education, Inc.
1345 Diversey Parkway
Chicago, IL 60614
(filmstrips, records, cassettes)

Smith, Kline & French Laboratories
1500 Spring Garden St.
Philadelphia, PA 19101
(booklet, books)

Spenco Medical Corp.
P.O. Box 8113
Waco, TE 76710
(pamphlets, posters, audiovisual materials)

Tane Press
2814 Oak Lawn
Dallas, TE 75219
(booklets, charts, filmstrips, etc.)

3M Company
Visual Products Division
3M Center
St. Paul, MN 55101
(teacher's guide, transparencies)

Trend House Publications
P.O. Box 2350
1306 W. Kennedy Blvd.
Tampa, FL 33601
(drug identification handbook)

Winston Products for Education
P.O. Box 12219
San Diego, CA 92112
(drug I.D. kits, flipcharts, slides, poster sets, mari-
    juana awareness packet, etc.)

Governmental

*Alcohol, Drug Abuse and Mental Health Administra-
    tion*
5600 Fishers Lane
Rockville, MD 20852
(pamphlets, booklets, etc.)

Federal Food and Drug Administration
5600 Fishers Lane
Rockville, MD 20852
(may contact regional offices for a variety of materials)

National Audiovisual Center
National Archives and Records Service
General Services Administration
Washington, DC 20409
(films, annotated catalogue of films)

National Clearinghouse for Alcohol Information
P.O. Box 2345
Rockville, MD 20852
(pamphlets, booklets, bibliographies, information, etc.)

National Clearinghouse for Drug Abuse Information
P.O. Box 1635
Rockville, MD 20852
(pamphlets, films, source books, etc.)

National Clearinghouse for Smoking and Health
Bureau of Health Education
Center for Disease Control
Atlanta, GA 30333
(newsletter, pamphlets, etc.)

National Institute on Alcohol Abuse and Alcoholism
5600 Fishers Lane
Rockville, MD 20852
(pamphlets, films, source books, etc.)

National Institute of Mental Health
5600 Fishers Lane
Rockville, MD 20852
(pamphlets, films, source books, etc.)

U.S. Department of Justice
Drug Enforcement Administration
Washington, DC 20537
(booklets, magazine, pamphlets)

Professional

American Alliance for Health, Physical Education and Recreation
1201 16th St., N.W.
Washington, DC 20036
(booklets, films)

American Medical Association
535 N. Dearborn St.
Chicago, IL 60610
(pamphlets, booklets, articles)

American Pharmaceutical Association
2216 Constitution Ave., N.W.
Washington, DC 20037
(over-the-counter drug book)

American School Health Association
P.O. Box 416
Kent, Ohio 44240
(articles, drug education teachers' guide, magazine)

National Education Association
1201 16th St., N.W.
Washington, DC 20036
(pamphlets, articles)

Public Service

Addiction Research Foundation
33 Russell St.
Toronto, Ontario, Canada M5S 2S1
(books, booklets, newsletter, films, cassettes, etc.)

Alcoholics Anonymous World Service, Inc.
P.O. Box 459
Grand Central Station
New York, NY 10017
(pamphlets)

Alcohol and Drug Problems Association of North America
Education Department
1130 Seventeenth St., N.W.
Washington, DC 20036
(pamphlets)

Al-Anon Family Group Headquarters, Inc.
P.O. Box 182
Madison Square Station
New York, NY 10010
(pamphlets, also Alateen materials)

American Cancer Society, Inc.
219 E. 42nd St.
New York, NY 10017
(information on tobacco)

American Heart Association
44 E. 23rd Street
New York, NY 10010
(information on tobacco)

American Lung Association
1749 Broadway
New York, NY 10019
(information on tobacco)

American Council on Alcohol Problems
119 Constitution Ave., N.E.
Washington, DC 20002
(pamphlets, booklets, charts, audiovisuals)

American Social Health Association
1740 Broadway
New York, NY 10019
(pamphlets, newsletter)

B'Nai B'Rith Youth Organization
1640 Rhode Island Ave., N.W.
Washington, DC 20036
(pamphlets)

Board of Social Ministry
Lutheran Church in America
231 Madison Ave.
New York, NY 10016
(booklet, filmstrip, resources)

Center for Mass Communication
Columbia University Press
136 South Broadway
Irvington, NY 10533
(alcohol, tobacco, drug films)

Cleveland Health Museum and Education Center
8911 Euclid Ave.
Cleveland, Ohio 44106
(drugs, smoking, alcohol education kits)

Do It Now Foundation
National Media Center
P.O. Box 5115
Phoenix, AZ 85010
(books, pamphlets, videotapes, records, leaflets, newsletter)

Drug Abuse Council, Inc.
1828 L St., N.W.
Washington, DC 20036
(evaluation, research, information, booklets)

Highway Safety Research Institute
The University of Michigan
Huron Parkway & Baxter Road
Ann Arbor, Michigan 48105
(alcohol materials catalogue)

Loma Linda University
Department of Health Education
School of Health
Loma Linda, CA 92354
(cartoon booklet, grades 6 to 8 teachers' guide)

Mental Health Materials Center
419 Park Avenue South
New York, NY 10016
(clearinghouse for films, videotapes, annotated directories, etc.)

Multicultural Drug Abuse Prevention Resource Center
8443 S. Crenshaw Blvd.
Inglewood, CA 90305
(booklets, minorities information and materials)

Narcotic Education Bureau
National Women's Christian Temperance Union
1730 Chicago Ave.
Evanston, IL 60201
(books, booklets, films, filmstrips)

Narcotics Education, Inc.
6830 Laurel St., N.W.
Box 4390
Washington, DC 20012
(films, filmstrips, books, pamphlets)

National Council on Alcoholism, Inc.
2 Park Ave.
New York, NY 10016
(pamphlets, books)

National Coordinating Council on Drug Abuse Education
1346 Connecticut Ave., N.W.
Washington, DC 20036
(newsletter, booklets, bibliographies)

National Congress of Parents & Teachers
700 N. Rush St.
Chicago, IL 60611
(booklets)

National Council on Alcoholism, Inc.
733 Third Avenue
New York, NY 10017
(pamphlets, books, slides, youth education)

National Safety Council
425 N. Michigan Ave.
Chicago, IL 60611
(pamphlets, booklets)

North Conway Institute
8 Newbury St.
Boston, MA 02116
(pamphlets, resource book, newsletter, etc.)

Pharmaceutical Manufacturers' Association
1155 15th St., N.W.
Washington, DC 20005
(pamphlets)

Public Affairs Committee, Inc.
381 Park Ave. South
New York, NY 10016
(pamphlets)

Pyramid
39 Quail Court
Suite 201
Walnut Creek, CA 94596
(newsletter, publications, services)

Rutgers Center of Alcoholic Studies
Publications Division
Rutgers University
New Brunswick, NJ 08903
(books, pamphlets, reprints)

Smart Set International
Division of Teenage American Freedom Fund
307 Maple Avenue West, #H-1
Vienna, VA 22180
(stickers, posters, newsletter, etc.)

STASH, Inc.
118 S. Bedford St.
Madison, WI 53701
(books, magazine, drug information, library services, etc.)

The National Council on Drug Abuse
8 South Michigan Av.
Chicago, IL 60603
(books, cassettes, films, reprints, newsletter)

The Proprietary Association
1700 Pennsylvania Ave., N.W.
Washington, DC 20006
(pamphlets)

United States Jaycees
Products Division
Box 7
Tulsa, OK 74102
(booklets)

Union of American Hebrew Congregations
Publications Department
838 Fifth Ave.
New York, NY 10021
(resource guide, cassette, poster set)

University of Oregon Medical School
Alcohol and Drug Section
Mental Health Division
Henry Building

309 S.W. 4th Ave.
Portland, OR 97204
(reprints and information)

University of Michigan
Audio-Visual Center
416 Fourth St.
Ann Arbor, MI 48103
(drug film rentals)

World Health Organization
Pan American Sanitary Bureau
525 23rd St., N.W.
Washington, DC 20037
(booklet, magazine, reprints)

Evaluation

The effectiveness of the formal education program will need to be evaluated by teachers and other school personnel. Consideration should be given to short-range and long-range procedures. A comprehensive discussion of evaluation is contained in Chapter 11; therefore no attempt will be made to duplicate that material. Instead time will be spent in trying to assist the teacher in terms of general functional procedures for the classroom.

The classroom teacher should perhaps give consideration to assessing these four areas: (1) the curriculum or curricula materials provided in drug education, (2) the course, or unit, on drug education when completed, (3) the achievement of established objectives, and (4) the resource materials provided. These items may be realistically evaluated by the teacher on a short-range basis. The long-range program should be planned by a committee of representative teachers.

The procedures for evaluation have to be determined by the teacher and by the material to be evaluated. Procedures might include subjective observations by teachers, parents, and nurses, the use of teacher-made tests on a pretest-posttest arrangement, checklists, and inventories.

Subjective teacher impressions as to completeness, serviceability, organization, and other related matters may form the basis for the evaluation of the curriculum. The drug course or unit itself might necessitate a device adopted from one in the in-service preparation part of Chapter 11.

The objectives probably should be assessed on a pretest-posttest basis, with the appropriate questionnaire or test prepared by the teacher. Chapter 11 has illustrative knowledge (cognitive) questions that may be adapted for any given classroom. It also contains suggested attitudinal questions for use in developing an inventory and several practice surveys for use on a pretest-posttest basis.

Resource materials may be evaluated by using the instruments found in Chapter 11.

These suggestions on evaluation are not meant to be comprehensive. They serve to illustrate possibilities for the teacher's assessment of the drug education program on a short-range basis.

Mini-courses

These are educational experiences for junior and senior high school students that may be elective or academic. They may include training as peer counselors or peer/cross-age tutoring as well as involvement in volunteer projects, independent studies, and other alternative activities. The courses may be conducted after school or during free periods and are voluntary. *Peer counseling* refers to the provision of services on a one-to-one or small group basis in which students listen, inform, refer, and help peers with the solving of problems. *Tutoring* experiences are conducted at the same grade level or at lower grade levels. An illustration of such a program is the one functioning in the Monticello Public Schools in Monticello, Arkansas, called "Drug Education Program, An Alternative Approach." Its purpose is to prevent or reduce drug abuse by providing students with experiences that offer greater satisfactions than drugs. The program includes these types of experiences as well as others:

1. Mini-courses—yoga, chess, karate, fishing, camping, motorcycling, rap sessions, drug education, charm training, and others
2. Independent studies in sciences
3. Teen involvement—work with fifth-grade classes to present positive self-image

4. Elementary school program—planned drug education for grades 1 through 6

Student informal education

The informal educational approach is a program of information, counseling, and guidance that is nondirective, voluntary, and generally has little structure. This latter aspect may not be quite true if young persons express a need for assistance, in which case some regularized, partially formal program may be necessary and established. The procedure involves both one-to-one and small group interaction sessions. It may also make provision for alternative activities that help individuals satisfy particular needs and interests. The informal educational approach can be extremely helpful for some drug experimenters in school but probably is most productive with periodic, compulsive, or relapse users. Empirical evidence indicates the formal educational program to have little impact on the experienced misusers and abusers of drugs, whereas the informal approach has possibilities for success if individuals want help.

The informal educational program must be complementary to the formal program. Both must be operative concurrently if drug education is to be truly preventive and reach all students effectively.

Informal learning occurs in diverse forms, in many places, under varying circumstances, and involves all kinds of people. This type of education lends itself to the involvement of peer groups. Schools must seriously consider the opportunity for student participation in such a service capacity of the drug program.

Informal education perhaps functions best if a resource person is provided to whom individuals can turn for help. This could be a teacher, counselor, student, psychologist, nurse, ex-addict, or anyone who is capable of effective communication with people. Schools are now employing specialists as drug counselors or drug coordinators to develop and implement programs. Informal education takes place anywhere—in a classroom, in a hall, on the street, in the school-yard, on the way home, or in a drop-in center in or outside the school or before or after school. It basically occurs when a person reaches out to someone else for information, guidance, or help, and it takes place wherever these people happen to be at the time. Informal learning could occur in a partially structured arrangement, such as a small group discussion in or out of school where attendance or participation is voluntary. It may take place in an unstructured arrangement on a one-to-one basis. Such sessions are often referred to as rap sessions.

Two organizational patterns for rap sessions are drop-in centers and hot-lines. The drop-in center is a place to meet and rap with an individual or a group. It may be located inside or outside the school. The drop-in center may be under school, community, or their combined supervision. These centers may employ specialized personnel who are capable of assisting with rehabilitation and treatment as well as providing crisis intervention and parent education. These centers should be initiated and operated with the cooperation of local police departments.

The hot-line is a telephone service, usually manned by students, or ex-addicts, or both, that provides information and guidance to young persons, parents, and others desiring assistance.

Alternative activities* may be focused on the individual or the community. Individual experiences may include sailing, sculpturing, crafts, and carpentry, among others. Community experiences may include career exploration and referrals, repair projects, landscaping projects, wilderness backpack trips, and mural painting at the library. Alternatives, Inc., Chicago, sponsors a school-based "rap" program and sponsors such community projects as newspaper recycling operated by high school students who receive work space, technical assistance, and financial support.

*See Cohen, A. Y.: Alternatives to drug abuse: steps toward prevention, Rockville, MD 1975, National Clearinghouse for Drug Abuse Information. Also see National Institute on Drug Abuse Alternatives, Washington, D.C., 1976, U.S. Government Printing Office.

Gallatin Council on Health and Drugs in Bozeman, Montana, provides big brother/sister programs, summer job seminars and placements, and leadership camps for fifth and sixth graders.

Illustrative programs

A variety of drug programs exist in United States schools. Those listed next provide illustrations of many of the components for drug education outlined in this chapter.

SPARK, New York City (School Prevention of Addiction Through Rehabilitation and Knowledge)

The services provided by this unique program are found in Table 7-11. In addition to a school district drug education coordinator, the ninety-six high schools have drug education specialists. Forty schools in the areas of highest drug abuse are also staffed by community workers. Helping the specialists are several thousand trained students. In nine high schools there are "intervention and prevention" centers staffed with a psychologist, social worker, guidance counselor, attendance teacher, classroom teacher, and two neighborhood workers (former addicts). Staff training involves reality therapy, humanistic education, and other group techniques.

Alameda County Schools, California

The Drug Education Center seeks to prevent substance abuse and is staffed by a director and six specialists. Its objectives are to help people examine their present quality of life and determine the most realistic quality for themselves. The services include working with educators, youth, community programs, and parents: values clarification, decision-making in subject areas, classroom management, teaching about drugs, counseling, curriculum developing, peer advisee training, workshops, communication skills, local resources, and an alcohol education outreach program.

PRIDE, Dade County Public Schools, Dade County, Florida

This drug abuse prevention program provides a county coordinator of substance education programs and six area drug resource specialists. Each school has its own drug specialist who implements an educational program that includes values clarification and aids students in making rational decisions, gain positive self-concepts, and develop a personal values system. Peer and cross-age counseling are conducted and a variety of alternative activities (yoga, macrame, meditation) are available. High school students may take an elective course that introduces

TABLE 7-11. SPARK Services*

	Offered to				
	SPARK staff	Students	Faculty	Parents	Community
Counseling					
One-on-one		X	X	X	X
Small group interaction sessions	X	X	X	X	X
Education					
Group leadership training	X	X	X		
In-service training			X		
Curriculum development		X	X	X	
Workshops		X	X	X	X
Referrals and emergency care		X		X	
Social, cultural, and recreational alternatives to drug abuse		X			

*Jaffe, A.: SPARK: School rehabilitation through drug prevention programs, Drug Forum **3**:137-147, Winter, 1974.

them to self-awareness, communication skills, decision-making, and values clarification.

Washoe County Schools, Reno, Nevada

The preventive substance abuse program is under the direction of a drug education coordinator. It consists of a curriculum for three levels of students in elementary, middle, and high schools. There is some emphasis on drugs and their effects but the focus is on values, emotions, community resources, and relations between physical and mental health including risk-taking, decision-making, and problem-solving. Small discussion groups of fifteen students each meet once or twice weekly for 20 to 25 minutes. Peer counseling, parent awareness, student feedback, and student-faculty human relations are also included. In high schools a comprehensive health education program is conducted and students may take a peer counseling class.

The Group School, Cambridge, Massachusetts

This school-based program is designed to help young people develop positive self-images, emphasizing the individual's ability to control one's own life. It is directed toward students from low income and working class backgrounds with the hopes of discouraging defeatist attitudes through an academic program which leads to a high school diploma. The program offers classes developed by staff and students, vocational training, and small group counseling. The school emphasizes democratic decision-making and student control.

Resource centers

Resource centers for drug education at federal, state, and possibly county or large school district levels are necessary if school drug education programs are to receive the necessary supplementary support to operate effective programs. Several hundred governmental and nongovernmental sources, including many commercial companies, organi-

zations, and agencies, are developing, distributing, and selling a variety of materials. These items include books, magazines, pamphlets, folders, films, filmstrips, tape cassettes, transparencies, drug kits, and numerous other teacher aids for use in community, teacher, student, and parent educational programs. In addition, new materials are being developed and made available. It is conservatively estimated that there are available for purchase or distribution:

2000 to 3000 books on drugs

3.5 million magazine and reference articles from hundreds of periodicals

20 to 25 newsletters and other special publications

200 to 300 films

Over 100 curriculum guides

3000 to 5000 pamphlets, folders, and other printed materials

300 to 400 catalogues of items

Also numerous filmstrips, cassettes, transparencies, and other aids

The quality of these items varies from poor to excellent. The mammoth problem confronting educators is not only to know what and where these materials are, but, more importantly, how good they are. These complications added to the emergence of new research data make keeping up to date and knowledgeable about drugs and suitable drug education materials an impossible task to manage for the teacher, the local school administrator, and other school personnel.

It is therefore recommended that state, county, and city departments of education, through their drug coordinators' offices, establish resource centers where all materials related to drugs can be catalogued and evaluated, and where a variety of information and help can be made available to teachers and schools upon request. It is further suggested that a newsletter be periodically distributed to school districts within the state to disseminate new information, new materials, and new ideas for school drug education programs.

At the federal level the National Clearinghouses for Drug Abuse Information, Alcohol Information, and Smoking and Health have served as coordinating agencies, making numerous materials and services available.

However, they have not provided the evaluation process so vital to educational programs, nor have they made known the items available from commercial and nonvoluntary sources. The National Coordinating Council on Drug Abuse Education has evaluated films, provided a bibliography, a drug education directory, a monthly newsletter, and other valuable aids, and is about to assess pamphlets, posters, and other items. However, their services are limited.

There is no model for the nature or conduct of the proposed drug resource center. The experience of school audiovisual centers could be useful in organization and operation. However, the services needed and proposed for drug education extend beyond the usual assistance made available by such offices in the past.

Roles of school and community resource personnel

For an educational program to function effectively, the personnel involved must have their roles and responsibilities clearly identified, efforts must be coordinated, and any anticipated problems must receive appropriate attention. The purpose of this section is to outline briefly the roles of drug coordinators, teachers, counselors, nurses, students, and community resource personnel.

Drug education coordinator, specialist, resource teacher

Schools throughout the United States have been designating individuals as drug education coordinators, drug education specialists, or drug education resource teachers, and by other titles at state, county, and local school district levels. This action is necessary if programs are to be launched and maintained. The numbers of such individuals found in schools is not known; however, a recent unpublished survey by the authors indicates that drug coordinators have increased to the point where 60% (twenty-six states) of the states reporting said that some districts in each state have employed or designated someone in this capacity. This same study revealed that 20% (nine states) of those re-

porting said that none were employed. By way of illustration, the state of Mississippi legislated funds so that a drug education specialist is provided for each school district. Dade County Public Schools, Florida, has identified a resource specialist in every junior and senior high school. At least five county school offices in California employ drug education coordinators, with most other county offices having designated someone with responsibility for the program. New York City Schools, as previously mentioned, has a drug education specialist in all ninety-six of its high schools. The qualifications and functions of these individuals are discussed in Chapter 11.

Teachers

The teacher's responsibility for formal and informal education will differ, depending on the grade level taught and the assignments provided by local schools and school districts. At the elementary level, formal education may be expected of teachers in all grades. Informally, every teacher becomes a counselor at some time. However, the specific function of the teacher when such help is needed may be to refer the student to someone else, such as the nurse or drug coordinator. At the secondary level, formal education may be organized into the direct or correlated pattern, and teacher responsibilities would become clear. At both elementary and secondary levels some teachers may be needed as drug education resource individuals for their respective schools. All teachers will need to be aware of student drug problems and be able to recognize signs and symptoms so they can identify and refer those individuals needing help to those who can assist them. At all grade levels, teachers should be concerned with the material contained in Chapter 9 regarding the school atmosphere and make efforts to utilize these suggestions in their classrooms.

Counselors and ombudsmen

Counselors and ombudsmen will most likely be primarily responsible for informal educational services. Modesto City Schools,

California, have employed ombudsmen in each of four high schools. Their specific activities are discussed in Chapter 8, but many of the comments in Chapter 9 are also appropriate for counselor implementation.

Nurses

The school nurse may act as a resource person in the formal educational program, as an occasional speaker to make classroom presentations, and she may also provide help in curriculum development. Informally, she has always been a health counselor and undoubtedly should extend this role to include the drug problem. The information and guidance that the nurse may provide for both students and parents is outlined in Chapter 8.

Physicians and psychologists

Physicians may help to provide medical aid and, with psychologists, may serve as counselors and offer guidance aid. In addition, these specialists can serve as liaisons with the community.

Students

It is axiomatic that students have an important role to play in the educational program. The students involved might include ex-addicts, drug users, former users, and "straights." Although the specifics still need clarification, the following are responsibilities that have been assigned to students in a number of schools:

1. Develop, administer, and tabulate questionnaires to determine the extent of drug use in the school.
2. Aid in curriculum development by helping to (a) identify needs and interests in drugs and (b) suggest course content.
3. Hold membership on school or school district drug advisory committee.
4. Speak or participate as a panelist, debater, or presenter in class and at parent and community meetings.
5. Review and evaluate drug education resource materials to be used in school.
6. Act as discussion leader for small groups

of students in elementary schools (fifth and sixth grades) and junior high schools.
7. Provide information, guidance, and counseling in rap centers and other places as well as peer counseling and cross-age tutoring.
8. Participate in the operation of hot-lines.
9. Develop recommendations for drug intervention and prevention activities in school.

Community resources

There are numerous speakers, experts, and helpers, such as physicians, pharmacologists, psychiatrists, parents, and ex-addicts, who are available to assist in educational programs, in addition to many agency and organization personnel. This source of assistance should be utilized by school districts in those capacities outlined in this chapter. One thought about ex-addicts reported by Miller needs consideration:

The advantage of using an ex-addict is that he can often establish rapport with students who tend to reject counseling attempts by teachers or law enforcement officials. But a word of caution: attempts to do 'the right thing' by hiring ex-addicts to run drug programs has made some schoolmen fair game for the flimflam man. A district in New Jersey was embarrassed last year when it discovered the chief of its drug prevention efforts, supposedly an ex-addict with a hatful of ideas for curbing narcotics abuse among teenagers was, in fact, still an addict. He was supporting his habit with the money the district paid him to run the program. Local or state narcotic officials can confirm whether someone is actually an ex-addict.*

DRUG EDUCATION FOR PARENTS

". . . without parental participation, school drug education programs will meet with only limited success."[23]

Schools must provide or stimulate community agencies to provide both formal and informal educational programs for parents. The drug abuse problems among young persons cannot be resolved without the help and support of parents. Such action, however,

---

*Miller, T. J.: Drug abuse: schools find some answers, Sch. Manage. p. 30, April, 1970.

may demand community support and co-ordination with society's many educational sources outside the school. The purposes of such instructional programs may be to help parents in the following ways:

1. Obtain understandings about children and youth
2. Improve communication between parents and young persons
3. Realize that their own characteristics, attitudes, and behavior affect children's participation in drug activities
4. Become aware of drug abuse as a social problem and particularly as a youth problem
5. Understand reasons why drugs are misused and abused
6. Understand the effects of drugs on the body
7. Identify the signs and symptoms of drug misuse and abuse
8. Become acquainted with sources of help for youth involved with drugs
9. Become aware of the laws relating to drugs
10. Recognize the parents' role in prevention, problem solving, communication, and creating a positive self-image
11. Understand the role of the school in the drug program and the parental support needed

Parent formal education

Planned sessions, seminars, study groups, or courses conducted for interested parents are all involved in parent formal education. These programs may be repeated if desired in an attempt to reach a broader segment of the adult population. They should be conducted at convenient times for parents and may tie in with existing adult organizations, such as the Parent-Teacher Association or Rotary Club.

The types of programs and the manner in which they are conducted should be dependent on such factors as the nature, size, diversity, needs, and locale of the audience. The programs might include speakers; panels; debate presentations involving knowledgeable and acceptable community leaders or representatives; group discussions with opportunity for free expression, including questions and answers; opportunities to meet and talk with young persons in the drug scene as well as ex-addicts; parent-student informal discussions; use of a television series prepared with school-community cooperation and sponsorship; field trips to rehabilitation and treatment resources; and student presentations and discussions.

Parent education is difficult and time consuming, especially if schools try to conduct a program alone. Therefore schools may wish to coordinate their efforts through one or more community groups who might be in a better position to reach the adult community. These community groups may be able to assume the primary leadership in this enterprise. Such action may be particularly necessary in low-income areas where parental communication may be more difficult to achieve. Schools working with community action groups may be in a better position to reach parents.

In attempting to help parents, the following preventive action should be introduced in educational programs:

1. Seek your child's trust and trust your child.
2. Get to know your child, encourage him to discuss his feelings, and try to understand them.
3. Help him to understand your feelings.
4. Take an honest interest in your child and his activities, his friends, and his friends' parents.
5. Help your child establish goals for himself.
6. Spend time together as a family.
7. Be firm, fair, consistent, and honest.
8. Maintain parental control and establish fair limits.
9. Help your child to understand that parental discipline is a form of concern and love.

Tom Gordon has developed a parent education program called P.E.T. (Parent Effectiveness Training) that has been used throughout the United States.[30] It consists of eight-session courses offered in private homes, schools, churches, and other locations. Parents are taught how to communicate and to resolve conflicts amiably and equitably. It uses the following techniques:

1. Understanding the roadblocks to communication—ordering, warning, exhorting, advising, lecturing, judging, praising, name-calling, interpreting, reassuring, probing, withdrawing
2. Door openers—such phrases are used as: "Tell me about it"; "Shoot, I'm listening"; "Let's hear what you have to say."
3. Active listening
4. "I" message—parents have the right to express feelings and opinions
5. Mutual problem solving—permits children to take more responsibility

Parent informal education

No guidelines or procedures have been established for conducting informal parent educational programs. Someone in each school or school district should act as a source of information and guidance upon parents' request. In any event, procedures should be established to provide this assistance.

Some suggested ways of helping are as follows:

1. Have a hot-line available for crisis intervention and emergencies. In some areas, this may be better provided by a community agency or organization.
2. Be knowledgeable about community resources to which parents can turn for assistance and guidance.
3. Prepare informational booklets or pamphlets about drugs and drug prevention for distribution to parents.
4. Utilize the mass communication media to disseminate information to parents about the services available to help youthful drug abusers.

REFERENCES

1. Arnold, M. R.: The trouble in drug education, Natl. Observer **10:**16, 1971.
2. Association for Supervision and Curriculum Development: Yearbook: perceiving, behaving, becoming, Washington, D.C., 1962, Association Press.
3. Bedworth, A., and D'Elia, J. A.: Guidelines for programs in drug education, J. Drug Educ. **1:**1-4, 1971.
4. Berlow, L.: Kids 'n drugs, Chapel Hill, N.C., 1971, School of Pharmacy, University of North Carolina.
5. Blavat, H., and Flocco, W.: A survey of a workable drug abuse program, Phi Delta Kappan **52:**532-533, 1971.
6. Blum, R. H., and others: Drug education: results and recommendations, Lexington, Mass., 1976, Lexington Books.
7. Brayer, H. O., and Carney, R. E.: Program for preventive drug abuse education using the concept of values and risk-taking, Coronado, Calif., 1969, Coronado Unified School District.
8. Byler, R.: Teach us what we want to know, New York, 1969, Mental Health Materials Center, Inc.
9. Carney, R. E.: Application of the RTAQ approach to a value-oriented drug abuse curriculum, Coronado, Calif., 1970, Coronado Unified School District.
10. Carney, R. E.: A report on the feasibility of using risk-taking attitudes as a basis for programs to control and predict drug abuse, Coronado, Calif., 1970, Coronado Unified School District.
11. Conceptual guidelines for school health programs in Pennsylvania, Harrisburg, Pa., 1970, Bureau of General and Academic Education, Pennsylvania Department of Education.
12. Cornacchia, H. J., and Staton, W. M.: Health in elementary schools, ed. 4, St. Louis, 1974, The C. V. Mosby Co.
13. Dearden, M. H., and Tekal, J. F.: A pilot program in high school drug education utilizing nondirective techniques and sensitivity training, J. Sch. Health **41:**118-124, 1971.
14. Dezelsky, T., and Toohey, J. V.: Are you listening to the lyrics? J. Sch. Health **40:**40-42, 1970.
15. Drug education in Maine, Augusta, 1970, Maine State Department of Education.
16. Edwards, G.: The prevention of drug abuse through increased human interaction, Garden City, N.Y., 1972, Innovative Designs for Educational Action, Inc.
17. Education Research Service Report, Drug Education: Goals, approaches, evaluation, Arlington, Va., 1975, ERS, Inc.
18. Emery, R. C.: Existentialism in the classroom, J. Teacher Educ. **22:**5-9, 1971.
19. Farias, H., Jr.: Mexican-American values and attitudes toward education, Phi Delta Kappan **52:**602-604, 1971.
20. Fraenkel, J. R.: Value education in the social studies, Phi Delta Kappan **50:**457-461, 1969.
21. Frankl, V. E.: Man's search for meaning: an introduction to logotherapy, Boston, 1963, Beacon Press.
22. Fromm, E.: Man for himself, New York, 1947, Rinehart & Co.
23. Galli, N.: How parents influence their children's drug attitudes and practices, J. Drug Educ. **4:**37-41, Spring, 1974.

24. Gallup, G. H.: Seventh Annual Gallup Poll of Public Attitudes Toward Education, Phi Delta Kappan **57:**227-241, December, 1975.

25. Gartner, A., and others: Children teach children, New York, 1971, Harper & Row, Publishers.

26. Glaser, F. B.: Misinformation about drugs: a problem for drug abuse education, Int. J. Addictions **5:**595-609, 1970.

27. Globetti, G.: Alcohol education in the schools, J. Drug Educ. **1:**241-248, 1971.

28. Goldstein, R., editor: The poetry of rock, New York, 1969, Bantam Books, Inc.

29. Goodstadt, M. S.: When is non-drug education drug education? The Journal (Addiction Research Foundation, Ontario, Canada) **5:**8-9, Dec. 1, 1976.

30. Gordon, T.: Parent effectiveness training, N.Y., 1970, Peter H. Wynden, Inc.

31. Guidelines for drug abuse prevention, Washington, D.C., 1970, Bureau of Narcotics and Dangerous Drugs, U.S. Department of Justice.

32. Hammond, P. G.: Why drug abuse education is failing in America, Speech given at Thirtieth International Congress on Alcoholism and Drug Dependence, Amsterdam, Sept., 1972.

33. Harmin, M., and others: Clarifying values through subject matter, Minneapolis, 1973, Winston Press, Inc.

34. Hochbaum, G. M.: Behavior modification, Sch. Health Rev. **2:**5-11, 1971.

35. Hochbaum, G. M.: Changing health behavior in youth, Sch. Health Rev. pp. 15-19, Sept., 1969.

36. Hochbaum, G. M.: Effecting health behavior, Presented at the Annual Meeting of the New York State Public Health Association, Buffalo, N.Y., May 23, 1967.

37. Hochbaum, G. M.: How can we teach adolescents about smoking, drinking and drug abuse? In Resource book for drug abuse education, Washington, D.C., 1969, National Institute of Mental Health, National Clearinghouse for Mental Health Information.

38. Hochbaum, G. M.: Learning and behavior—alcohol education for what? In U.S. Department of Health, Education and Welfare: Alcohol Education Conference Proceedings, Washington, D.C., 1966, U.S. Government Printing Office.

39. Hochbaum, G. M.: The problem of abuse of stimulants and depressants. In Hafen, B. Q., editor: Readings in drug use and abuse, Provo, Utah, 1970, Brigham Young University Press.

40. Imhof, J. E.: Drug education for teachers and parents, New York, 1970, William H. Sadlier, Inc.

41. Jacobsen, J.: Drug abuse and learning effects, Educ. Horizons **4:**97-104, 1970.

41a. Jaffe, A.: SPARK: School rehabilitation through drug prevention programs, Drug Forum **3:**137-147, Winter, 1974.

42. Junell, J. S.: Can our schools teach moral commitment? Phi Delta Kappan **50:**446-451, 1969.

43. Keniston, K.: Drug use and student values. In Resource book for drug abuse education, Washington, D.C., 1969, National Institute of Mental Health, National Clearinghouse for Mental Health Information.

44. Kurzman, M. G.: Drug education: boom or bust? Contemporary Drug Problems **3:**61-69, Spring, 1974.

45. Langer, J. H.: Educational approaches for drug abuse prevention education, Washington, D.C., 1970, Bureau of Narcotics and Dangerous Drugs, U.S. Department of Justice.

46. Lawler, J. T.: Peer group approach to drug education, J. Drug Educ. **1:**63-76, 1971.

47. Le Dain, G.: Interim Report of the Commission of Inquiry into the Non-medical Use of Drugs, Ottawa, 1970, Crown Copyrights.

48. Lewis, D. C.: Drug education, N.A.S.S.P. Bull. **53:**87-98, 1969.

49. Lewis, D. C.: How the schools can prevent drug abuse, N.A.S.S.P. Bull. **54:**43-51, 1970.

50. Lippit, R., and others: The cross-age helping package, Ann Arbor, Mich., 1972, Institute of Social Research, University of Michigan.

51. Loggins, D.: Clarifying values, what and how well? Health Education **7:**2-5, March-April, 1976.

52. Maslow, A. H.: Toward a psychology of being, New York, 1962, Van Nostrand Reinhold Co.

53. May, R., editor: Existential psychology, New York, 1961, Random House, Inc.

54. Meeds, L.: Education: key to the drug problem, Soc. Educ. **33:**664-666, 1969.

55. Mikeal, R. L., and Smith, M. C.: A positive approach to drug education, J. Sch. Health **40:**450-453, 1970.

56. Miller, M.: Drug education: a re-evaluation, J. Drug Educ. **1:**15-24, 1971.

57. Miller, T. J.: Drug abuse: schools find some answers, Sch. Manage. pp. 23-31, April, 1970.

58. Mullin, L. S.: Alcohol education: the school's responsibility, J. Sch. Health **38:**518-522, 1968.

59. Nagel, C. A.: Behavioral objectives approach to health instruction, J. Sch. Health **40:**255-257, 1970.

60. National Clearinghouse for Drug Abuse Information: Resource Book for Drug Abuse Education, ed. 2, Washington, D.C., 1972, U.S. Government Printing Office.

61. National Clearinghouse for Smoking and Health, National Center for Chronic Disease Control, U.S. Public Health Service: Classroom tested techniques for teaching about smoking, Washington, D.C., 1968, U.S. Government Printing Office.

62. National Institute on Drug Abuse: Doing drug education: the role of the school teachers, Rockville, Md., 1975, NIDA, Prevention Branch.

63. National School Public Relations Association: Drug crisis: schools fight back with innovative programs, Washington, D.C., 1971, Association Press.

64. New York State Department of Education: Drug education: a positive paper, J. Drug Educ. **1:**123-126, 1971.

65. Nowlis, H. H.: Communicating about drugs. In Resource book for drug abuse education, Washington, D.C., 1969, National Institute of Mental Health, National Clearinghouse for Mental Health Information.

66. Nowlis, H. H.: Drugs on the college campus, Garden City, N.Y., 1969, Anchor Books.

67. Nowlis, H. H.: Strategies for prevention, Contemporary Drug Problems 5:5-20, Spring, 1976.

68. Pertz, R.: Drug education and the law, J. Drug Educ. 1:157-170, 1971.

69. Plesent, E.: A community and its school's efforts to understand and deal with drug abuse, J. Drug Educ. 1:85-91, 1971.

70. Raths, L. E., and others: Values and teaching: working with values in the classroom, Columbus, Ohio, 1966, Charles E. Merrill Publishing Co.

71. Rees, F. D.: Teaching values through health education, Sch. Health Rev. 1:14-17, 1970.

72. Report of the Temporary State Commission to Evaluate Drug Laws, N.Y. State Document No. 11 (1974). In Education: scaling the problem down to size, Contemporary Drug Problems 4:83-92, Spring, 1975.

73. Richards, L.: Psychological sophistication in current drug abuse education, Presented at the Rutgers Symposium on Communications and Drug Abuse, Oct. 14, 1969.

74. Richardson, C. E.: Drug education: some insights and some analysis of a conceptual approach, J. Alcohol Educ. 16:1-7, 1970.

75. Rogers, C. R.: On becoming a person, Boston, 1961, Houghton Mifflin Co.

76. Rosser, J. M.: Values and health, J. Sch. Health 41:386-390, 1971.

77. Rucker, W. R., and others: Human values in education, Dubuque, Iowa, 1969, Kendall-Hunt Publishing Co.

78. Russell, R. D.: Some important ideas relating to the future of substances that modify mood and behavior, J. Alcohol Educ. 16:8-9, 1970.

79. Samuels, M., and Samuels, D.: Peer counseling, Miami, Fla., 1975, Fiesta Publishing.

80. Schaps, E., and others: Balancing head and heart: sensible ideas for the prevention of drug and alcohol abuse. Book 3: Implementation and resources, Lafayette, Calif., 1976, Prevention Materials Institute Press.

81. Simon, S. B.: Promoting the search for values, Sch. Health Rev. 2:21-24, 1971.

82. Suchman, E. A.: The hang-loose ethic and the spirit of drug use, J. Health Soc. Behav. 9:146-155, 1968.

83. Todd, F.: The school's role in alcohol education, Calif. Sch. Health 2:11-15, 1966.

84. Toohey, J. V.: Beatle lyrics can help adolescents identify and understand their emotional health problems, J. Sch. Health 40:295-296, 1970.

85. University of Nevada: A drug abuse prevention program for students, grades 4-6, project developed by the Research and Educational Planning Center, College of Education, Jan., 1971.

86. U.S. Dept. of Health, Education and Welfare, National Institute on Drug Abuse, Domestic Council on Drug Abuse Task Force: White Paper On Drug Abuse, Sept., 1975, Washington, D.C., 1975, U.S. Government Printing Office.

87. Vincent, R. J.: Selected instructional and behavioral objectives for a tenth grade drug education program, J. Sch. Health 41:310-313, 1971.

88. Vincent, R. J.: A ten-month comparison of the incidence of smoking marihuana at a midwestern university, J. Alcohol Educ. 15:25-34, 1970.

89. Wheelis, A.: The quest for identity, New York, 1958, W. W. Norton & Co., Inc.

90. Wolk, D. J.: Youth and drugs: guidelines for teachers, Soc. Educ. 33:667-674, 1969.

91. Yolles, S. F.: Prescription for drug abuse education, J. Drug Educ. 1:101-113, 1971.

92. Yolles, S. F.: Prevention of drug abuse education, Washington, D.C., 1969, National Institute of Mental Health, National Clearinghouse for Mental Health Information.

CATEGORICAL REFERENCES
Role playing

Chester, M., and Fox, R.: Role playing in the classroom, Palo Alto, 1966, Science Research.

Shaftel, F. R., and Shaftel, G.: Role playing for social values: decision making in the social studies, Englewood Cliffs, N.J., 1967, Prentice-Hall, Inc.

Hawley, R.: Value exploration through role playing, Amherst, Mass., 1974, Educational Research Press.

Magic circle

Lotecka, L.: We all get a chance to talk: the circle approach to affective/social education, McKeesport, Penn., 1974, MYCODA, Inc.

Bessell, H.: Methods in human development, activity guides (levels I-IV, level V), La Mesa, Cal., 1972, 1974, Human Development Training Institute, Inc.

Peer and cross-age tutoring/teaching

Gartner, A., Kohler, M., and Reissman, F.: Children teach children, New York, 1971, Harper & Row, Publishers.

Lippit, P., Lippit, R., and Eiseman, J.: The cross-age helping package, Ann Arbor, Mich., 1972, Institute of Social Research, University of Michigan.

Mainero, J., and others: A cross-age teaching resource manual, LaVerne, Calif., La Verne College.

Schell, L.: A comprehensive model of peer teaching in a general public school context, Berkeley, University of California.

Values clarification

Harmin, M., Kirschenbaum, H., and Simon, S. B.: Clarifying values through subject matter, Minneapolis, 1973, Winston Press, Inc.

Raths, L. E., Harmin, M., and Simon, S. B.: Values

and teaching, Columbus, Ohio, 1966, Charles E.
Merrill Publishing Co.

Rucker, W. R., Arnspiger, V. C., and Brodbeck, A. J.:
Human values in education, Dubuque, Iowa, 1969,
Kendall-Hunt Publishing Company.

Simpson, B.: Becoming aware of values, San Diego,
1973, Pennant Educational Materials.

Values and Decision-Making Program Teacher's Guides:
Understanding human behavior and readings in
human behavior (Grades 7, 8, 9, 10), Cleveland,
1972, Educational Research Council of America.

Peer counseling

Glasser, W.: Reality therapy: a new approach to psychiatry, New York, 1965, Harper & Row, Publishers.

Carkhuff, R. B., and Berenson, B. G.: Beyond counseling and therapy, New York, 1967, Holt, Rinehart
and Winston.

Samuels, M. and Samuels, D.: Peer counseling, Miami,
1975, Fiesta Publishing Corp.

Parent effectiveness training (P.E.T.)

Carkhuff, R.: The art of helping, Washington, D.C.,
1972, American Personnel and Guidance Association.

Gordon, T.: Parent effectiveness training, New York,
1970, Peter H. Wyden, Inc.

Group processes and interpersonal relationships

Schmuck, R., and Schmuck, P.: Group processes in the
classroom, Dubuque, Iowa, 1971, W. C. Brown Co.

Saz, S., and Hollinder, S.: Reality games, New York,
1972, The Macmillan Co.

Johnson, D. W.: Reaching out: interpersonal effectiveness and self-actualization, Englewood Cliffs, N.J.,
1972, Prentice-Hall, Inc.

Edwards, G.: Reaching out: the prevention of drug
abuse through increased human interaction, New
York, 1972, Holt, Rinehart and Winston.

DUSO (Grades K-4)

Dinkmeyer, D.: Developing understanding of self and
others manual, Circle Pines, Minn., 1970, American
Guidance Service, Inc.

Training/consultation resources*

The Athyn Group
1229 Western Savings Building
Philadelphia, Pennsylvania 19107
(215) 567-5755
(cross-age teaching, parent effective teaching, peer
counseling, role playing, value clarification)

*Center for the Study of Psychoeducational Processes
(Pep Center)*
9th Floor, Ritter Annex
Temple University
Philadelphia, Pennsylvania 19122

*Schaps, E., and others: Balancing head and heart:
sensible ideas for the prevention of drug and alcohol
abuse. Book 3: Implementation and resources, Lafayette, Calif., 1976, Prevention Materials Institute Press.

(215) 787-8084
(alternatives, cross-age teaching, values clarification)

Educational Research Council of America (ERC)
Rockefeller Building
Cleveland, Ohio 44113
(216) 696-8222
(curriculum materials in humanistic education, training and consultation in a variety of strategy and
subject areas)

Effectiveness Training Associates (ETA)
110 South Euclid Avenue
Pasadena, California 91101
(213) 796-6107
(parent effectiveness training, leader effectiveness training)

Human Development Training Institute
7674 University Avenue
LaMesa, California 92041
(714) 462-8230
(magic circle, peer counseling, role playing, conflict
management, and other strategies)

Institute for Reality Therapy
11633 San Vicente Boulevard, Suite 104
Los Angeles, California 90049
(213) 826-2690
(drug abuse prevention and humanistic education strategies)

Mid-Atlantic Training Committee, Inc. (MATC)
1500 Massachusetts Avenue, N.W., Suite 325
Washington, D.C. 20005
(202) 223-0582
(strategies, community/school organizing techniques,
evaluation, management and organization development, and team building)

National Humanistic Education Center
Springfield Road
Upper Jay, New York 12987
(518) 946-2206
(cross-age teaching, decision-making, value clarification
techniques, peer counseling, and others)

New England Center
Box 575
Amherst, Massachusetts 01002
(413) 549-0886
(alternatives to drug abuse, humanistic education
strategies, human development program, value clarification)

U.S. Office of Education Training Centers
Division of Alcohol and Drug Abuse Education
Room 2049, FOB 6
400 Maryland Avenue, S.W.
Washington, D.C. 20202
(prevention and education strategies including alternatives, cross-age tutoring, creative drug education,
role playing, and value clarification)

8
Drug services

School drug programs must include secondary prevention of drug misuse and abuse as well as provide guidance toward tertiary prevention in addition to the focus on primary prevention. Students participating in the drug scene and using drugs should receive aid that will interrupt the development of more serious problems or help to solve existing difficulties and help reduce or aid in the intelligent use of drugs. Students may need someone to talk with, to turn to in an emergency, or to ask about community resources. This assistance is identified as the drug services phase of the school program. It includes procedures and personnel necessary to (1) identify students using drugs, (2) give attention to crisis and other situations when students are under the influence of drugs, and (3) provide follow-up activities to help young drug users and abusers.

Previously evidence was presented indicating that a sizable segment of the student population was involved to varying degrees with an assortment of drugs. This data further revealed that the extent of drug usage was dependent on the drug selected. Although the reliability and validity of some of this information may be open to question, the data show that young people in school are using drugs. Some students have no problems, fewer have minor problems, and a still smaller number have more serious problems. This chapter, therefore, is devoted to those drug users who are in school, and special consideration will be given to those who are misusers and abusers. The information herein should help identify the various types of drug users so that they can receive counseling and guidance. It should also indicate where abusers can obtain treatment and, if necessary, rehabilitation. It is expected that such services, if provided, would not only have considerable impact in reducing the number of drug misusers and abusers in schools but would also help pupils find viable behavioral alternatives.

Participation of the schools in the drug services program identified herein is not meant to usurp the role of the home or of the community but rather to supplement and complement such efforts. In many areas of the nation, parents undoubtedly are looking to the school for such assistance. In addition, numerous community agencies can provide help that neither parents nor the schools can make available to pupils.

IDENTIFICATION OF DRUGS OF ABUSE

Brief attention will be given to the question frequently raised by teachers, administrators, and other school personnel: How can I identify drugs of abuse? Many school personnel feel that such information will help them protect students from using such drugs or aid in identifying drug users. Actually such drugs cannot be effectively identified by sight, taste, or smell because all drugs except marijuana can be found in tablet, capsule, powder, or liquid form and in varying colors and shapes. Even marijuana, which is usually smoked, can be found in candy, cookies, and tea. Identifying the drugs used by individuals is a difficult and complex problem. Most drugs can be correctly identified only by trained technicians using complicated laboratory techniques. Such qualified experts may be found in clinical laboratories, in medical schools, or in police departments. School personnel who feel these services are needed should seek out such resources in their own communities. In the event that drugs, or alleged drugs, are found on campus and it is necessary to determine if they are drugs of abuse, technical help should be solicited.

IDENTIFICATION OF DRUG USERS AND ABUSERS

Few tests exist that physicians or clinical specialists can use to detect drug use and abuse, but such procedures are normally not conducted in schools. Therefore, if schools are to aid young people, less exacting methods will be needed to identify drug misusers and abusers, particularly potential hard-core addicts. Secondary techniques can be used by school personnel to identify students using drugs and to guide these pupils to counseling services and rehabilitation or treatment assistance.

Some of the ways school employees may participate in locating drug misusers include the following:

1. Observe (a) signs and symptoms of the effects of drugs on student behavior, (b) personality characteristics of potential users, and (c) tell-tale evidence of use
2. Identify students taking prescribed medications at school
3. Self-identification of drug abusers
4. Peer identification
5. Clinical tests (for example, urine test for drugs)

Observable signs and symptoms
Effects of drugs on behavior

The most useful and perhaps the best way for school personnel to spot drug users, unless the students turn themselves in, is by observing behavioral signs and symptoms.

This method combined with the other procedures found herein will at best only give clues or suspicions of drug use. Actually, some symptomatic characteristics that are identified may not be due to drugs but to illness or depression resulting from emotional reaction. Drowsiness, apparent intoxication, and loss of appetite are symptoms of many diseases. Also the normal adolescent occasionally becomes moody, changes interests abruptly, loses interest in the opposite sex, skips school, and still may not be involved in the use of drugs. *There should be significant and recurrent behavioral and physical changes before suspicions are aroused.*

Unless students identify themselves as users or misusers, are subjected to the few clinical tests available, or are examined by clinical experts, *there is no accurate way of knowing whether a person is on drugs.* The pupil using drugs will usually endeavor to conceal the fact. He will generally, although not always, confine his involvement to after-school hours and weekends or absent himself from school. He may be evasive of questions. These factors complicate the identification process for schools.

School personnel should not be quick to draw conclusions about student drug use from observations of symptomatic behavior because of (1) the possible irreparable alienation that may result and (2) the hazard of infringement on the rights of pupils. Caution is the best advice to the observer.

Regardless of the procedure, or combination of procedures used, the matter of diagnosis is not within the capability or responsibility of teachers, nurses, or other school personnel. *Diagnosis should be left to physicians and clinical experts who are thoroughly familiar with the pharmacology of drugs and with the drug scene.* However, the observation of signs or symptoms of deviant behavior is within the capability of all school personnel.

General signs and symptoms. The general behavioral signs to look for in students who are drug abusers include the following:

1. Immediate observations
   a. Changes in attendance, discipline, academic performance, interest, legibility, neatness, cali-

ber of homework, attention; loss of interest in sports; failing memory

b. Display of unusual degrees of activity—excitement, boundless energy, excessive laughter, unusual talkativeness

c. Display of unusual inactivity—moodiness, depression, apathy due to questioning of values, drowsiness, lethargy

d. Deterioration of personal appearance and of concern for health habits—dress, loss of appetite and rapid weight loss, sudden increase in appetite

e. Unpredictable outbreaks of temper and flare-ups—nervousness, irritability, argumentativeness

2. Long-term observations

a. Wearing sunglasses at inappropriate times to conceal redness of eyes, constriction or dilation of pupils

b. Constantly wearing long-sleeved shirts or blouses to hide needle marks

c. Borrowing frequently from others or stealing to obtain money required to purchase drugs

d. Appearing frequently in out-of-the-way areas, such as closets, storage areas, or rest rooms; furtive behavior; fear of discovery

e. Association with known or possible drug users; evasive answers when questioned about nocturnal activities

f. Appearance of intoxication but no smell of alcohol, indicates possible involvement with marijuana or barbiturates

g. Adoption of use of "odd" words; different vocabulary

Specific signs and symptoms. Table 8-1 shows the specific physical and behavioral signs and symptoms of the commonly abused drugs. School personnel should be alert to observe these signs in pupils.

Personality characteristics of potential users

The literature reveals a great deal of information that would be useful or particularly helpful for predictive purposes. Helm,[13] when speaking about the predisposition to alcoholism, says that most alcoholics share the following characteristics:

1. Little tolerance for frustration
2. Difficulty in coping with stress or withstanding anxiety
3. Emotional tensions and conflicts, especially in family relations
4. Strong feeling of alienation from their community or family
5. High energy levels but poor impulse control

Raskin[31] has identified the following personality characteristics of drug users:

1. Passively dependent
2. Withdrawn
3. Rigidly compulsive
4. Anxious-insecure
5. Depressed
6. Distrustful
7. Aggressive
8. Emotionally unstable
9. Antisocial

TABLE 8-1. Specific physical and behavioral signs and symptoms

Drug	Physical	Behavioral
Depressants* Barbiturates (reds, redbirds, downers, goofballs), e.g., phenobarbital, Seconal, pentobarbital; tranquilizers	Signs of alcoholic intoxication, no odor of alcohol on breath; unsteady, stumbling gait; slurred speech; possible mental confusion, delirium, convulsions	Loss of interest in usual activities—school, family, etc.; quarrelsome disposition; drowsiness or sleeping in class; may appear disoriented; coma or deep sleep; if only small amount, relaxed, sociable, in good humor
Hallucinogens† LSD (acid, cubes, STP, DMT) psilocybin, mescaline,	Sit or recline in dreamlike trance; distortion of time and sense perceptions—sight, hearing, touch; increased heart rate and blood	Sit or recline in dreamlike trance; may experience fear, terror, grotesque distortion of visual and auditory stimuli and self-image

*Usually taken in the form of pills.
†Usually taken orally on impregnated sugar cubes, cookies, or crackers and in a group setting under special conditions to enhance effect; not usually in school.

TABLE 8-1. Specific physical and behavioral signs and symptoms—cont'd

Drug	Physical	Behavioral
peyote, nutmeg, morning glory seeds	pressure, dilated pupils, "goose-bumps"; not always euphoric; unpredictable flashback episodes possible	("bad trip"); hallucinations; may try to escape from group; may be anxious to relate experiences and "insights"; less apt to hide involvement
Marijuana‡ (pot, weed, grass, tea, hay, mary jane, hemp, hash)	Red, watery eyes; odor on breath or clothing similar to burnt rope; fingers show burns from smoking; increased appetite and desire for sweets	Behavior dependent on dose, psychological set of individual, and social setting in which the drug is taken; at lower doses—mild disinhibition; behavior patterns inconsistent, variable, and difficult to discern; at higher doses—behavior patterns more consistent, such as laughter, animation, drowsiness, possibly stupor, lack of coordination, impaired sense of time and distance, confusion
Narcotics Heroin (H, horse, smack, junk, snow), morphine, Demerol, codeine	Needle marks or scars over veins of inner surface of arm (mainlining) or over other parts of body; constricted pupils, do not respond to light; flushed face, red, watery eyes; redness and rawness of nostrils—sniffing heroin; loss of weight, appears emaciated; lack of pain	Lethargy, drowsiness, sleep, stupor, coma (deep intoxication); generally antisocial, shuns friends, classmates; may disappear from group; euphoria; hiding syringes, needles, bent spoons in locker
Solvents§ Glue, gasoline, lighter fluid, paint thinner, freon (pressurized cans), marker fluid, liquid shoe polish, tire patch cement	Runny nose and watery eyes (mucous membrane irritation); pungent odor of substance inhaled remaining on clothes and breath; nausea, poor appetite, weight loss (frequent user); poor muscular control; may appear intoxicated; may complain of double vision, ringing in ears, hallucinations	Drowsiness or unconsciousness after excess use; concealing rags, plastic or paper bags containing dried glue, model cement, or other solvents in student's belongings
Stimulants Amphetamines (bennies, speed, dexies, uppers, drivers, pep pills), cocaine (crystal)	Dilated pupils; tremor, unsteady hands; dryness of mouth and nose, bad breath (onion, garlic, alcohol), licks lips frequently; flushing, excessive sweating; prolonged periods without eating or sleeping (frequent user); enlarged pupils	Excessive activity, difficult sitting still, nervous, chain smoking; euphoria, liveliness, talkativeness followed by depressed mood and irritability, restlessness, argumentativeness; exaggerated self-confidence

‡Smoked rolled in cigarette paper (reefers, joints, sticks) or in Oriental-style water pipe, or pipe; cooked in brownies or cookies; unless under influence at observation, difficult to recognize; infrequent users may not show general symptoms.
§Usually inhaled by putting head in cellophane or paper bag.

10. Hypochondriacal
11. Attention-seeking
12. Symptoms of psychosomatic illness

Blum[1] claims that high-risk youth are behavioral problems at school, have mild conduct disorders, and lack self-confidence. In addition, they may be self-centered and self-indulgent, peer- and pleasure-oriented, heedless of the rights of others and lacking in discipline.

Robins and Guze[30] reported that alcohol problems in ghettos for blacks and whites occur when children are brought up in families that are broken, irresponsible, illegal, and contain adults with drinking problems.

Blum,[2] Smith,[34] Johnson,[19] and Jessor and Jessor[18] have all found correlates between intensity and variety of drug experiences with poor grades, classroom apathy, delinquency, and rebelliousness.

It appears evident from the available data that drug abusers have various adjustment problems that most likely have bearing on their exhibited behavior toward drugs. Teachers, nurses, counselors, and other school personnel need to be alert to the signs and symptoms of deviant behavior resulting from the failure of students to have their physical and psychological needs satisfied. These signs and symptoms may provide clues about potential drug users and abusers among children and youth. It has also been shown that schools may be able to help with these adjustment problems. Perhaps assisting students in finding their own identities and their own meaningfulness in life would be helpful. Chapter 9 provides further guidance and help.

Tell-tale evidence of use

Tell-tale evidence refers to those objects that indicate the presence of drugs. These objects serve merely as additional clues to be assembled in attempting to identify drug users and misusers in school. The following list of tell-tale evidence is not all-inclusive but merely illustrative of the possible materials that may be found in the possession of students, in lockers, and in other places on the school grounds:

1. Hypodermic syringe, needle, or equipment
2. Blackened or charred spoon
3. Eyedropper syringe (makeshift)
4. Cellophane, plastic, or paper bag with dried glue
5. Unprescribed pills and cough medicine
6. Solvents, especially glue
7. Special cigarette papers or pipes with odors other than tobacco
8. Purchase of expensive articles and unexplained possession of large sums of money

Taking prescribed medicines at school

Permitting students who need medication, even though prescribed, to come to school creates a variety of problems that have not always been easily resolved. Whether a teacher, nurse, or other school official should be responsible for remembering to administer the substance, or for reminding the student to do so, has been the biggest hassle created. Students who come to school with such conditions as anemia, coughs, diabetes, hyper- or hypothyroidism, allergy, or epilepsy are usually readily identified. Parents generally inform schools of their children's conditions and seek the school's assistance with prescribed medications. Due to the legal complications involved, many school districts have developed general policies and procedures for handling such situations. When an emergency arises, such as a diabetic coma, and schools have been informed as to the student's condition, they are better able to cope with the situation.

One issue that has received considerable newspaper publicity recently is whether amphetamines should be used to calm hyperactive, or hyperkinetic, children despite their prescription and the general consensus of medical people as to their value. This controversy came to light in June 1970 when it was reported that 5% to 10% of the elementary schoolchildren in Omaha, Nebraska, received such treatment. Someone then concluded that apparently some 500,000 pupils in grades 1 to 6 in the United States were receiving amphetamines. With the present drug problem in society, a variety of people, including legislators, began to question this use of amphetamines because it added further complexities to a major social problem. The matter became more involved when additional individuals challenged physicians' diagnoses and still others made claims that children were being unnecessarily quieted when the real problem was that they were bored with their classes.

It is not the purpose of this book to take a stand for or against the use of amphetamines or stimulants for hyperactive children. We wish rather to indicate the complexity of the drug problem faced by schools even when certain drug users have been identified. A second purpose is to provide limited understanding about the hyperkinetic child.

Laufer[23] states that medication for hyperactive students has been used quite often in recent years. The condition itself (generally referred to as "cerebral dysfunction") is associated with the abnormal functioning of the part of the brain that controls automatic, involuntary processes. It is believed to have many possible causes, including genetic factors, birth process difficulties, illness, hemorrhage, emotional problems, and delay in maturation. The symptoms of this condition are overactivity, distractibility, impulsiveness, variability, unpredictability, emotional sensitivity, explosive irritability, and repetition of the active behavior. Hyperactivity causes problems in learning and may be extremely upsetting to other students and teachers. Stimulating drugs, including Dexedrine, Benzedrine, Ritalin, and Tofranil, have been prescribed for treatment, and in clinical experience the medications have had desirable effects on the hyperkinetic condition.

Peer identification

Occasionally students who are concerned about their friends and their friends' drug habits will give teachers and other school personnel information revealing that these friends are taking drugs. This information should be turned over to the individual in school who is best qualified to communicate with such students in an effort to provide assistance and guidance.

Peer identification should be looked upon as a means of helping students with problems and not for any other purpose. In addition, information received should be held in strict confidence and young people who provide it should understand that it will be treated this way.

Self-identification of drug abusers

A fourth, and unquestionably the best, procedure for locating drug users is to motivate users to identify themselves. As stated earlier, observations or other methods for discovering drug-involved students may not be reliable and at best are only indicators. Therefore, if young people could be stimulated to seek help on their own, the possibility of combating the drug problem would be greatly improved. To accomplish such a goal is no easy task; some of the methods used will be discussed later. At the moment it is sufficient to say that every school will need someone with whom students feel they can communicate. Whether this is a teacher, nurse, counselor, or someone else, such an individual must not only be well informed about the drug scene and knowledgeable about youth and their problems but also should be easily, readily, and frequently available when requested to rap with students. He should be willing to render aid when called upon for help. Some schools have delegated one person to serve in the capacity of an ombudsman—a kind of mediator for student problems and a counselor for students involved with drugs. Ungerleider and Bowen[38] recommend the ombudsman approach and have reported its successful use in the Campbell Union High School District, San Jose, California. Numerous schools have since employed such individuals.

Should school personnel wish to motivate drug-using students to make their own decisions about the need for help, a list of considerations prepared by Dr. Allen Y. Cohen[4] might be made available. Dr. Cohen states that if students wish to find out if the danger line has been crossed they might use the following checklist:

1. Increase in concentration problems
2. A failing memory
3. Decrease in mathematical ability
4. Creeping paranoia, feelings of persecution, or thinking that certain people or institutions are becoming hostile toward you
5. Exaggerated feelings of self-confidence or increased underlying feelings of inferiority
6. Passivity, loss of energy, or lack of desire to do anything except "lie back and groove"
7. Difficulty in speech; feeling you cannot form thoughts into words
8. Increasing hang-ups in close relationships, especially with parents and with the opposite sex
9. Greater impressionability; flying off the handle easily
10. Feelings of futility about life and hopelessness about your own future
11. A total denial on your part that drugs might be harmful for you

Clinical tests

Although blood tests may be used to locate drug abusers, urine testing is the current clinical procedure to determine if drugs are present in the body. Heroin, amphetamines, barbiturates, and other drugs, except marijuana and LSD, are tested in this manner. Currently there are no readily available clinical tests to identify these latter two drugs if present in the biological fluids of the body.

Technical help is necessary to analyze urine. Samples are collected and sent to a laboratory where two procedures may be used. The thin-layer chromatography test is less expensive and less sensitive but will also produce fewer false positives. The free radical analyzation test (FRAT) is more expensive and more sensitive but provides a high incidence of false positive results.

The presence of alcohol can be detected in two ways. A rough but simple method is the breath, or balloon, test, which determines the percentage of alcohol present. A more accurate method is to analyze the blood, but this involves clinical help.

Clinical testing information is discussed because a few individuals have advocated its use in the school program. We disagree with such a proposal for these reasons:

1. There are better ways to help students or to persuade them to voluntarily seek aid than to use such demeaning procedures on suspected drug users. This action would increase distrust in students rather than establish rapport.
2. There is a legal question about the infringement on the rights of individuals unless the tests were voluntary and approved by parents. However, should permission be granted, there is still doubt about the appropriateness of using this procedure in schools.
3. Such procedures may not be necessary because the number of compulsive and relapse users of most drugs is not very large, except possibly in some schools. Hence the cost might be too high in terms of the results.

WHAT TO DO FOR ABUSERS

There are perhaps four situations when school personnel may need to act and, in some cases, to act quickly, with regard to drug users who have been identified through any or all of the procedures previously outlined. These situations vary in their immediacy for action and are categorized as follows in descending order of importance.

1. *Emergencies and crisis intervention.* Drug use that creates a serious condition, perhaps involving life and death, depending on the drug used, is an emergency and requires crisis intervention. In an emergency situation a person may have taken an overdose of barbiturates, narcotics, or other drugs. It is a matter of life and death, and medical aid is needed quickly; the person may be unconscious. Other cases in need of prompt attention include diabetic coma, LSD bad trip, toxic psychosis or flashbacks, or student "freak-

out" suicide threats. These are serious, life-threatening situations, but they may not demand as quick action as the situations previously described. All of these conditions may occur in schools but only on rare occasions.

2. *Under the influence.* When a student is under the influence of a drug it will be obvious because he will be nauseous, drowsy, overstimulated, or otherwise unable to function. The youth may be causing a disruption in school; he may be drunk on alcohol, drowsy or sleepy on barbiturates, or very high on marijuana.

3. *Suspected of being under the influence.* Some of the signs of drug use will be evident in the student but they may not not be clear. These signs may result from the use of alcohol, marijuana, stimulants, barbiturates, or other drugs.

4. *Self-identification.* When under the influence, the student may voluntarily seek help from someone in school.

All of these four situations should be included in the policies and procedures established for a given school or school district. In Chapter 11 policies and procedures will be discussed.

In addition to the aforementioned, there will be other students not under the influence who have been suspected of using drugs and who will need aid. They will not require quick action, however. Ways to help these students will be covered later in this chapter.

With regard to the procedures to follow in emergency and crisis intervention ("hurry") cases, no attempt will be made here to provide extensive details as to "what to do" but merely what are the necessary essentials. When specific, detailed information needs to be included in policy and procedure statements, school personnel should consult medical and other sources in the community.

Emergencies. When a person is unconscious due to drugs or for whatever reason and has stopped breathing, this is a "hurry case" in first aid and immediate action must

be taken. Such action probably must occur within 5 minutes if the person is to survive and brain damage due to the lack of oxygen is to be prevented. An emergency demands the prompt start of artificial respiration with the concurrent call for medical aid. A physician, or an ambulance for transportation to the hospital, or both may be summoned. School policies should govern the exact procedures to follow. Parents need to be notified as quickly as is feasible. Whenever possible, as a secondary action, the cause of the unconsciousness should be determined by asking people who may have witnessed the action or through tell-tale signs that may be available. This may aid the physician in treatment.

Crisis intervention. The nature of the crisis intervention action will depend on the drug taken and the extent of the crisis. In all cases medical aid should be summoned, parents should be notified, and tell-tale evidence should be located to try to determine the drug used.

Stimulants. A speed "freak-out" is similar to a bad trip with LSD but more difficult to handle. It may be obvious by these acute signs: anxiety, paranoid feelings, rapid speech, repetitive ideation, muscle tremor, and occasional toxic hallucination. Someone should stay with the victim and help to reassure him and relieve anxieties.

Barbiturates. An overdose of barbiturates is a serious matter, especially since withdrawal without medicine is more violent and dangerous than heroin withdrawal. The drug disinhibits (like alcohol) and the release of suppressed behavior can create a serious and explosive situation. If taken in conjunction with alcohol, barbiturate overdose may be extremely serious and could lead to death due to the synergistic depressant action of the two drugs. If a large dose has been taken within 2 hours, the victim is conscious, and you are awaiting medical aid, it may be advisable to induce vomiting. Be cautious of the hazard of aspiration of vomitus material following this procedure.

Hallucinogens. Three types of situations may occur with hallucinogens: bad trips, toxic psychosis, and flashbacks. In all cases help is needed due to the anxiety reactions created.

1. *Bad trips.* Be sure to rap with the person on a bad trip and try to talk him down. Be supportive and friendly; help the person feel warmth and acceptance. Talk about what he wants to talk about and assure him that what is happening will vanish when the drug wears off. Try to make him relax and go with the trip.

2. *Toxic psychosis.* The state of toxic psychosis produces anxiety characterized by panic, excitement, and paranoia and is due to large doses of the drug. You still must talk the person down and let him know that the experience is due to the drug and will wear off. Remain with the individual at all times.

3. *Flashbacks.* With hallucinogens it is possible to have a sudden recurrence (flashback) of a previous, probably bad, trip complete with anxiety reactions and perception distortions yet independent of any drug use. You still must talk the person down and point out that the drug has taught him to react improperly to these illusions.

Under the influence. If a student is inexplicably demonstrating abnormal behavior and is unable to function at school, yet his vital signs indicate no immediate danger, parents should be notified. The student should be removed from the classroom and placed where he can be observed by a nurse, teacher, principal, or other person while awaiting the parents' decision as to disposition. Perhaps medical consultation is advisable; it should be suggested to parents when they are contacted. The parents should come for the student; if this is not possible, the student should remain under supervision and be taken home or to a physician's office.

Suspected of being under the influence. A student whose behavior indicates that he is under the influence of a drug (a little high) but still functioning within the normal school setting should be referred to the person delegated to implement school procedure in such instances. Suspension, expulsion, consulta-tion with parents, or any other action should receive careful consideration. No precipitous action should be taken (Chapter 10).

Self-identification. If a student reports his use of drugs to someone in school, and if he is under the influence, any of the procedures outlined in this section may need to become operative. If the case is one that does not involve quick action, the procedure for students under the influence would be appropriate.

FOLLOW-UP PROCEDURES

Having identified some of the drug users and abusers, including those suspected of or admitting to drug use, the school must decide what to do about helping these students. It is futile to merely locate students with problems unless something is done for them. More importantly it will be necessary to offer assistance not only to those who may seek help but to all others who are referred to school personnel for aid. The decision to provide help should be based on the school's desire to fulfill its educational obligation, that is, to provide opportunities so students can profit most from their experiences. This necessitates that pupils be at their highest levels of wellness. The use of drugs may interfere with the attainment of these states of well-being. Thus schools must be involved in the resolution of drug problems. The services rendered to help students will be referred to as follow-up procedures. They include counseling and guidance, use of community resources, and adjustment of school programs.

Counseling and guidance

The phrase "counseling and guidance" has many meanings, but it will be used here in the context of providing educational assistance mainly through a variety of informal educational procedures identified in Chapter 7. Some aid may also be forthcoming from the formal educational program previously described. Counseling and guidance refer to the efforts made to provide understanding, to make interpretations about the drug problems students face, and to try to help solve these problems when desired. Counseling and guidance involve the interaction of school personnel with students and parents in a variety of settings. The purpose is to assist in formulating action plans.

Providing drug counseling

It is becoming clear that each school needs to have at least one person who is assigned the responsibility of drug counseling. This individual may involve others, including students, to help provide aid, but he is held accountable for the availability of such services. Ungerleider and Bowen[38] call such an individual an ombudsman, others identify him as a drug counselor, whose responsibilities might include:

1. Establishment of procedures for identification of users and abusers
2. Availability and accessibility to students for information and guidance upon request through rap sessions or small group procedures
3. Aid in the development and implementation of follow-up procedures
4. Aid in the development of policies and procedures
5. Liaison with school personnel such as teachers, nurses, pyschologists, and principals
6. Management of in-service programs when necessary
7. Crisis intervention when necessary
8. Liaison with community institutions, including the police and the courts
9. Parental guidance and assistance
10. Aid in developing the drug curriculum and instructional program or as a resource when requested

The counselor may or may not be the administrator in charge of the total school drug program. This is a decision that each local school district must make. The counselor should not be confused with the drug education resource individual mentioned in Chapter 7. Although such a name is appropriate for the drug counselor, the former name generally identifies the person who aids teachers in the formal educational program. However, Chapter 10 provides information about administrative structure that should be considered.

The ombudsman, or counselor, should essentially possess these characteristics:

1. Be an approachable person who is able to communicate easily with students and is understanding of student problems, culture, and concerns
2. Be readily available and accessible whenever needed
3. Be willing to talk and not preach; be willing to listen and not dominate the conversation
4. Be honest and truthful in approach; one in whom students can place trust and faith
5. Not be using illegal drugs himself
6. Not be afraid to discuss drugs or anything else: sex, search for life's meaning, etc.
7. Have some preparation and ability to recognize emotional disorders, to offer guidance, and to refer students to the school nurse, psychologist, or to a community resource
8. Be knowledgeable about the drug scene, especially in the youth culture, and know how to assist those drug users and abusers who desire help
9. Can work well with school personnel and community people, including parents
10. Be interested and willing to help young people with drug problems

When school districts may find it impossible to locate ombudsmen, or counselors, with these qualifications, it will probably be necessary to select likely candidates from within the school system. There are three basic qualifications such individuals should possess: (1) the ability to communicate with students, (2) acceptance by students, and (3) a sincere interest in wanting to help young people. To further prepare these individuals, schools should encourage participation in a wide variety of activities, including attendance at workshops and conferences, visitations to and discussions with people working in the drug scene, meetings, and involvement with the police.

In counseling young people about drugs, Frykman[14] has identified these guidelines that may be helpful:

1. Keep all confidences a sacred trust
2. Offer help so it can be easily refused or accepted
3. Wait patiently until the person wishes to make contact and to identify with you; do not force the relationship
4. Concentrate on the articulated problem, even when you become aware of far deeper ones
5. Seek to understand the problem as he sees it, not as you see it
6. Show positive support in his struggle and interest in what he has to say
7. Try not to solve things for him; help him instead to come to some conclusion as to how to solve the problem himself
8. Gently steer the conversation toward what he is obviously leaving out; do not finish sentences for him
9. Be aware that he senses or imagines your response because of past experience with helping agents

Several additional thoughts to be considered by the counselor when dealing with students with drug problems are those expressed by Dorsey and Silverman[6]:

1. Encounters with drug users may be difficult for many reasons; the user may be confused about the need for help and be reticent to seek help
2. Students frequently engage in a reconnaissance of the counselor prior to overtly asking for help
3. Both the drug user and the counselor encounter each other with certain expectations, biases, and fears
4. The student seeking help may be uncertain about what help is
5. The student may be afraid of being "busted"
6. The student may not trust the counselor

Numerous schools are using students to help with counseling in a variety of ways, including *peer counseling* and *cross-age tutoring*, identified in Chapter 7. Students, whether they have been addicts or not, have been available for one-to-one relationships, in small group discussions, at drop-in centers, and on hot-lines. How successful such procedures have been has not been fully ascertained.

The procedure for counseling used in the Palo Alto Unified School District in California utilizes drug counselors who have been chosen by the students because they can be trusted and because students can communicate with them without fear of reprisal. Each school has a group of drug specialists among whom are teachers, administrators, psychologists, and counselors. This team has been exposed to a special in-service training program. The members are free to respond to student needs in the manner they deem appropriate and effective. They are provided with released time from teaching or other responsibilities during the day if students require help.

Illustrations of types and procedures

The types and procedures of counseling in drug problems have assumed a variety of forms that have been used in an informal setting. The procedures used have included any or all of the following: drop-in, rap, or informational centers (on or off school grounds) run by school personnel, students, or both; peer-group activities in which high school students visit junior high schools, or junior high schools visit fifth and sixth grades or through peer counseling, and rap with students; hot-lines on or off campus for student and parent use; school newspapers, special bulletins, and other communication procedures in schools; special notices to parents; and counseling with students or parents or both.

Various combinations of the types and procedures of counseling have been used in programs throughout the country. Programs in California, North Carolina, Ohio, New Jersey, and New York are illustrative of the efforts being made.

Project Adelante, Pueblo, Colorado. This is a community-linked program designed to deal mainly with poor Chicanos, blacks, and whites and their problems. The primary function is to provide positive alternatives for negative behavior through counseling at the Drop-In Center, drug education discussions, activities and recreation, youth and adult workshops in values clarification, day care programs, and others.

Kitsap County Council on Youth, Inc., Bremerton, Washington. This is a community-oriented program that offers counseling therapy to strengthen communication for youth and their families. These services are enhanced by a drop-in center, recreation, and other activities. A youth council serves in both a treatment mode and as a programmatic board of advisers.

Innovative Youth Services of Racine, Inc., Racine, Wisconsin. This is a program designed to provide preventive counseling for youth who feel that they are exhibiting behaviors not conducive to their personal growth and development. It offers a 24-hour hot-line, counseling, rap groups and peer group activities, referrals, and crisis intervention. The role of the staff advisor is one of support; the young people are the program.

Fayetteville Public Schools, Arkansas. Fayetteville has a school-based program that seeks to prevent negative behaviors through such strategies as decision-making skills, values clarification, alternatives to drug abuse, and improved self-esteem. The Teen Involvement facet of the program (fifth graders) is organized and run by teen counselors.

Teen-Peer Facilitator Program, Gainesville, Florida. This is a school program that involves one full-time paid employee and twenty-five full-time volunteer students. It seeks to deal with the problems of negative self-concepts, clarifying values, and developing decision-making skills through a Big Brother/Big Sister program, tutoring, rap groups, and developing friendships.

Shalom/Operation Discovery, Philadelphia. This is an inner-city program designed to help youth avoid becoming involved in drug abuse by improving their school ability, to prepare youth for community leadership, to encourage creative potential, and to strengthen their sense of control over their own lives. These goals are met through counseling and various workshops in communication skills, values clarification, and human relations.

Monterey, California. A Drug Information and Youth Crisis Center has been established to inform or counsel young people and adults about drugs and related problems. The program includes education, detoxification, and rehabilitation. More specifically, the center provides the following services: (1) a 24-hour switchboard with immediate referral for medical or psychiatric assistance, (2) consultation with existing agencies, including schools, for improving drug education, (3) a library of resource materials and training aids for educators and agencies, (4) continuing institutes for the training of those involved in drug education and counseling programs for drug users and their families, and (5) rehabilitation, job placement, and follow-up contact whenever possible.

Rap Place, Lewiston, Maine. This program offers peer and professional counseling as well as a 24-hour crisis service, a weekly radio program, part-time job and babysitting referral services, and in-school decision-making groups. The staff is composed of teenagers and young people in their early twenties.

Josephone County Council on Drugs, Grants Pass, Oregon. This county outreach program offers social seminars, a state-wide newsletter on substance abuse, a 9-week series of radio shows, high school peer counseling, 24-hour hot-line, and other services. Youth volunteers are responsible for the hot-line and the high school peer groups.

Use of community resources

Schools will discover that after the counseling and guidance phase, some students will require the assistance of available community agencies. Pupils and parents may need help in identifying and locating local resources. Therefore the personnel assisting students and parents must know about the various private psychotherapists, private physicians, public and private hospitals, hotlines, guidance and outpatient clinics, mental health centers, city and county agencies, religious organizations, and other services. Personnel should conduct surveys of resources available in their communities. Liaison and communication should be established with these agencies so that referrals and assistance with the school program become possible.

The nature and extent of community resources has greatly increased in recent years but will depend on location. Schools centered in metropolitan areas may have more such resources than those in rural areas. In probably all cases the supply will fall short of the need. This should induce schools and school districts to take the initiative and motivate the forces in the community to provide a variety of service centers, particularly in ghetto areas. Thus the schools and the community can work together in a common cause.

Adjustment of school programs

School districts must be cognizant of the student's welfare when determining action to be taken with drug abusers and must consider the school's basic function, which is educational, in reaching any decision to suspend or expel students. Schools should try to keep students in school, perhaps through innovative approaches, or should attempt to provide educational services wherever pupils may be—in jails, juvenile halls, or other correctional institutions. Schools located in low-income areas or in predominantly ethnic minority neighborhoods will need to give special attention to these matters.

Chapters 6 and 7 identified and briefly described a number of educational alternatives that provide clues to some of the adjustments to which schools must give consideration. These procedures included alternative education in terms of alternative schools, as well as mini-courses and alternative activities. Chapter 9 provides additional school modifications in the school atmosphere that are important to students. They include student alienation and unrest, pupils' physical and psychological needs, and creation of humaneness as appropriate to meet the differential needs of student drug misusers and abusers.

One adjustment method used in Fresno, California, is an alternative to suspension or detention for students found on campus with alcohol and/or drugs, or when it is felt students need intense, early, education intervention. Students are referred by principals, vice-principals, deans, counselors, school psychologists, and others to a special course which they must attend once monthly for 2 hours for the school calendar year. The content includes information, personal and peer dynamics, decision-making, values clarification, and alternatives to drugs.

In a Sacramento high school, students discovered smoking receive a 3-day suspension unless they agree to attend a "Five Day Clinic to Stop Smoking" developed in cooperation with the County Medical Society. Parents are expected to accompany students at the 1½-hour sessions. The program includes information, films, lectures by a physician, helpful advice by a psychologist, and discussions. Students are asked to control diets, fluid intake, and breathing habits. Although suspensions have dropped there is no evidence compiled to show a decreased incidence of smoking. However, reports from a mail survey showed that 70% to 80% had made a decision to stop smoking.

Alternative school movement

In the past 10 years the enormous growth of the alternative school movement has occurred and is illustrative of a procedure that has been attempted to provide more meaningful, self-satisfying, and motivating education for young people. The types of schools that have emerged are:

1. Open schools—individual and learning organized around interest centers in class or a building
2. Schools - without - walls — Philadelphia Parkway's program (Chapter 9)
3. Learning centers—concentrated in one location and available to all students in the community, e.g., magnet schools, career-education centers, vocational and technical schools
4. Continuation schools—drop-out centers, reentry programs, pregnancy-

maternity centers, evening and adult schools, street academies

5. Multicultural schools—bilingual, with open enrollment
6. Free schools—greater freedom for teachers and pupils; nonpublic alternative schools
7. Schools-within-schools—mini-schools, satellite schools; may be related to other six types previously mentioned

These schools generally provide options for students, parents, and teachers; are committed to be more responsive to student needs; have a more comprehensive set of goals and objectives; are more flexible and more responsive to change; are more humane to students and teachers; and have fewer rules and bureaucratic restraints.

Deal[5] reported on a study of two high schools in California in which the alternative approach had problems with implementation. The difficulties arose because both teachers and students were unable to cope with the change from one of authoritative control to one of unlimited freedom. At first, great enthusiasm was exhibited on the part of everyone, but after a while, gloom and dissatisfaction developed. Chaos seemed to be the rule and the procedure whereby every policy decision had to have a democratic consensus was traumatic. The conclusion was that success was possible but an organizational design needed to be established that would facilitate rather than impede educational goals.

The Brown School, Louisville, Kentucky. This open school has a multicultural curriculum developed around learning centers within the school and learning activities in the community. Students assume greater responsibility for their own learning. Many classes are nongraded. The high school curriculum is problem-centered.

St. Paul Public Schools, St. Paul, Minnesota. This school system has developed a network of learning centers that provide for the voluntary integration of students and offer the following educational opportunities: automotive, aesthetic, foreign language, elementary career, black minority culture, resource laboratory, and others.

New York City schools. Two programs for addicts are operative, each of which is an innovative approach to education. One deals with the addict in a special school setting; the other works with established treatment facilities.

Alpha School, a special public school, seeks to rehabilitate former addicts while they continue their high school education. It is located in a two-story former milk plant and houses sixty students, most of whom were high school drop-outs. Students spend 1 year at this school, take equivalent high school work, and receive intensive counseling before returning to their regular schools. Once back in their own schools these students are expected to help counsel their peers about drug use.

An extensive project exists whereby programs leading to a high school equivalency diploma are available within the city's narcotic treatment centers, including Daytop Village, Odyssey House, Lagos, city hospitals, and prisons. The program includes remedial reading, mathematics, counseling toward returning to school, a "college discovery" project, vocational guidance aimed at developing salable skills, and help with obtaining jobs after rehabilitation.

• • •

Other approaches to adjustment include the Opportunity School in San Francisco, Project Community in Berkeley, California (Dr. William Soskin, director), and the Summerhill School in England. These schools do not focus on drug problems and drop-outs, although they are probably acquiring many drug-involved students. Rather they try to provide a meaningful, interesting, stimulating, functional type of education. The atmosphere is freer; there are no rigid dress codes and the importance of time schedules and attendance is minimized or eliminated. Teachers are not looked upon as authoritarians but as facilitators of education. Programs are tailored for individual differences and interests and often dove-tail employment opportunities. Much use is made of the community. In a sense, these are schools without walls. Informal and open discussions on any world topics or social programs are possible. Thus the attempt is not to deal with drugs per se, but with individuals and their needs.

SUMMARY

In summary, three essential points are significant:

1. Identification of student drug misusers and abusers is not a simple procedure. Where recurrent signs and symptoms appear, pupils should be referred to physicians or clinical experts thoroughly familiar with the pharmacology of drugs for assistance.
2. Schools should provide one or more individuals who communicate easily with students and especially with drug misusers and abusers.
3. Help to students with drug problems includes knowledge of the community resources and adjustment of school programs.

REFERENCES

1. Blum, R. H., and others: Drug education: results and recommendations, Lexington, Mass., 1976, Lexington Books.
2. Blum, R. H., and others: Horatio Alger's children, San Francisco, 1972, Jossey-Bass, Inc. Publishers.
3. Bowen, H., and Schroeder, W.: Drug abuse handbook, Campbell, Calif., 1970, Campbell Union High School District.
4. Cohen, A. Y.: Decisions about drugs, paper presented in Juneau, Alaska, 1970.
5. Deal, T. S.: Why alternative high schools failed, Stanford, Calif., March, 1975, Stanford University.
6. Dorsey, D., and Silverman, M.: Counseling of students who use drugs, Calif. Sch. Health 4:15-20, 1968.
7. Drug abuse: a reference for teachers, Trenton, 1969, New Jersey State Department of Education.
8. Drug Abuse Council: Drug abuse control: administrative guidelines, Los Angeles, 1970, Los Angeles City Schools.
9. Drug abuse: escape to nowhere, Philadelphia, 1967, American Association for Health, Physical Education, and Recreation, and Smith, Kline & French Laboratories.
10. Drug crisis: schools fight back with innovative programs, Washington, D.C., 1971, National School Public Relations Association.
11. Drug education handbook, Denver, 1970, Alcoholism and Drug Dependence Division, Colorado Department of Health.
12. Drug education in Maine, Augusta, 1970, Maine State Department of Education.
13. Dyer, W., and Vriend, J.: Understanding and counseling the chronic drug user, J. Drug Educ. 5:23-35, 1975.
14. Frykman, J. H.: A new connection: an approach to persons involved in compulsive drug use, San Francisco, 1971, Scrimshaw Press.
15. Guber, B.: Management of students suspected to be under the influence of drugs, Calif. Sch. Health 4:9-11, 1969.
16. Helm, S. T.: Predisposition to alcoholism. In Resource book for drug abuse education, Chevy Chase, Md., 1969, National Institute of Mental Health, National Clearinghouse for Mental Health Information.
17. Hubbard, H.: Drug treatment and prevention: Hope House Inc., Albany, N.Y., N.A.S.S.P. Bull. 54:95-105, 1970.
18. Jessor, R., and Jessor, S. L.: Adolescent development and the onset of drinking; a longitudinal study, Institute of Behavior Science, University of Colorado, May, 1974 (Monograph).
19. Johnson, B. D.: Marijuana users and subcultures, New York, 1973, John Wiley & Sons, Inc.
20. Jorgensen, J.: An alternative to suspension for smoking, Phi Delta Kappan 57:549, 1976.
21. Land, H. W.: How a parent can teach his child about drugs, Today's Health 49:42-45, 1971.
22. Land, H. W.: What you can do about drugs and your child, New York, 1969, Hart Publishing Co., Inc.
23. Laufer, M. W.: Medications, learning and behavior, Phi Delta Kappan 52:169-170, 1970.
24. Leviton, D.: Crisis intervention by the health educator, Sch. Health Rev. 1:22-36, 1970.
25. Miller, C. M.: Crisis intervention and health counseling: an overview, Sch. Health Rev. 1:15-17, 1970.
26. Montgomery County Mental Health Association: A county mental health association's hotline, Sch. Health Rev. 1:27-30, 1970.
27. Moorehead, C.: Drug inspections welcomed, Times Educ. Suppl. 2900:5, 1970.
28. National Institute of Drug Abuse: A catalogue of alternatives for young Americans, Rockville, Md., 1975, Prevention Branch, Alcohol, Drug Abuse, and Mental Health Administration, Department of Health, Education, and Welfare.
29. Pavey, S.: Crisis intervention by the counseling psychologist, Sch. Health Rev. 1:18-21, 1970.
30. Robins, L. N., and Guze, S. B.: Drinking practices and problems in urban ghetto populations. In Department of Health, Education and Welfare: Recent advances in studies in alcoholism, Washington, D.C., 1972, U.S. Government Printing Office.
31. School board policies on drug education and drug use, Waterford, Conn., 1971, National School Boards Association.
32. Seccombe, W.: Illusionogenic crisis and effective intervention, Int. J. Addictions 8:11-14, 1971.
33. Smith, D. E., and Bentel, D. J.: Drug Abuse Information Project, Fourth Annual Report to the Legis-

lature, San Francisco, 1970, University of California, San Francisco Medical Center.

34. Smith, G. M.: Rebellious behavior predicts drug use, reported in the Social Seminar Newsletter SCAN, July, 1973.

35. Smith, V. H.: Alternative schools: the development of options in public education, Lincoln, Neb., 1974, Professional Educators Publications, Inc.

36. A teacher resource guide for drug use and abuse, Lansing, 1970, Michigan State Department of Education.

37. Teacher's resource guide on drug abuse, Harrisburg, 1969, Division of Public Health Education, Pennsylvania Department of Health.

38. Ungerleider, J. T., and Bowen, H. L.: Drug abuse and the schools, Am. J. Psychiatry **125**:105-111, 1969.

39. The voluntary health agency, Sch. Health Rev. **1**:36, 1970.

40. Winston, S. L.: Drug counseling: a workshop with a purpose, Clearing House **44**:227-228, 1969.

9

School atmosphere

Some teachers are great. . . . They put bandages on my hurts—on my heart, on my mind, on my spirit. Those teachers cared about me, and let me know it. They gave me wings.

THOUGHTS OF A DROP-OUT[31]

Educational effectiveness is directly related to the atmosphere found in schools. How well students learn is not solely dependent on the imparting of factual information nor on the physical aspects of the environment, such as textbooks, resources, and buildings. Hartman[33] says learning involves the perceptions, interests, and feelings of learners. Thus any educational institution must consider the social-emotional aspects and the attitudes and interactions of students, teachers, parents, and others. The climate and the learning that takes place in schools are affected by how people feel, believe, and value as well as how people treat each other. People must be concerned with individuals and not just subject matter. School personnel should treat students with kindness and humaneness. Borton adds, "I believe that what a student learns in school, and what he eventually becomes are significantly influenced by how he feels about himself and the world outside."[2]

What happens inside people and is not readily apparent in tangible form but is reflected in people's attitudes may truly be a reflection of the school climate or the school atmosphere. School personnel must really care about students in order to provide security, happiness, independence, individuality, freedom to make decisions, interest, desire to learn, equality of opportunity, freedom from bias and prejudice, fair and just actions, and involvement. Smith and Luce[44] best describe this atmosphere in the title of their book, *Love Needs Care*. They say we need to care about people to provide love. Glasser[15] says that schools must not only become more personally involved with students but they must (1) emphasize thinking over memorization and must have success with less failure; (2) provide a curriculum relevant to children's needs outside of school; and (3) help young people assume responsibilities for their own behavior. In essence, schools must be concerned with developing the attitudes, feelings, and behaviors of their students. The school climate may contribute to or detract from the achievement of this goal.

The atmosphere found in schools in the United States today is best reflected in the selected statements that follow. Glines has said: "Present conventional schools are the most inhumane institutions in America. They closely rival the prisons; the only difference is that after 3:00 P.M. and on weekends we let the prisoners escape."[16]

The National School Public Relations Association reports a comment made in the *Washington Post* by Terry Beresford on the school

244

situation: "A rigid and outdated public school system in which students are treated with distrust and often with hostility helps create for youth a climate in which escapism, rebelliousness, defiance of rules and risk-taking—all typical adolescent behavior—are given added appeal, and drug use becomes a kind of rite of initiation for passage out of childhood or out of the established order."[8] The National School Public Relations Association also claims: ". . . majority of youth are bored with their education and find schools neither meaningful nor exciting."[8] Dearden quotes this remark as having been made by a student: "Teachers seem more interested in whether we chew gum, sit in our assigned seats, or have sideburns, than they do in relating to us as human beings and students."[6]

If these comments are representative of the school atmosphere, they provide some clues to why many youth are bored with schools and with education. They provide leads to the reasons for student unrest. The lack of meaningful and challenging education as well as the overly conforming and constricting nature of many schools may be factors contributing to youth's disenchantment and encouraging them to seek escape through the use of drugs. Providing a school climate conducive to the greatest learning and helpful in reaching some of the root causes of drug misuse and abuse depends on these three factors: (1) student alienation and unrest, (2) physical and psychological needs of pupils, and (3) humaneness in the school.

STUDENT ALIENATION AND UNREST

Numerous young people have feelings of disaffection for the school, the home, and the community. Alienation with and unrest in society exists among many junior high and high school students. Although the extent of student alienation and unrest is not known today, it has occurred with sufficient frequency and intensity to warrant attention and study. It may provide clues to the drug problem.

Alienation has various meanings but herein it refers to the reaction to, and even the rejection of, the accepted values, goals, and institutions that have normally been characteristic of America as youth attempt to find self-identity. Such feelings result in disenchantment, dissatisfaction, and unhappiness with programs, teachers, parents, and social conditions, and lead to unrest and possibly rebellion among some young people.

The problems of alienation and unrest involve psychological, social, and possibly spiritual and ideological factors that affect youth. King[24] writes that Erikson says the major psychological task of the adolescent is to form a stable identity so that he can successfully pass into adulthood. The conditions for this transition to take place, for the adolescent to find this identity, can occur if (1) there exist meaningful adult roles—the greater the number found in a meaningful social context the smoother the transition is likely to be; (2) there are clearly defined transition points, or social activities, to facilitate the transition; and (3) there is stability and consensus about the value system of society—it must provide acceptable answers to the questions: Why am I here? What meaning is there to my life? How do I relate to others? Where am I going after death? Such questions have spiritual overtones and applications.

The transition of youth through adolescence is likely to be crisis oriented and to lead to upheaval and rebellion, depending on the stability of the existing social conditions. Today the social structure is undergoing a variety of changes and modifications, including shifts in political power, the explosion of knowledge, the economic structure, the family organization, the availability of increased leisure time, and the value system. In addition, there is considerable confusion and fuzziness regarding how society expects youth to behave in the adult role.

Not all students feel a sense of crisis. The majority are able to adapt to the changing conditions and to make the transition into adulthood. However, attention must be given to those who are unable to meet the situation easily, to those who encounter problems, and to those who turn to a magical solution to life's problems through the use of drugs.

The social changes taking place in this world are challenging the military complex and war, the establishment and its bureaucracy, big business and its control over man, the dichotomy of affluence and poverty in the world, technology and its destruction of nature and man, materialism and secularism, the political system, intellectualism and the knowledge explosion, prejudice and bias, inequality, civil rights, and other values. Young people have discovered that their lives have been outlined and determined by others rather than by their own experiences, their own self-searching, and their own listening to life. They desire opportunities to experience life on their own and to be free to make decisions and changes by themselves. They do not wish to have everything programmed in a prescribed curriculum or predetermined by schools, parents, or society. They desire and need opportunities to grow up by themselves, to act responsibly, to work closely with seriously concerned adults, and to participate in other meaningful ways.

The problem of alienation has existed for a long time among the impoverished, the minorities, and the rejected. However, the present alienation is coming from the average, affluent, and adjusted American as well as from the fortunate, talented, and privileged individual. Keniston[23] says the "new" alienation is not the bottom one-third of the population concerned with poverty, exclusion, sickness, oppression, lack of choice, and lack of opportunity; it is found among those who have every possible advantage. Alienation is bound up with the technological society in which we live.

The National School Public Relations Association[8] reports that high school student unrest and protest are related to the following factors:

1. Racial issues and the black student's commitment to the renaissance of his people—demand for more black teachers, guidance counselors, and administrators; recognition of black identity, pride, and culture

2. Dress and grooming regulations—miniskirts and maxilocks
3. School smoking rules and the cafeteria
4. Censorship and regulation of school papers, the scheduling of sporting events, and social events at school
5. Lack of student voice in rule-making and in determining school policies and curriculum
6. The open versus the closed campus
7. Need for new student organizations
8. Dissatisfaction with the school program and personnel—teachers who neither like their jobs nor students; worthless counseling programs; lack of relevant curriculum; class groupings; grades; examinations; homework
9. Staff members who contribute to unrest by
   a. Tending to talk rather than listen
   b. Imposing primarily white, Anglo-Saxon value systems on students
   c. Tending to overemphasize rules, regulations, and other rigid controls
   d. Seeing pupils not as individuals but as groups
   e. Tending to "turn-off" students who display deviant behavior in terms of class performance, grooming, and dress
   f. Locking students into categories of ability or aptitude
   g. Tending to convey through a look, tone of voice, or gesture "silent contempt" for some deviant characteristic of the student

Wynne[48] claims student unrest is not only the product of war, poor teaching, racism, and poverty. He has additionally identified the following reasons:

1. Diminishing work experience—students remaining in school longer than at any period of history and hence having little contract with adults except those in the immediate family
2. Increase in suburban living, resulting in reduced contacts among intergeneration people
3. Development of shopping centers; advent of modern transportation resulting

in fathers going farther away to work and children having less contact with fathers or perhaps not even knowing what father does

4. Diminishing of the extended family such as grandparents, uncles, aunts, and the like, resulting in less contact with sympathetic adults

It should be evident that the school atmosphere is not the only factor contributing to student alienation and unrest but is one of several social forces that can have a definite effect on pupil behavior. Undoubtedly it is one of the contributing causes of the use and misuse of drugs. The school atmosphere is directly related to effective learning. Keniston[22] states that the type of student who is prone to use drugs is the "disaffiliate," the one who rejects the prevalent American values. Kohn and Mercer[25] support this view, saying that drug use and the attitudes toward drug use may be related to a left-right, rebellious-authoritarian dimension of sociopolitical ideology. These same authorities report similar findings by Zinberg, McGlothin, Blum, Geber, and Suchman, who indicate a greater tendency to drug use among student political activists, those opposed to restrictions on individual freedom, those exhibiting sociocultural alienation, individuals who are rebellious to authority, those opposed to parents, and individuals who reject conventional values.

Gottlieb[18] says the use of drugs is not only an attempt at personal adjustment but also a personal reaction to maladjustment. He reasons that the poor have always been discriminated against and have had difficulty in achieving economic and familial stability. Therefore delinquency and drugs are a part of life for the poor because such people are born to pessimism, futility, mistrust, negativism, and quick pleasures. Thus the young ghetto person turns to drugs to get away from unpleasant reality.

According to Keniston[23] these signs help to identify the alienated outlook of students:

1. A distrust of commitment—rejection of the American culture, rejection of group activities, realization of the futility of civic and political activities, a hesitancy to act

2. A pessimistic existential viewpoint—future looks dark and unclear, anxiety about the world, belief that meaning can only be created by the individual, finding it impossible to communicate, belief in the universe as chaotic, unstructured, and meaningless

3. Showing anger, scorn, and contempt

4. Quests for the esthetic—desiring awareness experience, living for today, interested in self-expression, creativity, passion, emotion, and feeling, being a social outsider

PHYSICAL AND PSYCHOLOGICAL NEEDS

Physical, psychological, or emotional needs of children and youth must be considered in order to provide the most productive school atmosphere. The fulfillment of these wants helps young people develop and maintain a high level of mental health. Chapters 6 and 7 introduced formal and informal educational attention to this important concept. It is necessary to provide understanding of causative factors of the drug problem. Needs play a significant role in the preventive health program. Opportunities must be offered for the fulfillment of these needs if schools are to aid in preventing the misuse and abuse of drugs.

Physical needs include food, air, water, warmth, rest, sleep, clothing, and freedom from disease and from other health hazards. Schools may find it advisable to provide free breakfasts and lunches for needy students, to maintain a comfortable and safe environment, to establish procedures to protect, maintain, and promote the health of their students, and to prepare rest and relaxation facilities and activities for those needing such relief. These actions are not meant to replace the functions or responsibilities of the home or the family as the primary sources of such need fulfillment, but rather to assist in a complementary capacity. When the home is unable to supply adequate food, clothing, or sleeping quarters, the school may find it necessary to help care for these student wants, especially in the inner city areas. The school acts in loco parentis and has both a legal and a moral responsibility to utilize its resources in helping to satisfy the physical needs of pupils and to assist in the improvement of learning.

More importantly perhaps, and more complex to satisfy in schools, are the psychological or emotional needs.[4] These provide children with the feeling of self-worth, self-esteem, or self-image that is extremely important to personal adjustment. They generally include the following:

1. Affection—love
2. Security—to belong, to have roots, to have protection
3. Acceptance as an individual—free of prejudice and bias, concerned about individual differences
4. Achievement—success experiences, recognition; schools with "less failures" concepts
5. Independence—to be a creative and developing person, to be on one's own, to act under one's own guidance and direction, to make decisions, to be self-expressive
6. Authority—guidance and direction by adults
7. Self-respect—courteous, fair, and just treatment

Failure on the part of the students to adequately satisfy their physical and emotional needs may result in deviant behavior. Psychological and social maladjustments in children and youth may occur and may be manifested in behavior contrary to normal. Such social-emotional disturbances may exhibit themselves in terms of:

1. Overtimidity—withdrawing, crying easily
2. Overaggressiveness—bullying, quarreling, boisterousness
3. Excessive daydreaming—persistent inattentiveness
4. Excessive boasting or showing off
5. Poor sportsmanship
6. Undue restlessness—habit tics, stammering, nail-biting

7. Frequent accidents or near-accidents
8. Abnormal sex behavior
9. Difficulty in reading or reciting
10. Failure to advance in school at normal rate
11. Stuttering or other forms of difficulty
12. Lying, stealing, cheating
13. Resistance to authority, constant complaints of unfairness
14. Unhappiness and depression
15. Gradual deterioration and marked sudden drop in educational achievement
16. Lack of interest or motivation
17. Constantly seeking attention or popularity

Glasser[14] says identity is related to the psychological wants of individuals and is a basic human need. If a child cannot find success identity, he will follow the pathway to failure identity. Therefore the deviations previously identified may not have serious implications when they first appear, but if they persist could become significant problems. The individual will be hampered in achieving the identity necessary to attain the psychological maturity needed in adulthood.

In speaking of needs Maslow[30] places human needs in a hierarchy. At the bottom, he says, are the physiological needs (hunger, thirst). Next are the safety needs, followed by love, affection, and belonging, then personal esteem, and finally self-actualization. Self-actualization refers to becoming what one is capable of becoming. Maslow states that needs at the lower levels must be satisfied before higher needs emerge. Hence few people achieve self-actualization.

Blum[3] and others in Chapter 8 provided evidence to support relationships between the use of drugs and student maladjustments. Schools, and especially teachers, must therefore make efforts to prevent such deviant conditions from occurring by providing an environment where young people feel secure, wanted, and loved, experience success, are treated fairly and justly without bias and prejudice, are involved, and are free to express themselves openly. Teachers should observe signs and symptoms of abnormal behavior as previously described and be aware of the appropriate action to take if such signs appear. The instructional program must be motivating and meaningful, and the school must engage teachers and counselors who are interested in children and youth. This kind of a school atmosphere is necessary to provide the help needed to attain emotional maturity so that students can acquire a high level of mental health and thus be able to cope with the problems of society. Such an atmosphere will help divert young people from seeking escape through the drug scene.

CREATING HUMANENESS IN SCHOOLS

"A commitment to humanism calls for a shift in thinking from self to learner . . . to be less concerned with what we do and much more concerned with what happens in the hearts and minds of those we do things to."[33] A spiritual, ideological concept involving a moral issue and relating to learning and the learning process is emerging. It is being labeled "humanism" or "humaneness" and is an important part of the school atmosphere. Humaneness has special significance because of its relationships to preventing student maladjustments and in turn to drug misuse and abuse. The humaneness need has resulted from the many rapid changes that have been and are taking place in society, including technology, science, and the knowledge explosion. A series of important questions have been raised in education regarding the nature of educational goals and of the process used to achieve such goals. Junell asks, "Is rational man our first priority? Have we placed too much faith in the power of the intellect, while tragically disregarding humane values? Does public education owe its responsibility to the intellectual-academic world, or to the emotional-social one?"[21] René Dubos[26] has said that science alone cannot be trusted to determine the future of man and his civilization. Krutch[26] has remarked that science cannot make value judgements and therefore can tell us only what can be done, never what we ought to do. Foshay queries, "Is the function of the schools to

make a citizen or to serve the person, to make a man?"[39] He adds that social criteria are necessary but not sufficient for humane purposes.

Humaneness or humanism has not been clearly defined in the literature and therefore has a variety of meanings. Some of the key words used to express the term include trust, self-reliance, options, human relationships, freedom, justice, equality, alternatives, values, self-reliance, friendship, and decision making. Foshay[39] has said it is to pursue humane ends in a human form. Combs[39] refers to humane people as those concerned with the feelings, beliefs, values, attitudes, and understandings of others. When humaneness is applied to learning or to education, Maslow[30] refers to it as self-actualization, achievement of those interests that are uppermost in the hierarchy of needs. He believes that we live by our personal commitments, from which the individual derives a value system that motivates his behavior. Learning therefore is related directly to the learner. What actually takes place stems from a person's own innovations, interests, and commitments, which are internal. The emphasis on the educational process, therefore, should be to make learning become self-directed. Achievement of self-directed learning is dependent on the human atmosphere in classrooms and in the school. This atmosphere includes tolerance, friendliness, respect for the individual, freedom of choice, self-expression, decision making, and other such considerations.

The basic goal of humanism in education is to make learning so interesting that the student will say, "I want to go to school." It becomes the teacher's role to aid the student in the search, or achievement, of self-actualization. Thus the student seeks to identify himself and to become a unique entity. To achieve this, teachers must constantly help the student increase the understanding about his feelings and attitudes and aid him in the expansion of his self-awareness. It is clear that self-awareness requires help from the teacher, especially through interpersonal relationships and communications. The process of bringing about self-valuing is referred to as creating humaneness in schools.

There is no magic formula to apply in developing the concept of humaneness in schools, but perhaps the suggestions that follow will provide specific ideas that teachers, administrators, and others may find stimulating and useful:

1. Maximize individual learning through recognition of individual differences in terms of uniqueness, potential, and achievement by providing opportunities for self-direction and self-management, by allowing for independent student and individual progress, and by creating special programs and curricula—Head Start, Upward Bound, and others.

2. Encourage and increase student involvement in the educational process through their participation in curriculum development, surveys, evaluation, development of policies, and open-forum discussions, through encouraging freedom of expression and choice, and in other ways.

3. Make the curriculum, instruction, and experiences meaningful and relevant to the needs of the student and of society. Permit flexibility of subject matter, including discussion of controversial areas.

4. Prepare instructional objectives in behavioral terms that deemphasize the mere acquisition of factual information.

5. In the instructional program, efforts should be made to make success inevitable.

6. Grades and grading procedures should become noncompetitive and noncomparative in order to reduce the pressures that arise. Instead consideration should be given to nongrading techniques based on individual evaluation methods and utilizing performance criteria.

7. Permit and encourage openness in classrooms, including freedom of expression, experiences, choices, and a variety of alternative opinions or data to make student decisions possible.

8. Teachers should try to act humanely in all relationships with students. They should express the feelings and attitudes of joy, anger, laughter, and sadness that anyone would experience. Students should be ac-

cepted as they are and not as someone wishes them to be. Tolerance should be exercised in terms of dress, appearance, errors, ability, and achievement.

9. School personnel should develop trust in students as individuals. They should show interest in their pupils and should be understanding. They should treat students honestly, fairly, justly, and without bias or prejudice.

10. Encourage increased and improved communications between school personnel and students. Administrators might tour the buildings more frequently and talk with students. Teachers might have lunch with pupils on occasion.

11. Students should be listened to more frequently and more intently. When listening, school personnel should do so with interest, making no attempt at judgments or evaluations. They should listen for positive thoughts rather than disagreements and for the general ideas expressed rather than the details.

12. In junior and senior high schools flexible class scheduling may be used.

13. Disciplinary procedures should be reviewed in terms of their intent. Are they punitive or are they in the best interest of the students?

14. Teachers need to be involved to a greater extent in school affairs and should have opportunities for freedom of expression and decision making regarding curriculum, instructional practices, and other procedures.

15. The atmosphere of the school should be open for both teachers and students; freedoms should be given every consideration and the climate should be one of warmth, friendliness, and security.

Special humane consideration must be given to the poor minority and inner-city children and youth who attend schools. Washington states: "Too often deprived children encounter in the school an institution out of touch with the reality they know. All too often such factors diminish rather than enlarge the child's view of himself and his world. Children learn not what they are told but what they experience. The child who is hostile, insecure, and unsuccessful needs to know adults who are secure, successful and free of hostility."[39] She further says that the student who comes to school with the frustration and unappeased physical and emotional needs found in a life of poverty and often compounded by prejudice expects the same rejection that he has learned from society. Educators therefore must develop approaches to these compelling needs, especially for the poor minority youth.

These hypotheses for teacher-student-group relationships need consideration:
1. The student self-concept is a significant factor in his ability to learn.
2. The student must be valued as an individual.
3. Every child wants to succeed.
4. The student's belief in himself must be nutured if he is to grow emotionally and intellectually.
5. True learning will take place only if the student is an involved participant in the process.
6. The power structure and the learning situation must be understood and used to advantage because the child needs both the support of peers and the opportunity to differentiate himself from others.

However, to implement the suggestions identified will involve radical changes in schools today. That such changes are possible may be demonstrated in the very liberal approach to the application of the concept of humaneness found in four schools and one school district. Broad provision is made for freedom of thought and action, with the goal being that students will achieve self-actualizations toward learning. These attempts focus on the belief by certain authorities that schools need not have walls. The development of alternative education and activities described in Chapters 6, 7, and 8 are outgrowths of modifications needed in school curriculums. These illustrations may be especially useful among minority youths, drop-outs, and those in deprived areas. Drug abusers could profit by experiences in these schools.

The Summerhill School in England is a small, private institution that has no requirements, rules, homework, regulation, roll-taking, grades, texts, or social conventions.[10] The theory behind this approach is that a free child is a happy child and eventually becomes a responsible child. There is the feeling that true discipline comes from the self.

The Benjamin Franklin Parkway High School in Philadelphia comprises 60% black and 40% white students and also stresses much freedom and individual initiative.[19] It is a school that apparently has no schoolhouse. It says its place of learning is anywhere and everywhere. Students may be admitted with parental consent simply by showing interest. The students must meet the same requirements for graduation as in any other city school. The emphasis in the school is on making students self-reliant, self-directed, and responsible individuals who will be worthwhile members of society. The students are placed in groups of 15 with one full-time faculty member assigned to each group. The humanistic atmosphere is one of tolerance, friendliness, optional dress (no codes), with teachers and students on a first-name basis, attendance optional, people accepted as they are, no grades, no rigid requirements, no competitiveness, smoking permitted, no strict authority or discipline, and no limits on personal freedom. Students and faculty discuss together what they want to know, or learn, and teachers explain to students what they need to know. Teachers write evaluations of students' work but give no grades.

The Wilson School in Mankato, Minnesota, reaches students from ages 3 to 19 and has tried to develop a humane school.[16] It operates under these main provisions: students choose their own instructors, select their own adviser-counselors, plan their own course of study through individual conferences, have no required classes, follow an open-campus policy, may go home if nothing interesting is being offered because attendance is optional, have no established number of courses to take or required length of time to complete them, and are evaluated in terms of learning objectives through conferences with instructors and parents. The program is individually diagnosed and prescribed for each student but there are no graduation requirements. Also, students are encouraged to take as much work outside the school as possible, including trips with parents, work in local governments and in hospitals, and other experiences.

New York City has used the so-called "street academy" approach to attract dropouts or push-outs from their schools. This involves a three-tiered, privately funded and controlled school system that is geared to meet immediate and long-range needs of students. Thirteen street academies have been organized in which small groups of students meet with several teachers and streetworkers in storefront centers to study everything from Eldridge Cleaver to Plato. The pace and curriculum are set by the teachers and students according to the specific needs and interests of the individuals. Harlem Prep, on the third tier, offers a college preparatory program.

•   •   •

In summary, it should be evident that the school atmosphere may play a significant role in the drug misuse and abuse problems of those students prone to abuse drugs; the atmosphere is important in facilitating effective learning. To help prevent drug difficulties and to obtain the best results from the learning process, it is important that schools be cognizant of (1) the reasons for student alienation and unrest, (2) the physical and psychological needs of pupils, and (3) the significance of creating humane schools. The data reveal that there is much work ahead if schools are to develop the atmosphere necessary for student self-actualization in self-directed learning. When students in large numbers, including drop-outs and other nonachievers, begin to say, "I want to go to school," such a goal will show evidence of realization.

REFERENCES

1. Alschuler, A. S.: Humanistic education, Educ. Technol. 10:58-61, 1970.
2. Borton, T.: Reach, touch and teach: student concerns and process education, New York, 1970, McGraw-Hill Book Co., Inc.
3. Blum, R. H., and others: Horatio Alger's children, San Francisco, 1972, Jossey-Bass, Inc., Publishers.
4. Cornacchia, H. J., and others: Health in elementary schools, ed. 4, St. Louis, 1974, The C. V. Mosby Co.
5. Dearden, M. H.: Adolescent drug abuses—a problem of interpersonal relations and school organization, J. Drug Educ. 1:205-215, 1971.
6. Dearden, M. H., and Jekal, J. F.: A pilot program in high school drug education utilizing non-directive techniques and sensitivity training, J. Sch. Health 41:118-124, 1971.
7. Dorr, R.: Sensitivity training, Sch. Health Rev. 1:38-40, 1970.
8. Drug crisis: schools fight back with innovative programs, Washington, D.C., 1971, National School Public Relations Association.
9. Education USA Special Report: Individually prescribed instruction, Washington, D.C., 1968, National School Public Relations Association.
10. Emery, R. C.: Existentialism in the classroom, J. Teacher Educ. 22:5-9, 1971.
11. Erikson, E. H.: Identity: youth and crisis, New York, 1968, W. W. Norton & Co., Inc.
12. Frankl, V. E.: Man's search for meaning, New York, 1959, Washington Square Press.
13. Gerzon, M.: The whole world is watching: a young man looks at dissent, New York, 1969, The Viking Press, Inc.
14. Glasser, W.: The effect of school failure on the life of a child. In National Association of Elementary School Principals: The elementary school: humanizing? dehumanizing?, Washington, D.C., 1971, National Education Association.
15. Glasser, W.: Schools without failure, New York, 1969, Harper & Row, Publishers.
16. Glines, D. E.: Creating humane schools, Mankato, Minn., 1971, Campus Publishers.
17. Goodman, P.: High school is too much, Psychol. Today 4:25-26, 1970.
18. Gottlieb, D.: Alienation and rebellion among the disadvantaged, Paper presented at the fourteenth Annual Conference of Mental Health Representatives of State Medical Societies, sponsored by the American Medical Association Council on Mental Health, Chicago, March 15, 1968.
19. Greenberg, J. D., and Roush, R. E.: A visit to the "school without walls," Phi Delta Kappan 51:480-484, 1970.
20. High school student unrest, Washington, D.C., 1969, National School Public Relations Association.
21. Junell, J. S.: Is rational man our first priority? Phi Delta Kappan 52:147-151, 1970.

22. Keniston, K.: Drug use and student values, Paper presented at the National Association of Student Personnel Administrators Drug Education Conference, Washington, D.C., November, 1966.
23. Keniston, K.: The uncommitted: alienated youth in American society, New York, 1965, Dell Publishing Co., Inc.
24. King, S. H.: Youth and society, Paper presented at the Annual Convention, National Congress of Parents and Teachers, San Diego, Calif., May 21, 1968.
25. Kohn, P. M., and Mercer, G. W.: Drug use, drug-use attitudes, and the authoritarianism-rebellion dimension, J. Health Soc. Behav. 12:125-131, 1971.
26. Krutch, J. W.: A humanist's approach, Phi Delta Kappan 51:376-378, 1970.
27. Lee, W. S.: Human relations training for teachers: the effectiveness of sensitivity training, Calif. J. Educ. Res. 21:28-34, 1970.
28. Levy, N. J.: The use of drugs by teenagers for sanctuary and illusion, Paper presented at the symposium on *Our Youth: Apathy, Rebellion and Growth* at the Carnegie Endowment International Center, New York, November 12, 1966.
29. Malcolm, A.: Drug abuse and social alienation, Today's Educ. 59:28-31, 1970.
30. Maslow, A. A.: Motivation and personality, New York, 1954, Harper & Row, Publishers.
31. McLeod, A.: Growing up in America: a background to contemporary drug abuse, Rockville, Md., 1973, National Institute of Mental Health.
32. Meeds, L.: Drug abuse as a reaction to the stresses of growing up, Sch. Health Rev. 1:3-5, 1970.
33. Moustakas, C.: Personal growth: the struggle for identity and human values, Cambridge, Mass., 1969, Howard A. Doyle Publishing Co.
34. National Association of Elementary School Principals: The elementary school: humanizing? dehumanizing? Washington, D.C., 1971, National Education Association.
35. Prettyman, R. L., and others: Drug abuse and the school scene, Sci. Teacher 35:45-47, 1970.
36. Protest in the sixties, Ann. Am. Acad. Polit. Soc. Sci. vol. 382, March, 1969.
37. Randolph, N., and Howe, W.: Self-enhancing education: a program to motivate learners, Palo Alto, Calif., 1966, Sanford Press.
38. Roszak, T.: The making of a counter culture, Garden City, N.Y., 1969, Anchor Books.
39. Scoby, M. M., and Graham, G., editors: To nurture humaneness: commitment for the 70's, Washington, D.C., 1970, Association for Supervision and Curriculum Development.
40. Siberman, C. E.: Crisis in the classroom: the remaking of American education, New York, 1970, Random House, Inc.
41. Simmons, J. L., and Winograd, B.: It's happening: a portrait of the youth scene today, Santa Barbara, Calif., 1966, Marc-Laird Publications.
42. Simon, S., and others: The day the consultant looked at our grading system, Phi Delta Kappan 51:476-479, 1970.
43. Small, G. R.: Humanism in education, Clearing House 43:195-197, 1968.
44. Smith, D. E., and Luce, J.: Love needs care, Boston, 1970, Little, Brown & Co.
45. Suchman, E. A.: The hang-loose ethic and the spirit of drug use, J. Health Soc. Behav. 9:146-155, 1968.
46. Wertheimer, P. A.: School climate and student learning, Phi Delta Kappan 52:527-530, 1971.
47. Wright, T. H.: Learning to listen: a teacher's or a student's problem? Phi Delta Kappan 52:625-628, 1971.
48. Wynne, E.: Student unrest re-examined, Phi Delta Kappan 53:102-104, 1971.
49. Yablonsky, L.: The hippie trip, New York, 1969, Pegasus.
50. Yearbook 1966: learning and mental health in school, Washington, D.C., 1966, Association for Supervision and Curriculum Development.
51. Yolles, S. F.: Prevention of drug abuse. In Resource book for drug abuse education, Chevy Chase, Md., 1969, National Institute of Mental Health, National Clearinghouse for Mental Health Information.

10

Coordination of the school drug program

For the school drug program to function efficiently, the segments—education, services, and atmosphere—must be coordinated. Interrelationships that exist between the segments must be clarified and an administrative organization must be established in order to mold the various aspects of the program into a smoothly functioning, effective operation that will have impact on children and youth. Thus coordination as herein described will refer to (1) resolving administrative problems, (2) establishing the administrative organizational structure, (3) developing policies and procedures, (4) financing the program, and (5) providing in-service preparation.

Although this chapter will focus primarily on matters relating to local schools and school districts, a number of problems and matters pertaining to national and state activities will also briefly be considered.

ADMINISTRATIVE PROBLEMS

There are a variety of administrative problems in need of attention at the national, state, and local levels in the United States. Several have not been adequately or appropriately answered for a number of years. Such omissions unquestionably are important contributing factors to the failure of drug programs and their lack of impact on young people to date. Without consideration of these issues, the activities for effective drug programs will continue to be unsuccessful.

At the national level, four major problems need attention: (1) coordination of agency efforts to resolve the drug problem, (2) continuing financial support for state programs, (3) improved clarity and implementation approaches of prevention programs, and (4) lack of program evaluation.

1. There is need for the coordination of efforts of the variety of federal agencies. Until the passage of the Drug Abuse Office and Treatment Act of 1972, a number of agencies were independently involved in drug education, treatment, rehabilitation, training, and research programs and were separately funded. The creation of SAODAP (Special Action Office for Drug Abuse Prevention) in 1971 resulted in the appointment of a Special Consultant to the President who had authority over all federal programs and activities, irrespective of the nineteen agencies that ran them. This office was expected to coordinate, evaluate, and help improve services. However, on June 30, 1975, SAODAP ceased to function as a White House Coordinating Agency. Today, the following are the primary agencies involved in the drug problem: The Alcohol, Drug Abuse, and Mental Health Administration (ADAMHA) is an agency of the Public Health Service, U.S. Department of Health, Education and Welfare (DHEW) that renders services in prevention, control, and treatment of alcohol abuse and alcholism, drug abuse, and mental and emotional illness. It is the umbrella organization

of the National Institute on Alcohol Abuse and Alcoholism (NIAAA), the National Institute on Drug Abuse (NIDA), and the National Institute of Mental Health (NIMH). All four of these offices are independently budgeted and operate generally in the same fashion. The Office of Education (OE) is involved in drug education and is part of the DHEW but is not related to ADHAMHA. The Drug Enforcement Administration (DEA) is part of the Department of Justice and is responsible for law enforcement. In addition, there are a number of other agencies participating in drug abuse prevention programs.

2. The adequacy and continuance of federal support to state educational agencies may be crucial if drug education programs are to be maintained and survive. The discontinuance of funds, especially for the Office of Education, has unquestionably caused a number of states to end state level programs, although numerous states have budgeted funds from their own sources for these services. A recent unpublished survey of state drug education coordinators in the United States which we conducted indicated that funds are not prevalent at the federal level and may be diminishing at the state level. In 1975, twenty-seven states allocated funds to state drug education offices that averaged $136,000, with seventeen states having no funds provided. Nine of these states indicated that moneys budgeted were less than those received in 1974, while five states said they had their funds increased.

The funding problem is compounded by a dichotomy of philosophy and action. The Office of Education has been allocated no funds for 1977, yet NIDA advocates primary prevention to be its main focus of activities. In addition, large sums of money are being provided for law enforcement and treatment and rehabilitation, with little or no funds for education. A further complexity to the problem is the allocation of sizeable sums of money in recent years for programs dealing with alcohol and alcoholism.

3. Although the National Institute of Drug Abuse has recently more clearly defined prevention and indicated the importance of primary prevention, the need for further clarity of meaning and the search for effective approaches to implement the definition continues. In addition, the disrepute into which drug education has fallen in recent years because of its cognitive emphasis raises the question of which approach or approaches to follow. NIDA, OE, and numerous authorities have promoted affective education, with little or no cognitive aspects as the strategy to follow. Many programs have been focused in this direction as a result. Yet Schapps[15] and Blum[1] have provided evidence that a combination of information and attitudes may have positive impact on students. Unquestionably there is need for greater experimentation and the development of model programs such as the one outlined in this text before clarity of meaning of prevention and definition of approaches will be known.

4. Increased quantitative and qualitative evaluation programs that address themselves to the impact of programs on young people must be financially supported and actively promoted by federal, state, and local agencies. This matter has not received adequate attention; further information is provided in Chapter 11.

At the state level these problems are the more significant ones in need of attention:

1. The question of the provision of adequate financial and other support for drug education as broadly defined in this volume by the single state drug agencies that have been organized to provide leadership and coordination for the total program (an improvement over the federal arrangement)

2. Whether the five regional training centers provided by the Office of Education at the national level will render adequate preparation of school teams to give the leadership necessary to develop and implement programs

3. The need for special emphasis on the problems of children and youth from the minorities and inner cities continues, despite the inauguration of a number of interesting programs

4. The support for the expansion and implementation of parent training programs
5. The determination of the most effective approaches to be used in schools
6. Difficulties and possible apathy in demonstrating the impact of programs on young people in terms of affective and action goals, as well as cognitive objectives

At the local level these critical administrative factors for program implementation are in need of resolution if effective school drug programs are to emerge:

1. Commitment by school districts to drug programs
2. Delegation of administrative responsibility for programs
3. Determination of school personnel responsibilities and qualifications
4. In-service training of personnel in specific terms (when, how, where, what, who, and funds available)
5. Place of drug education in the curriculum and amount of time to be permitted for it at various grade levels; nature of drug education and the place and time in the formal and informal program in the curriculum
6. Financial support for personnel and resources
7. Role of the school in community action
8. Involvement of students, parents, community organizations, agencies, and other individuals, including the police

ADMINISTRATIVE ORGANIZATION

In order for the administrative problems outlined to receive consideration for resolution and if a school drug program is to have a chance of success, an organizational structure consisting of basically two essentials is necessary. These are (1) somone delegated with the responsibility to direct and conduct the drug program and (2) an advisory drug committee. Such an administrative arrangement is also necessary at federal and state levels.

At the federal level, a variety of agencies have been identified that have been bud-geted funds and have selected directors to provide leadership to develop and conduct programs. Responsibilities and services have been defined, and many such organizations have advisory committees in operation.

At the state level practically all states have appointed a coordinator of drug programs with direct responsibility to the governor. In addition, the receipt of federal funds by state offices of public instruction and the assurance that such funds will be continued for several more years have resulted in the designation of an administrator for drug programs in every state and territory in the United States. Many of the larger states have employed several staff members. In California, drug coordinators have been designated for each county within the state. Although the functions of these leaders vary, they generally include the following:

1. Creating awareness of the problem of drug abuse among school and community personnel
2. Providing in-service training for teachers, administrators, counselors, and parents
3. Curriculum development or implementation or both
4. Coordination with other state agencies
5. Research and development of new techniques and evaluation
6. Providing resource information and materials

Many states have also established advisory committees whose members include other state agencies, teachers, administrators, counselors, students, parents, and a variety of community representatives.

A number of the large school districts in this country are employing administrative personnel, identified as drug coordinators, drug education coordinators, drug program directors, and by other names, on a full-time basis with responsibility for drug programs. The frequency and extent of such action is not known. Where such specialists are found, there may also be a committee, comprising people from the school and from the community, to provide help with the program. Although no established criteria serve as guidelines in the selection of a coordinator, these personal attributes should be sought:

1. Is approachable by students
2. Is able to communicate easily with young people, teachers, and administrators
3. Has the ability to accurately articulate student concerns
4. Has interest in and empathy for children and adolescents
5. Is a good listener
6. Is able to work successfully with others, including community resource and agency personnel
7. Is familiar with the drug scene or is willing to acquire such understanding

No attempt has been made to specify the responsibilities of drug coordinators. However, sufficient information is given here for individual school districts to establish such functions locally.

In Mississippi funds have been provided for drug education specialists for each school district in the state. Qualifications include a teaching certificate, 1 year of teaching, and a 2-week training course. Duties include planning, initiating, and assisting teachers in the alcohol and drug curriculum, serving as a resource person, aiding in the development of peer groups, and supervising in-service programs. The emphasis is on values, self-concept, and decision making.

In the Dade County Schools of Florida, a resource specialist is found in every junior and senior high school to assist teachers in obtaining necessary materials, counseling parents, aiding students to locate rehabilitation agencies, organizing student involvement programs of alternative activities, training students as peer counselors, establishing "rap" rooms, and conducting teacher and parent communication programs.

The establishment of a school drug advisory committee is not only valuable at the federal and state levels but has special significance at the local level. It is usually the motivating force behind programs and serves as the bridge between the schools and the community. The composition of this committee must be determined in each school district, but it should comprise a variety of school and community representatives, including students and parents. Responsibilities will differ, but the following are suggested functions:

1. Help develop procedures for identifying drug users and abusers.
2. Prepare procedures for referral and treatment of students using drugs.
3. Encourage the development of a comprehensive educational program.
4. Aid in efforts to coordinate the school, home, and community.
5. Aid in the development of parent education programs.
6. Support and encourage in-service programs.
7. Help prepare and determine school policies and procedures.
8. Aid in the selection of the drug coordinator.
9. Provide assistance in conducting surveys to determine the extent of the drug problem among students.
10. Assist in the selection of instructional resource materials.
11. Help design procedures for evaluating the drug program.

POLICIES AND PROCEDURES

Schools and school districts need written policies and procedures for the total drug program (education, services, atmosphere, and coordination) that (1) clearly identify the actions that school personnel may take, (2) establish the lines of authority, and (3) determine the responsibilities of all staff members. Without such statements, the boards of education, superintendents of schools, teachers, counselors, and other personnel may be unfairly obligated to handle drug problems when they are not assured of school support or are unclear about what action is to be taken. Cooperative effort on the part of both schools and law enforcement agencies in developing policies is needed if the confusion regarding the handling of students who violate the law and of other related matters is to be clarified.

In the development and implementation of

administrative guidelines, school personnel should consider the students' welfare and positive therapeutic approaches to pupils' problems first rather than turn to punitive solutions. It is most important that schools make the effort to find alternatives to legal action for student drug offenders. It is felt by some that the school's authority and responsibility should be confined to student actions on school property or during regular school-sponsored activities. However, it may be necessary to extend this responsibility to relations with police, probation departments, community organizations, jails, and other agencies as long as the purpose is focused on the education of the individual.

Whenever action is to be taken regarding students, schools should consider each case on its own merit and in regard to the total behavior of the individual. In addition, procedures regarding drugs should be established whereby all avenues for correction and rehabilitation within the school setting are exhausted prior to considering suspension or expulsion. This latter action should be a "last resort," taken only when all possible efforts to help have failed.

The "hard line" approach in dealing with drug users may seriously impair the possibility of meaningful dialogue between students and school personnel regarding drugs. Such a policy undoubtedly leads to distrust, suspicion, and withdrawal by students. It ignores the argument that punishment treats the symptom and not the cause, thereby complicating the problem of rehabilitation. However, school officials agree that pressure must be brought to bear on pushers of drugs, with less severe treatment applied to those students who are only users of drugs.

In all cases involving drugs, the school principal will probably play the major role. Before making a decision, however, he should obtain as much information as possible by consulting with teachers, counselors, nurses, physicians, parents, and friends. The principal is the one who will have to interpret the policy and make adjustments in its application when necessary. This interpretation should be governed by sympathy and understanding so that any action taken will aid in the rehabilitation and continued education of students.

The policies and procedures established by school districts should cover the entire school drug program. More specifically they should include:

1. The educational phase
2. The services phase, identifying drug users and abusers and what to do for abusers in emergencies, crisis intervention situations, students under the influence, and related conditions
3. The school atmosphere and the role of school personnel
4. Coordination of the total program with attention to law violations involving possession, sale, and other matters related to drugs whether they occur on campus or during school-related activities or off campus and not under school supervision but where schools may intervene upon request of parents, the police, or others

Material in Chapters 7 to 9 also provides information that needs to be included in the policies and procedures to be established. The following material additionally considers important student relations as well as the legal and law enforcement aspects of handling students involved in drugs.

Guidelines

These questions, many of which have been developed by the Salinas Union High School District, California, may provide assistance in determining the role of the school in handling students involved with drugs:

1. Must drug or narcotic offenses be committed while the student is under the supervision of the school for school officials to become involved?
2. What is the school's position when drug offenses are committed off campus and not under school supervision?
3. How should schools handle a student who is referred to the office by school personnel because he is under the influence or in possession of a drug or narcotic?
   a. Should the parents be notified by the school?
   b. Are there situations in which the parents may not be notified?
   c. Should juvenile authorities be notified?
   d. Should the school treat the student?

4. How should schools handle a student who voluntarily reports to the office, admits use of a drug or narcotic, and requests assistance with his problem?
   a. Should the parents be contacted if the student objects?
   b. Should juvenile authorities be notified?
5. What standards of evidence should the school use in determining whether a student has wrongfully used, sold, or been in possession of prescribed drugs or narcotics?
   a. Police record?
   b. Probation or court record?
   c. Should the school take action without due process (punitive or protective suspension)?
6. Should the school recommend professional counseling for students identified as drug users?
   a. With parental consent?
   b. Without parental consent?
   c. What agencies? Law enforcement? Probation? County medical department? Specialist employed by the school district? Others?
7. What are the legal responsibilities of the district and of school personnel?
8. How are confiscated drugs to be handled by school personnel?
9. What is to be done when outsiders are found dealing with drugs in school?
10. How can conflicts between enforcement agencies and the schools be resolved?
11. How should law enforcement personnel be handled when they come to school?
12. Should undercover policemen be used in schools to search out drug traffic?

Suggested areas to include in policies

When specific policies and procedures are being established, a school drug abuse advisory committee should be formed to assume the responsibility for developing a proposal to be placed before the school board. There are no prescriptions regarding the composition of committee membership; however, the committee should have broad representation, including students, parents, and community representatives. The committee should obtain advice from legal sources and the police in the preparation of proposals. The suggestions that follow may be used in the preparation of policies and procedures.

It should be noted that the legal concept of "in loco parentis," which has given schools parental responsibility over students, appears to be changing, is being replaced, or will be replaced by the principle of "student rights." The question of the infringement of the rights of minors is being challenged by recent court and legal actions. By way of illustration, state laws permitting students to receive venereal disease and contraceptive counseling as well as drug abuse guidance without parental approval are being passed in many states. In addition, the questions of due process, consultation with a lawyer, avoidance of self-incrimination, identification of civil and legal rights of children, and the cross-examination of hostile witness are being considered by the courts. In an attempt toward clarity, school districts have prepared lists of student rights.

Suspension* and expulsion. The laws of each particular state in regard to suspension and expulsion need to be given consideration. However, these thoughts should help:

1. Resort to suspension or expulsion only after careful study of all the facts and when no other approach is found to be feasible.
2. Only after due process is supported by records of testimony and not simply hearsay or supposition evidence should a student be suspended or expelled.
3. Contact parents as soon as possible to discuss appropriate action. A student showing an emotional or psychological problem should be directed to help.
4. The evidence must be definite and concrete that the student's behavior will interfere with the maintenance of discipline and the learning process of other students in the school or with the student's own physical or mental health.
5. Reputable advice from a variety of sources must indicate such action to be in the best interest of the student in terms of his intellectual and social development.
6. Advise the student as to vocational and other educational opportunities that he may be required or encouraged to pursue and that may be useful in his gaining readmission.

---

*See Chapter 8 (p. 240) for alternatives to suspensions used in Fresno and Sacramento, California.

Rights of students with regard to search. Federal laws permit school authorities the "reasonable right to inspection of school property and premises" even though such areas have been set aside for the exclusive use of a particular student. Hence inspection of student lockers and their contents is permissible when the evidence supports such action. However, such search usually may not include individual belongings (pockets, purses, etc.). The right to inspect becomes a duty when parents surrender their children to the public schools (in loco parentis) and expect certain safeguards to occur. Inspections should not be undertaken without careful thought and then only for clearly compelling reasons.

In New York City these guidelines are in force:

1. School personnel may search lockers, closets, desks, and similar areas under school control "at any time."
2. A teacher seeing a student "in possession" of narcotics or a hypodermic instrument may immediately search the student or place him under a citizen's arrest for search by the police.
3. A teacher may also search any student who, in the "opinion" of the teacher, is "reasonably suspected" of possessing drugs or drug instruments. Reasonable suspicion is more than mere suspicion and should be based on "concrete personal observations," or at least on "apparently reliable" information from other students.
4. Information from student informants may be the sole basis for a search if the informant has, in the past, given information that has proved to be "consistently accurate" in two or three separate instances.
5. Indiscriminate searches are to be avoided. Although they are "not per se illegal," they offend everyone's "sensibilities" and undermine the status and credibility of school authorities.
6. All personal searches are to be made by school personnel, with police to be called in only for protection.

In New York City the last regulation takes on added significance because of a decision by the New York State Supreme Court in the case of a teacher searching a youth suspected of possessing narcotics. The court said the teacher, acting in loco parentis, or in the place of a parent, needed only a "reasonable suspicion" to justify the search, although a policeman in the same circumstances would be bound by stricter standards of search and seizure. The case involved the arrest of a 16-year-old youth for the possession of a hypodermic needle and related equipment discovered by a teacher during a search. The court agreed, in a 2-to-1 decision, that a school official stood in the place of a parent with regard to the pupils in his care. They said the official had an obligation to protect the children from harmful and dangerous influences, which would include narcotics.

Rights of students with respect to questioning. The following rights of students must be honored:

1. Notice of charges—specific charges to be made at any hearing should be given in advance to parents or to the individual defending the student.
2. Right to counsel—student may be represented by his parents or legal counsel at any hearing.
3. Right to cross-examination and confrontation—parents and others may do so.
4. Privilege against any degree of self-incrimination—parents and others should know that, according to the Fifth Amendment, students may refuse to answer questions that might incriminate themselves.
5. Right of transcript of proceedings—a copy should be available to student and parents.
6. Right of appellate review—case can be reviewed by a higher authority.

Personal records. The question of whether or not to record the drug incidents of students should receive careful study. If they are to be recorded, they should be kept in a separate folder for the exclusive use of school officials in developing constructive plans for student rehabilitation. They should not be part of the student's permanent record, and access to this information should be limited to specifically designated persons.

Readmission. Any student suspended or expelled because of drug-related problems should have the right to be readmitted. The decision should be based on a review of (1) the steps taken to seek solutions to the problems that were the basis for the suspension and (2) the medical and psychiatric records from treatment and rehabilitation agencies and other available records. School authorities should be assured that an honest attempt has been made by the student to deal with the problem while in school. It may be necessary to establish a review board.

Confidentiality and police relations. "Most schools are uncertain about their role regarding privileged communication—whether the drug-using youngster who confides in a school representative should be reported to his parents, the police or even the school administrator."[22] The teacher, counselor, or other school official often faces the dilemma of wanting to assist students by establishing communication and trust and yet trying to resolve the question of possibly breaking the law. In order to protect himself, the individual often feels obligated to report confidential information to some authority.

It is clear that teachers, counselors, and others need to feel secure when relating to a drug-involved student and must display confidence when in this role. Policies and procedures should be clearly established so that when a student confides to a school official that he or she is using drugs, that individual is able to be honest and forthright with the student. He should try to help the student understand the full ramifications of this involvement and motivate him or her to a decision for positive action.

The law on confidentiality is vague in some states, except for such persons as doctors and lawyers. However, courts[17] in several states say that merely failing to inform public authorities about felonies that may, or may not, have been committed is not breaking the law. In Connecticut[16] the law states that any professional employee who in good faith discloses, or does not disclose, such professional communication shall be immune from any liability, civil or criminal. In Maryland[23] these legal protections are operative:

1. Whenever a student seeks help about a drug problem from a teacher, counselor, administrator, or other individual, no statement made by the student or observations of the educator are admissible in any court proceeding.
2. Educators do not have to inform parents about students seeking help about drug problems, nor must they divulge the identity of students.
3. Any young person, including those under 18 years of age, may receive treatment for a problem of drug abuse without parental consent, and the physician is not legally bound to inform the parents.

It is important to consider the role of the school as focusing on the welfare of the student. Therefore this consideration should enable confidentiality to become a tool with which the school may better fulfill its educational function. Breaking the trust of the student who reveals confidential information will shut off communication at a time when it may be vitally needed.

Counselors recognize that any information given to them during an interview usually constitutes hearsay evidence and is, therefore, not ordinarily admissible in court. However, there are exceptions to this rule and it is clear that schools must establish policies and procedures regarding this important matter or should obtain interpretations as to the legal provisions of confidentiality applicable in their individual communities.

At times schools may wish police to conduct investigations of students suspected of drug activities, or police themselves may wish to investigate. When drugs are being sold on campus, it will be necessary to take action and to work with the police to apprehend the pusher and to confiscate the drugs. In addition, police may be willing to turn over suspected drug abusers to the schools for guidance and help. Police may offer to assist with the school educational and guidance programs. They may be of help in the decision on confidentiality. In any event, schools should appoint one person to establish liaison and to coordinate actions between the police and the schools.

Counseling, guidance, and rehabilitation. The follow-up procedures schools establish to help students should include counseling, guidance, and rehabilitation (Chapter 8).

Undercover policemen on campus. The question of using undercover policemen on campus to ferret out drug pushers is not easily resolved. Apparently parents would prefer this arrangement to having dope pushers sitting in classes with their children. However, certain students believe that police spies may produce attitudes of tension and mistrust, resulting in greater student unrest, which is not necessary in the school setting. The decision to use policemen must be weighed carefully in terms of the severity of the drug problem. Basically, an undercover operation should be the action of last resort in attempting to handle the drug situation and should only be instituted when all other means to resolve the problem have been explored and rejected.

ILLUSTRATIONS OF SCHOOL DISTRICT POLICIES AND PROCEDURES

The policies and procedures from the Newton Public Schools, Massachusetts, and the Los Angeles City Schools, California, have been selected to serve as illustrations. No attempt has been made at evaluation. These policies and procedures represent two approaches that schools and school districts may find useful.

Newton Public Schools, Massachusetts

Procedure for drug abusers

1. As soon as a student is positively identified as a drug abuser in the school, or as one who engages in drug traffic in the school, the principal will send him home after notifying the parents, inviting them in for an appointment to explain the issue (a copy of the letter should go to the superintendent). The understanding will be that the student must remain under the constant surveillance of the parents while he is at home. At this point the principal will notify the Supervisor of Attendance (using only one person as the liaison between the schools and the police should reduce the communications problem) who in turn will informally notify the police of the action taken by the principal.

2. The student will be readmitted to the school only after he has had both a physical and a psychiatric clearance. The physical evaluation can be done either by a private physician or the Newton Department of Public Health. The psychiatric evaluation can be done privately by the Newton Mental Health, Massachusetts General Hospital, or some other comparable agency. If these facilities are not available, the school psychiatrists will do the evaluation. Whenever private physicians, psychiatrists, or other evaluating personnel have completed their work, they should send their reports to the Chief Psychologist of the Division of Pupil Personnel. The physical and psychiatric clearance will be an assurance that the student has enough stability to re-enter the mainstream of school activities.

3. If the student is unable to get clearance after a reasonable period of treatment, the principal shall then forward a recommendation to the School Committee that they drop the boy or girl from the school roster. The action would be a last resort, with recognition that the student's removal by no means solves his problem.

Obviously, before step one can take place the student drug abuser must be identified. To do this, each teacher will be asked to pass on any information (fact or hearsay) to the principal. Once the principal has collected enough information and proof, he may then take step one as recommended; otherwise he will continue to receive and sift the information. No one should minimize the importance of the principal's role in this very sensitive position.

The relationship between the schools and the police must be very close and continuous. Each agency has to extend itself more than they do at present. The schools must not withhold information on the grounds that the police are interested only in law enforcement. On the other hand, the police must be sensitive to the schools' interest in the student's therapy, and must not act hastily without consultation with the school authorities. The life of the boy or girl must be paramount in the minds of the members of both agencies.

The schools and the police can gain the confidence of the parents by the judicious handling of individual cases. Surely, if the parents see that both the police and the schools have compassion and concern for their children, they will respond positively toward any efforts of the public agencies. Perhaps the knowledge that public and private agencies within the community are working cooperatively on the problem will help to allay the fears of parents whose children are caught up in the use of drugs.

Los Angeles City Schools, California*

USE—Pupil suspected of being under the influence of drugs, narcotics, or other harmful substance.

I. Determination of need for medical attention
   A. Evaluate observable symptoms.
   B. Provide for examination by school nurse or physician.
   C. Interview pupil, if he is coherent, in presence of an adult witness.
      1. Question pupil regarding amount and type of narcotic consumed or substance used.
      2. Attempt to determine if pupil is in possession of drug, narcotic, or harmful substance.
      3. Confiscate all physical evidence obtained as a result of investigation.
         a. Seal evidence in an envelope bearing the name of the pupil from whom it was confiscated, the date and time it was confiscated, and the signature of the person who confiscated it.
         b. Provide law-enforcement agency with all confiscated evidence.
   D. Provide for an appropriate period of observation in a supervised, non-classroom environment.
   E. Inform parent or guardian of reasons for the investigation even is pupil is found *not* to have been involved with illegal drugs, narcotics, or other harmful substances.
   F. Refer to procedures outlined below under II if symptoms develop which indicate a need for emergency medical attention.

II. Provision for necessary emergency medical attention
   A. Provide needed attention.
      1. Call ambulance, in accordance with emergency procedures listed on "Accident Instructions" card, or
      2. Call law-enforcement agency, or
      3. Send pupil, accompanied by a certificated employee, to authorized medical facility listed on "Accident Instructions" card, if procedure listed in 1 or 2 above is not followed.
   B. Notify parent, guardian, or authorized person listed on pupil's "Emergency Information" card.
      1. Call as soon as possible after emergency arrangements have been made.
      2. Request that school be informed regarding pupil's progress.
   C. Notify law-enforcement agency if such notification was not made when emergency arrangements were completed.
   D. Conduct a thorough investigation by interviewing witnesses and/or pupil's associates and examining school records.
   E. Report information, limited to obvious symptoms, to the school nurse or physician for recording on pupil's confidential "Health Record" card.
   F. Suspend pupil, and schedule conference with parent and pupil after emergency medical attention has been provided and pupil has recovered from the incident.
   G. Consider taking one or more of the following additional actions:
      1. Provide for a rehabilitation program within the local school, including the use of one or more of the following: medical supervision, individual and/or group counseling, parent education, opportunity class, opportunity program, etc.
      2. Utilize district guidance, counseling, health, and attendance services with appropriate regard for confidentiality and use of privileged information.
      3. Provide information, in accordance with district policy, to parent or guardian regarding availability of public and private resource agencies for rehabilitation. . . .
      4. Provide for inter-school adjustment (e.g. opportunity transfer, opportunity school).
      5. Notify Los Angeles County Probation Department or California Youth Authority regarding the drug involvement of pupils whose cases are active with these agencies.

---

*From Drug Abuse Council: Drug abuse control: administrative guidelines, Los Angeles, 1970, Los Angeles City Schools.

6. Refer to school physician for recommendation regarding possible need for medical exclusion.

III. Procedures when emergency medical attention is not indicated

A. Evaluate observable symptoms.

B. Provide for examination by school nurse or physician.

C. Interview pupil in presence of an adult witness.

1. Question pupil regarding amount and type of drug or narcotic consumed or of harmful substance used.

2. Attempt to determine if pupil is still in possession of drug, narcotic, or harmful substance.

3. Confiscate all physical evidence obtained as a result of investigation.

a. Seal evidence in an envelope bearing the name of pupil from whom confiscated, the date and time it was confiscated, and the signature of the person who confiscated it.

b. Provide law-enforcement agency with all confiscated evidence.

D. Provide for a limited period of observation in a supervised non-classroom environment.

E. Refer to procedures outlined above under item II (A through G) if symptoms indicate a need for emergency medical attention.

F. Utilize the following procedures for pupil if no further symptoms are discernible and is not involved in possession or sale:

1. Inform parent or guardian, and consult with law-enforcement agency at the time of incident. (If pupil does not have a known history of drug abuse nor significant delinquent behavior, further involvement by law-enforcement agency may not be necessary unless additional information is obtained relative to the incident and such action is in the interest of pupil and school.)

2. Schedule an early conference with parent and pupil at school.

3. Consider suspension of pupil, pending formulation of an individualized plan to aid in the solution of pupil's drug abuse problem.

4. Refer to IIG above for additional follow-up procedures, and verify pupil's participation in a rehabilitation program.

G. Determine all related aspects of incident by interviewing witnesses and/or pupil's associates and examining school records for background information.

H. Report information, limited to obvious symptoms, to the school nurse or physician for recording on pupil's confidential "Health Record" card.

POSSESSION—Pupils suspected of possessing drugs, narcotics, or other harmful substances which are illegal or have the potential for abuse

I. Determination of pupil involvement

A. Interview pupil in presence of an adult witness.

B. Request pupil's cooperation in conducting a search of his person and possessions.

1. Search may include pupil's lockers and other locations at school where it is suspected that illegal drugs, narcotics, or other harmful substances may be hidden.

a. The search should be made by a school administrator or his delegated certificated representative in the presence of an adult witness.

b. The search should not be conducted by a security agent unless the pupil has been placed under arrest.

c. Security agents should not be present when searches are conducted by other school personnel.

2. Law-enforcement agency should be notified if the pupil continues to be uncooperative after a reasonable effort has been made to gain his cooperation. (A reasonable effort may include requesting parental assistance in gaining pupil's cooperation.)

C. Determine all related aspects of incident by interviewing witnesses and/or pupil's associates and examining school records for background information.

D. Confiscate all physical evidence obtained as a result of investigation.

1. Seal evidence in an envelope bearing the name of the pupil from whom it was confiscated, the date and time it was confiscated, and the signature of the person who confiscated it.

2. Provide law-enforcement agency with all confiscated evidence.

E. Inform parent or guardian of reasons for the investigation even if pupil is found *not* to have been in possession at school of illegal drugs, narcotics, or other harmful substances.

II. Procedures when possession is established
   A. Notify law-enforcement agency.
   B. Notify parent or guardian.
      1. If an arrest is made and the pupil is removed from school, a representative of the law-enforcement agency should notify the parent or guardian prior to the time that the pupil would normally return home from school.
      2. A member of the school staff also may notify the parent or guardian if a pupil is in the custody of a law-enforcement agency.
   C. Suspend pupil, and schedule an early conference with parent and pupil.
   D. Examine pupil's records to aid in determining an appropriate course of action, which may include one or more of the following:
      1. Provide for a rehabilitation program within the local school, such as medical supervision, individual and/or group counseling, parent education, opportunity class, opportunity program, etc.
      2. Utilize district guidance, counseling, health, and attendance services with appropriate regard for confidentiality and use of privileged information.
      3. Provide information to parent or guardian in accordance with district policy regarding the availability of public and private resource agencies for rehabilitation. . . .
      4. Provide for inter-school adjustment (e.g., opportunity transfer, opportunity school).
      5. Notify Los Angeles County Probation Department or California Youth Authority regarding the drug involvement of pupils whose cases are active with these agencies.
      6. Request [Area] Superintendent to initiate expulsion proceedings [when facts warrant such actions].
   E. Follow procedures referred to in "Sale" section (item II) if it is established that the pupil sold or furnished a dangerous drug, narcotic, or other harmful substance to another person, or persons.

SALE—Pupils suspected of selling or furnishing a dangerous drug, narcotic, or other harmful substance to another person, or persons.

I. Determination of pupil involvement
   A. Interview pupil in presence of an adult witness.
   B. Request pupil's cooperation in conducting a search of his person and possessions.
      1. Search may include pupil's lockers and other locations on campus where it is suspected that illegal drugs, narcotics, or other harmful substances may be hidden.
         a. Search should be made by a school administrator or his delegated certificated representative in the presence of an adult witness.
         b. Search should not be conducted by a security agent unless the pupil has been placed under arrest.
         c. Security agents should not be present when searches are conducted by other school personnel.
      2. Law-enforcement agency should be notified if the pupil continues to be uncooperative after a reasonable effort has been made to gain his cooperation. (A reasonable effort may include requesting parental assistance in gaining pupil's cooperation.)
   C. Determine all related aspects of incident by interviewing witnesses and/or pupil's associates and examining school records for background information.
   D. Confiscate all physical evidence obtained as a result of investigation.
      1. Seal evidence in an envelope bearing the name of the pupil from whom it was confiscated, the date and time it was confiscated, and the signature of the person who confiscated it.
      2. Provide law-enforcement agency with all confiscated evidence.
   E. Inform parent or guardian of reasons for the investigation even if pupil is found *not* to have been selling or furnishing a dangerous drug, narcotic, or other harmful substance to another person, or persons.
   F. Follow procedures referred to in the sections on "Use" and/or "Possession" if it is determined that pupil was involved in use and/or possession.

II. Procedures when sale is verified
   A. Notify law-enforcement agency.
   B. Notify parent or guardian.
      1. If an arrest is made and the pupil is removed from school, a representative

of the law-enforcement agency should notify the parent or guardian prior to the time that the pupil would normally return home from school.
2. A member of the school staff also may notify the parent or guardian if a pupil is in the custody of a law-enforcement agency.

C. Suspend pupil, and schedule an early conference with parent and pupil.
1. Provide information, in accordance with district policy, to parent or guardian, regarding the availability of public and private resource agencies for rehabilitation. . . .
2. Inform parent or guardian that pupil will continue to be suspended pending further investigation and final disposition of the case.

D. Request [Area] Superintendent to initiate expulsion proceedings when facts warrant such action.

ROLE OF SCHOOL PERSONNEL

The entire school staff has responsibility for the drug program. Counselors' functions have been covered in Chapter 9 and drug coordinators, specialists, and resource individuals are identified in this chapter. The duties of psychologists, social workers, and other personnel will need identification. We will now provide what is essentially to be expected of the primary personnel.

1. Superintendent and school board
   a. Provide commitment to a school drug program.
   b. Approve policies and procedures.
   c. Provide funds for a drug coordinator and for conducting the drug program.
   d. Delegate appropriate authority for the development and implementation of the program.
2. Principal
   a. Manage the overall drug program.
   b. Assist in motivation, implementation, and evaluation.
   c. Aid in home and community communication.
   d. Assure compliance with state laws in school policies and procedures.
   e. Help in the selection of qualified teachers.
   f. Encourage and support in-service programs.
   g. Make concerted efforts to improve the school atmosphere.
   h. Give primary consideration to student welfare before taking disciplinary action in drug cases.
3. School physician (where available)
   a. Aid in identifying drug users and abusers.

b. Serve as liaison with home and community resources.
   c. Assist particularly in the development and implementation of the drug services program.
   d. Serve as a resource person in planning and developing the drug education curriculum and instructional program.
4. School nurse
   a. Be primarily responsible in the drug services program.
   b. Advise both students and teachers regarding drug problems and program.
   c. Respond to emergency situations in schools.
   d. Act as liaison between phyicians, school, home, and community resources.
   e. Serve as a resource person in curriculum development and in the instructional program.
5. Teacher
   a. Help identify drug users and abusers through observations of symptomatic behavior.
   b. Be familiar with procedures for handling students with drug problems.
   c. Provide school atmosphere conducive to learning.
   d. Conduct drug instructional program.

FINANCING

Perhaps the most crucial aspect of any drug program is the availability of funds for development and implementation. Without financial aid for schools, especially in this tight money period, no program can be planned or made operative. Without federal funds it is questionable whether the wide variety of school programs now under way would ever have been started or could be maintained. It is estimated that it takes at least 3 to 5 years for drug programs to become operational and firmly established if adequate funds are provided and other administrative factors previously identified receive attention. Therefore, unless federal funds are available and state monies are continued and expanded for a number of years, many programs now functioning will suffer or disappear. State and local aid since 1970 has increased substantially, having been substituted for minimal federal support. The result has been that numerous drug programs are underway. However, there is evidence that these funds also may be diminishing. Apparently the focus on drug education within states is less intense than it was from 1970 to 1976. These factors support the position that drug education must find a place in the curriculum where it has permanency. The proposals in Chapter 7 provide suggestions for such an arrangement.

The availability of funds in itself does not assure quality programs. The achievement of quality necessitates the commitment of school boards to drug programs, qualified personnel to conduct these programs, and other factors described in this text. Our major concern, therefore, is to motivate school districts to give high priority to conducting programs that are effective in the lives of children and youth. This book is a result of our concern.

Financial support for drug programs, primarily educational, has come from three governmental levels—federal, state, and local school districts.

Table 10-1 indicates the total federal drug abuse prevention funding that has been provided to the various governmental agencies since 1971 and includes an anticipated budget through 1977. Although a number of other national organizations have made grants and awarded contracts to state education agencies and local schools, the primary source of such financial aid over the years has been the Office of Education (OE). Table 10-1 reveals that the education or prevention component of the drug problem was given low priority since the percentage of total budget allocations was comparatively small.

One of the first sums of money awarded to OE was $3.5 million in 1970 under the Educations Profession Development Act. Each state department of education and territory in the United States was awarded between $40,000 and $210,000, depending on population, to develop educational programs primarily for training teachers and to establish a state office. Approximately $500,000 was used to establish four National Training Centers in Drug Education in the United States (we directed the one in San Francisco) and to establish the National Action Committee (an advisory group to the Office of Education). Before such funds were avail-

TABLE 10-1. Total federal drug abuse prevention funding (in millions of dollars)*

	FY 71 actual	FY 72 actual	FY 73 actual	FY 74 actual	FY 75 actual	FY 76 estimated	TQ estimated	FY 77 estimated	Total FY 71-77
SAODAP	—	1.5	39.9	27.3	13.0	—	—	—	81.7
DHEW	69.7	193.1	255.1	349.4	320.1	338.4	46.4	359.0	1,931.2
NIDA	56.2	116.7	181.4	272.9†	220.1	232.2	21.2	247.8	1,348.5
NIMH	—	—	—	4.5	5.2	4.2	—	4.3	18.2
NIH	—	—	—	3.3	3.0	3.2	—	3.5	13.0
SRS	3.6	58.0	53.0	54.0	79.0	88.0	23.0	94.0	452.6
OE	5.4	13.0	11.9	5.7	4.0	2.0	—	—	42.0
OHD	4.5	5.4	8.8	9.0	8.8	8.8	2.2	9.4	56.9
OEO	12.8	18.0	‡	—	—	—	—	—	30.8
VA	1.1	16.2	27.7	30.3	33.2	36.7	9.4	38.0	192.6
DOD	1.1	58.7	73.0	68.6	64.0	61.3	14.3	57.8	398.8
Justice	40.3	36.5	33.5	34.5	26.6	46.4	6.7	24.3	248.8
State	—	1.0	1.0	0.9	0.7	0.8	—	0.8	5.2
HUD	8.7	13.0	6.3	1.6	2.9	4.0	0.9	4.8	42.2
USDA	—	2.5	1.9	1.8	1.6	1.6	—	1.0	10.4
Other federal¶	0.2	1.4	2.9	2.8	9.0	3.5	1.3	4.0	25.1
Total	133.9	341.9	441.3	517.2	471.1	492.7	79.0	489.7	2,966.8

*From Cline, S., and Goldberg, P.: Governmental response to drug abuse; the 1977 federal budget, Washington, D.C., 1976, The Drug Abuse Council, Inc.
†High because of a supplemental received in FY 73, and not obligated until FY 74.
‡Total of $23.0 million included in NIDA funds.
¶Includes amounts of less than $1 million each year in DOL, DOC, CSC, DOT, ACTION, other.

able, a number of projects in schools and school districts had been financed under the Bureau of Higher Education Act, Title I, and the Elementary and Secondary School Education Act, Titles III and V. These direct state allocations to provide for state drug education coordinators and program support continued through 1974, when they were terminated. The Office of Education also supported a series of state, college, and community projects for a number of years since 1971.

Some of the Office of Education money in 1972 was used to establish regional training centers with these functions: (1) training and technical assistance to educational systems and some community projects, and (2) technical assistance to state drug education departments, single state drug agencies, and state departments of alcoholism. Training programs were the predominant services available through the seven regional centers that had been established throughout the country. Seven-member community teams were awarded $5,000 for a 10- to 13-day session at one of the regional centers to train them as leaders to be able to develop and implement programs. Five-member school teams comprising a teacher, counselor, administrator, and two others (possibly a student) were allowed up to $10,000 (minigrants) for a 10-day training session at one of the centers. The program consisted of the development of communication skills, community organization, program information, building a team model, interpersonal relations, and action planning. Up to $6,000 of the sum awarded to schools could be used to pay a third of the salary of a full-time drug coordinator for one year. There is no question that these training programs did a great deal to stimulate the development and introduction of programs into school systems. However, by 1975, only school teams were being trained in the five remaining regional centers. In 1976, Office of Education funds were further reduced and the services provided were limited to the teams that had been trained in the previous years with some aid to state agencies and innovative projects.

Table 10-1 indicates that the Office of Education will be phased out of the drug education program since no funds are scheduled for allocation. Yet sizeable sums of money are to continue for law enforcement and treatment and rehabilitation. It should be clear where the federal emphasis has been in recent years. Is it any wonder that educational programs have not had much impact on students to date?

Further reflection on the federal allocation for drug education shows that the OE budget for 1976 was less that 0.5% of the total funds allocated. During the 6-year period of 1971-1976, the Office of Education averaged 1½% per year of the monies provided by Congress. It should be obvious that federal funds to state agencies and schools has been very limited. Dr. William Harvey, Director, NASCO West-Drug Abuse Treatment Center, St. Louis, Missouri, when testifying before the U.S. Senate Hearings on Alcohol and Narcotics in 1975, summed up the situation accurately when he said: ". . . federal drug abuse prevention effort has been inadequate. . . . It is neglected in funding . . . in visibility."

In the past few years, many states have supported drug education programs and have assumed the financial burden when federal funds were terminated. Table 10-2 identifies the state funds allocated to state drug education offices in 1975; the average amount was $137,000. Five states provided $450,000 on the average; however, there were seventeen states that had no monies allocated.

The conclusion that may be reached from the financial picture described is that drug education is becoming less important and lower in priority at both the federal and state levels, despite the continued rise in the misuse and abuse of drugs in the United States. It raises the question: How can schools help young people without adequate funds?

It is appropriate to add that federal authorities have recognized the alcohol problem. In 1975, approximately $135 million was appropriated, and $130 million was made available to national agencies. Approximately 70% of these funds were delegated to treat-

TABLE 10-2. State funds allocated to state drug education offices, 1975 (44 states)*

Amounts (thousands)	States		Number of state changes from 1974			Estimated average state funds (thousands)
	Number	Percent	Up	Down	Same	
0	17	38	—	—	—	—
1-5	0	—	—	—	—	—
6-10	1	2	1	—	—	8
11-20	2	5	—	1	1	15
21-50	10	23	5	2	3	35
51-100	6	14	1	4	1	75
101-300	3	7	1	1	1	200
Over 300	5	11	4	1	—	450
Totals	44		12	9	6	137

*Estimated total funds to twenty-seven states, $3,688,000; one state received $600,000.
From Cornacchia, H. J., and Smith, D. E.: Unpublished survey of U.S. State Drug Education Coordinators, 1976.

ment and rehabilitation; the amount to prevention and education was quite small.

IN-SERVICE PREPARATION

Despite the numerous in-service programs for school personnel that have been conducted in the last few years, there is still a great need for continuance and expansion in this area. Many individuals have not been reached to date and a great deal of new research on drugs and new approaches to treatment and rehabilitation are appearing in the literature, making it necessary to keep individuals up to date with current information through periodic refresher meetings or in other appropriate ways. Therefore the material presented in this section is designed to supply ideas for the content and presentation of a variety of orientation programs for those individuals needing an introduction to the drug scene and of updating and growth programs for those in need of such assistance.

Despite the in-service programs that have been conducted, confusion and lack of understanding still exist regarding the nature of the school drug program that is effective. The conceptual model developed herein is unique in its organization for schools. Implementation is needed if an impact on young people is to occur. Many school programs continue to be fragmented and have de-

veloped in piecemeal fashion without clarity of purpose.

The information that follows is intended to provide suggestions and ideas for those with responsibility for conducting in-service programs for school personnel.

Participants

Programs may be prepared for a variety of school and community people. The schools may desire to include such school personnel as board members, superintendents, assistant superintendents, principals, teachers, counselors, and school nurses; students; and community individuals, including parents, policemen, lawyers, physicians, psychiatrists, and health department staff members. It may be advisable to have small meetings just for counselors, school nurses, or teachers, depending on the problem facing the school. If the gathering is a first in-service meeting for sensitization purposes, it may be advisable for a variety of school personnel, students, and community representatives to participate. The goals to be achieved should determine which groups will participate.

Objectives

The goals for in-service programs should not only be cognitive in emphasis but also affective and action oriented if at all possible. Thus concern should be given to the attitudes and practices of those in attendance as well as the knowledges and understandings that they should acquire. In addition, emphasis should be given to the spectrum of health, including physiological, pharmacological, social, psychological, and spiritual aspects. These objectives should be adapted according to the nature of the audience, the length of the meeting, and other factors. By way of illustration, a session for school board members and superintendents might try to arouse their interest in and make them feel the need for a drug program that deals humanely with drug users and abusers. A program for teachers may stress cognitive, affective, and action aspects but may also be concerned with the improvement of communication and decision-making skills in the classroom.

To be specific, an all-inclusive coverage of the drug field is provided in the following overall purposes, from which the appropriate goals may be selected for any given program. These purposes are stated in behavioral terms and are categorized so as to be of practical help in establishing objectives for in-service programs.

1. Cognitive domain
   a. Explain the nature, extent, and significance of the drug problem in society, especially relative to children and youth in the ghetto areas.
   b. Identify the national, state, and local drug laws.
   c. Identify the pharmacological, psychological, sociological, and possibly spiritual effects of drugs on man and society.
   d. Recall the nature of the community organization for effective drug abuse programs.
   e. List the community resources available to help drug abusers.
   f. Explain a variety of significant school drug education programs.
   g. Describe a variety of ways to effectively communicate with children, youth, and the community in order to effect behavioral and attitudinal changes.
   h. Identify a variety of approaches used and community resources available for rehabilitation and treatment of drug users and abusers.
   i. Identify symptomatic behavior of students who may be misusing and abusing drugs.
   j. Explain the growth and development charac-

teristics as well as the physical and emotional needs of children and youth.
   k. Recall the school district's policies and procedures for handling drug abusers.
   l. Identify the physical and psychological needs of children and youth and understand the relationship of these needs to drug misuse and abuse.
2. Affective domain
   a. Appreciate the reasons why youths misuse and abuse drugs.
   b. Be interested in developing ways to make the community more aware of the need for drug education programs in schools.
   c. Feel more sympathetic toward young people and the stresses and problems facing them in society.
   d. Feel more sympathetic toward young misusers and abusers of drugs.
   e. Believe that a school drug program is necessary.
   f. Feel the need for greater student involvement in school drug programs, including peer and cross-age counseling.
   g. Value the need for a school atmosphere conducive to learning.
   h. Believe that the stress on students to develop values is necessary in the educational program.
   i. Desire to meet the needs of students and provide success experiences.
3. Action domain
   a. Assess and help others to analyze the drug culture in schools and in society.
   b. Organize the community resources to support, assist with, and improve school drug education programs.
   c. Help pupils identify alternative learnings and activities to drug use.
   d. Develop a humane classroom atmosphere in school.
   e. Plan and develop a curriculum in drug education for grades K through 12.
   f. Involve students to a greater degree in school drug programs.
   g. Participate in the development of drug education curricula using the concept approach.
   h. Demonstrate a variety of techniques for evaluating the school drug program.
   i. Evaluate and select drug instructional materials.
   j. Provide competent guidance assistance for student drug users and abusers.
   k. Provide leadership in the development of policies and procedures for the school drug program.
   l. Demonstrate improved skills in the counseling and guidance of drug users and abusers.
   m. Develop and improve school drug programs.
   n. Prepare others to develop, promote, and improve school drug programs.
   o. Help students in their search for identity and for self-actualization in learning.
   p. Demonstrate a variety of effective drug education teaching techniques.

q. Conduct peer counseling and peer and cross-age tutoring training for students.
r. Provide classroom experiences in decision-making, coping, and self-image skills for students.
s. Individualize learning to meet the needs of students and to provide success experiences.
t. Help students solve problems and stressful conditions.
u. Work with parents to provide understandings about children and youth.

Essential program components

The following brief outline provides in capsule form those essential components, the content, to be included in a total school drug program. In-service programs can utilize whatever portions of the following that are deemed appropriate:

1. Physiological or pharmacological aspects—drug classification, definitions, types, methods of administration, form available, effects on body, and medical use
2. Psychological aspects—why drugs used and abused, alternatives to drug use, personalities predisposed to use of drugs, growth and development characteristics, physical and psychological needs of children and youth, characteristics of abusers and potential misusers, and self-image and self-esteem concept
3. Sociological aspects—nature and extent of drug problem (including inner city areas), youth drug culture, youth alienation and unrest, factors affecting drug use, rehabilitation and treatment, the courts and the law, controls and prevention, history of drugs, and religion and drugs
4. Spiritual aspects—value systems, moral implications, and humanism
5. The school drug program
   a. Education (drug and mental health)—curriculum development, problems, techniques of teaching, resources, youth involvement, parent education, and alternative education and activities
   b. Services—identification of abusers, counseling and guidance, community resources, and adjustment of programs
   c. Atmosphere—mental health needs, student unrest, and creating a humane atmosphere
   d. Coordination—problems, administrative organization and advisory committee, drug coordinator, and policies and procedures
   e. Evaluation
6. Communication procedures—group processes, youth involvement, peer counseling and tutoring, peer values and pressures, community awareness, use of multimedia approach, and decision-making, problem solving, and coping
7. Community resources and activities including parent involvement

Activities and experiences

It is recommended that a variety of activities and experiences be provided, with opportunities for selection by participants if individual needs are to be satisfied. This may not be possible where training sessions are of 1 and 2 days' duration, where sufficient staff help is not available, and where community and other resources are limited. Nevertheless the concept of using different approaches is important in planning for in-service programs. These suggestions are not meant to be exhaustive in nature but rather illustrative of ideas that have been workable:

1. Large group sessions—speakers, panels, and debates
2. Small group sessions to:
   a. Discuss speaker presentations
   b. Exchange ideas
   c. Air biases, prejudices, and views regarding the drug scene, drug users, youth unrest, and other issues
   d. Meet, communicate with, and even challenge youthful drug abusers in or out of the drug scene
   e. Learn techniques of improving communication
   f. Be exposed to a variety of communication exercises and games; values clarification, decision-making, coping
   g. Participate in a variety of formal and informal discussions
   h. Be involved in problem solving centered on those problems introduced by participants, using such techniques as role play and psychodrama
3. Field trips—halfway houses, juvenile detention centers, community clinics, youth "drop-in" centers, mental hospitals, drug treatment units, courtrooms covering drug cases, the drug street scene, rock music houses, and other community resources concerned with drug rehabilitation and treatment
4. Discussions with youths, drug users and abusers, and ex-addicts
5. Utilization of community resource speakers—police, lawyers, judges, physicians, pharmacologists, psychiatrists, sociologists, and psychologists or, where speakers are not available, videotapes or audiotapes (Check with local medical centers and other community resources for materials.)
6. Film series, "The Social Seminar," developed by the National Institute of Mental Health (Address: Box 2305, Rockville, Maryland 20852.), "Inside-Out," and others
7. Time for individuals and groups to view films (see Chapter 7), evaluate resource materials, or read independently whenever possible
8. Workshop periods for curriculum development,

program planning for teachers, development of evaluative instruments, development of policies and procedures for school districts, and other activities

9. Pretests and posttests of participants' knowledge and attitudes (Suggestions and ideas may be found in Chapter 11.)
10. Group process activities[9] to improve communication and awareness skills
    a. Experimental
       (1) Communication exercises—a person speaks precisely to an audience and the speech is taped and played back to check points covered
       (2) Simulated experiences of acceptance and rejection;[10] role playing
       (3) Exercises to increase skill in observation and listening
       (4) Exercises using group resources
    b. Group processes
       (1) Sensory stimulation—exploring and discovering the refreshing and relaxing appeal of the multimedia process, including hi-fi records, tapes, TV, films, and psychedelic lights
       (2) Peer-group pressure—participants sit in a circle and leader asks for a volunteer to walk inside circle. As person walks, leader asks if someone wishes to join him. Stroller is encouraged to describe feelings of being alone inside circle. Leader continues to ask if anyone will join stroller, to help him out. As participants in inner circle are added, they are asked to describe their feelings and opinions about themselves and the group. Exercise continues until leader stops to review and analyze the participants' remarks (discourse tends to correspond closely to discourse of drug users [inner group] and nonusers [outer group]).
       (3) Breaking down formalized structures—provide different seating arrangements and organization of conference each day; rearrange chairs; sometimes have speaker address from lectern or sitting on floor for meetings; occasionally move into the community, etc.
       (4) Illustrations of frustrations
       (5) Role playing
       (6) Introduction to DUSO and Magic Circle or other approaches

Organizational arrangement

When possible, and provided the in-service session is to continue for 2 to 3 days or more, it is advisable to provide a "live-in" experience. This is an arrangement where all participants are involved in close proximity for a specific period of time at a pleasant location that is removed from the general work routine. A place should be selected that is relaxing and comfortable, and where participants can communicate during the major part of the day. The live-in experience offers an excellent opportunity to be informal, to dress optionally, to get to know participants better, including the students attending, and to discuss many topics that may not be presented in the planned sessions. Opportunities for social and recreational activities should be provided. The live-in experience is a functional, unusual, and effective way to bring about human relationships. It is a continuous training session during which a great deal of work can be accomplished. If a live-in is not possible, sites for in-service training should be selected that will permit informality, comfort, and limited sociability.

There is no single best length of time for a training session. How long it lasts should be determined on the basis of the goals to be achieved and a variety of other logistical factors. It may meet for 1 to 3 hours once a week for 2 or more weeks, 4 to 6 hours for 1 day, 8 to 16 hours over 2 or 3 days (weekend), 1 week, 2 weeks, or longer. To take advantage of the many activities previously identified and to feel somewhat knowledgeable about the drug scene, perhaps a 2-week live-in session, or a comparable series of experiences, is the minimum training to be received. This is especially true if the trainees are to assume leadership roles in schools. Shorter periods might be workable but the attitudinal effect of the drug scene and the possibility of field trips become difficult to realize in short, periodic meetings.

When possible and desirable, the session might be offered through a local college or university so that credit toward a degree or in lieu of class hours could be obtained.

Evaluation

Periodic assessment of the training session, or the in-service program, should take place. Suggestions and illustrations of procedures that might be usable are given in Chapter 11.

REFERENCES

1. Blum, R. H., and others: Drug education: results and recommendations, Lexington, Mass., 1976, Lexington Books.
2. Colorado Interdepartmental Committee on Alcohol and Drug Abuse: Progress report to Colorado General Assembly, Denver, 1971, Colorado Drug Education Program, State Department of Health, Education, Institutions and Social Services.
3. Colorado State Department of Education, Colorado drug abuse education program: an interdepartmental project—training workshop, Colorado, December 6-11, 1970.
4. Drug abuse: a reference for teachers, rev., Trenton, N.J., 1968, Division of Curriculum and Instruction, New Jersey State Department of Education.
5. Drug Abuse Council: Drug abuse control: administrative guidelines, Los Angeles, 1970, Los Angeles City Schools.
6. Drug abuse programs: a guide to federal support, report series no. 7, Washington, D.C., 1971, National Institute of Mental Health, National Clearinghouse for Drug Abuse Information.
7. Drug crisis: schools fight back with innovative programs, Washington, D.C., 1971, National School Public Relations Association.
8. Finlater, J.: The drug scene: the scope of the problem faced by the schools. In Teaching about drugs: a curriculum guide, K-12, Kent, Ohio, 1970, American School Health Association.
9. Hamilton, L. D.: Drugs: what can the schools do about the problem? Educ. Canada **10**:30-36, 1970.
10. How to plan a drug education workshop for teachers, Washington, D.C., 1969, National Institute of Mental Health, National Clearinghouse for Mental Health Information.
11. Langer, J. H.: School-law enforcement cooperation. In Guidelines for drug abuse prevention education, Washington, D.C., 1970, Bureau of Narcotics and Dangerous Drugs, U.S. Department of Justice.
12. National Institute on Drug Abuse: Beyond the three R's: training teachers for affective education, Washington, D.C., 1975, U.S. Government Printing Office.
13. National Institute on Drug Abuse: Doing drug education: the role of the school teachers, Washington, D.C., 1975, U.S. Government Printing Office.
14. Report of the Ad Hoc Committee on Drug Abuse, Dallas, 1970, Superintendent of Schools, Dallas Independent School District.
15. Schapps, E., and others: Primary prevention research: a preliminary review of program impact studies, Walnut Creek, Calif., 1976, Pyramid Project.
16. School board policies on drug education and drug use, Washington, D.C., 1971, National School Boards Association.
17. School drug policies: a guide for administrators, Boston, 1969, Division of Curriculum and Instruction, Massachusetts Department of Education.
18. Stamford Public Schools, Connecticut: Curriculum guide for drug abuse education, Chicago, 1971, J. G. Ferguson Publishing Co.
19. A statewide plan for drug abuse prevention education in Arizona, Phoenix, 1971, Arizona State Department of Education.
20. Tate, C. P.: In-service education for teachers, Sci. Teacher **37**:49-50, 1970.
21. Teacher's resource guide in drug abuse, Harrisburg, 1969, Division of Public Health Education, Pennsylvania Department of Health.
22. Ungerleider, J. T., and Bowen, H. L.: Drug abuse and the schools, Am. J. Psychiatry **125**:1691-1697, 1969.
23. Wiggins, X.: Public schools and drug education: report of a conference, Atlanta, 1972, The Southern Regional Education Board.

PART FOUR

CONCLUSION

11
Evaluation

The total school drug program and its component parts that have been described in this book should be periodically assessed to determine the extent to which objectives have been achieved. It is necessary to know the extent of the impact of prevention efforts on children and youth. It is important to discover whether programs are in need of modification to determine whether they should continue to be offered or financially supported.

It is unfortunate that the evaluation process has not received adequate attention by those individuals having responsibility for the many preventive drug programs now in operation in the United States. The Educational Research Service[10] said, ". . . evaluation appears to be the weakest and least developed area in school drug programs." In addition, not much is known about the impact of such efforts on young people. Peterson,[19] Goodstadt,[1] Louria,[15] Schapps,[23] the Drug Abuse Council,[13] Randall and Wong,[21] Smart and Fejer,[25] and Blum,[1] have all indicated that little evaluation is underway, and limited information is available that indicates whether drug prevention programs are effective. The Drug Abuse Council of Washington, D.C., discovered that only eighteen of thirty-nine state boards of education had a uniform drug education policy for their school systems, and less than one-half of these policies were evaluated for results. Thirty-two boards left the decisions for evaluation up to local school systems, which in turn permitted individual teachers to determine what actions to take. This data con-

firms the findings of an unpublished survey we conducted of forty-four state drug education coordinators. It revealed that the establishment and following of evaluation procedures by school districts was found in 2% in most schools; 14% in many schools, 59% in some schools; 11% in no schools; and 14% were unknown.

What data are available in regard to the effectiveness of drug prevention reveal limited positive results. Smart and Fejer[25] state only a few studies have inquired about drug usage, while Blum[1] says he knows of no decline in drug use attributable to drug education. Although Berberian and Thompson (1974) reveal that some rate of increase in drugs occurred in older students, there was an increase in use by younger students. The SPARK program in New York City, using after-school counseling for students with serious drug problems, has given some promising results. There were desirable student behavioral changes—a reduction of absenteeism by 28%, disciplinary problems by 49%, major subjects failed by 39%, and increase in grades by 8.5%. Smart and Fejer[25] and Goodstadt[1] report that knowledge improvements are possible but that attitudes and drug use changes are ineffective. Blum[1] and Schapps[23] claim cognitive and affective (values clarification) emphasis may have some positive effect. Randall and Wong[21] and Blum[1] state that long-term impact of the various educational procedures is not known. Burkett[2] says there is no research regarding the effectiveness of alcohol education programs. Neeman and Meenan[17] reveal that of fourteen anti-smoking campaigns, some have had only minor and many produced no effect. The unpublished survey of state drug education coordinators that we conducted (Table 11-1) supports the evidence that the effectiveness of programs is questionable. It reveals that in 12 to 25% of the states, many, most, or all school drug education programs have had an impact on students.

The complexity of the drug program, the newness of its emergence (although many have appeared in recent years), the lack of available devices, and the limited attention paid to the development and use of instruments make it difficult to provide a comprehensive program of evaluation. However, an attempt will be made to define the scope of what is to be assessed, to state some guiding principles of operation, to introduce a variety of illustrative devices, and to provide several sources for other instruments.

SCOPE

The nature of the drug evaluation program should include the total program as well as the segments of drug education, drug services, the school atmosphere, and coordination. The following outline (see Chapter 6) illustrates the areas that may be focused upon in the evaluation process.

I. The total school drug program
II. The educational program
  A. Effects on students
    1. Formal education
      a. Objectives—cognitive, affective, action domains
      b. Content
      c. Methods or pupil learning activities
      d. Resource materials
      e. Course or unit of instruction
      f. Teacher, counselor, or administrator
      g. Patterns of organization—direct, correlated, alternative education
      h. Mini-courses—peer counseling, cross-age tutoring
    2. Informal education/counseling, alternative activities, and others; goals, cognitive, affective, action domains
  B. Effects on parents
III. The services program
  A. Appropriateness of drug user identification procedures
  B. Adequacy of procedures for handling drug users and abusers
  C. Effect of guidance and counseling on the rehabilitation of students
  D. Adequacy of community resources to aid students
  E. Effect of school program adjustments on students in terms of learning and drug abuse problems
IV. The school atmosphere
  A. Effect on student alienation and unrest
  B. Extent of success in satisfying physical and emotional needs
  C. Impact of humane school atmosphere on learning and on the control and prevention of student misuse and abuse of drugs
V. Coordination of the program
  A. Effectiveness of the drug coordinator
  B. Value of school drug advisory committee
  C. Adequacy of financial aid
  D. Effectiveness of organizational structure
  E. Usefulness of established policies and procedures
  F. In-service program values and effects

Table 11-1. State drug education coordinators' opinions of effectiveness of drug education programs in the United States (forty-four states)

Grade level	All	Per-cent	Most	Per-cent	Many	Per-cent	Some	Per-cent	None	Per-cent	Un-known	Per-cent
Primary	1	2	5	11	5	11	13	30	2	5	18	41
Intermediate-middle	0	0	4	9	6	15	16	36	1	2	17	38
Upper-junior high	0	0	3	7	5	11	19	43	0	0	17	39
Senior high	0	0	3	7	2	5	18	41	2	4	19	43

PRINCIPLES OF EVALUATION

The general guiding principles that will be helpful in evaluating the school drug program will be identified within these headings: (1) how to evaluate, (2) who evaluates, (3) when to evaluate, and (4) problems in attempting to conduct an evaluation program.

How to evaluate

Schools should utilize a variety of procedures to determine present status of program drug use and abuse, and others, for baseline purposes, and to discover the progress made toward the achievement of desired goals. Such procedures may include observations by teachers, students, counselors, and others; checklists; questionnaires; self-tests; pretests and posttests; opinionnaires; practice inventories; and analysis of records. The evidence obtained can be of a subjective nature when it is collected in empirical form, or it can be of an objective nature, so that it may be statistically analyzed through the use of mechanical devices or by other quantitative means. Whenever possible, objective evidence should be acquired but subjective data may be the only kind obtainable because appropriate instruments are not available or because of other inhibiting factors.

A broad spectrum of assessment methods to gather both quantitative and qualitative data should be used. Educational evaluation processes all too frequently merely attempt to discover how many of something exists or to answer the following questions: Do we have a program? Are there qualified teachers? Are there adequate resource supplies? It is imperative that evidence be obtained to determine the effectiveness of the drug program. Evaluation should attempt to determine what impact the program has had on students to be qualitative. This is more difficult to achieve and may be an impossible process at atimes, especially if behavioral objectives in the educational program have been established. Nevertheless, such data are necessary to best demonstrate accountability. What a program does to students is more relevant than determining how much of something a school may possess.

A number of illustrative evaluation instruments are found later in the chapter. However, certain relevant weaknesses may be evidenced including the reference of the instruments to local situations. There are few standardized instruments available at this writing and there are no known devices to assess the individual drug program components categorized as services, atmosphere, and coordination. (See "Criteria for Evaluating the School Drug Program," p. 284.) Schools, school districts, and school personnel therefore should utilize or adapt those instruments found in this chapter in addition to devising methods to meet their own local needs.

It is advisable for school districts to periodically employ expert help to develop reliable or valid instruments or to help with the evaluative process.

Who evaluates

Students, school personnel, including teachers, counselors, administrators, and nurses, and the community, especially parents, should be involved in assessing the school drug program. The individuals who should participate will be selected depending on the goal or goals to be achieved.

It should be stressed that students may provide such useful services to teachers or administrators as (1) responding to questionnaires to determine the effect of classroom educational experiences; (2) helping to assess the value of films and pamphlet materials to be used, or purchased, for the drug educational program; (3) conducting surveys of student drug misuse and abuse and in other ways (the Drug Abuse Council provided research grants of $2500 to high school teams to investigate the drug scene in schools and communities and to examine drug education programs); (4) aiding in determining the meaningfulness of the content of the drug education program; and (5) aiding in determining whether teachers and counselors have the ability to communicate with students effectively. Students should be included in the evaluative process.

One of the functions of the school drug advisory committee may be involvement in evaluation. This committee may participate in the development of procedures, support the need for assessment, or decide to delegate this responsibility.

When to evaluate

Frequently it has been said that evaluation is a continuing process; there is a beginning, but no end. Such a statement applies to the school drug program.

Realistically, no evaluation program of great intensity and length can continue over an indeterminate period of time. However, teachers, administrators, and others should at least minimally participate in the periodic assessment of their activities. The nature and degree of intensity together with the frequency of what takes place will differ depending on the time available, the people involved, the nature of the program, and numerous other variables. In the classroom the teacher might well consider pretesting and posttesting behaviors during a course or unit related to drugs, or merely use personal observations to find results. In the school or school district, short- and long-range goals should be established to assess the various segments of the total drug program. Most evaluative studies to date have been for limited periods of time, with only meager information about long-term effects.

In any event consideration must be given to the establishment of a time period over which the entire program will be measured. In addition, evaluation may occur at each grade level or grade level group (primary, intermediate, upper, or high school). The specific procedures, timing, personnel involved, and other matters should be determined at the local level to meet local needs. Drug programs should include provision for the evaluation process and receive consideration in their developmental stages.

Problems in evaluation

One significant problem in drug education programs is the community expectation in some areas that a dramatic reduction in the numbers of students using, misusing, or abusing drugs should take place after relatively brief instructional programs. Knowl-

edge of the difficulties in the process of behavioral change indicates that the achievement of such a goal is impossible. In addition, the strength of the social forces and factors outside the school—television and other mass media, peer influence, adult use of drugs—makes it clear that schools by themselves cannot solve this widespread drug problem. In fact schools may not be able to have much effect at all. They may be able to aid in the limited reduction of some drug use and help in the more intelligent use, but support and cooperative assistance from the total community are needed for even partial success.

The question may be raised as to whether young people are to be turned off of all drugs, including aspirin, alcohol, and tobacco. Therefore it is important that the goals established in school drug programs be reasonable in their potential for achievement, clearly defined, and within the limitations of the funds, facilities, resources, teacher competencies, and learning atmosphere available.

A second problem in evaluation is the assessment of action domain goals when much of the student behavior involving drug use and misuse occurs outside the school setting. Such actions are unobservable and difficult, if at all possible, to assess. Therefore expecting schools to turn pupils off drugs in any dramatic fashion after only 1 or 2 years of conducting drug programs is unreasonable. Schools will find it difficult to know what they have achieved in this regard. This is not to imply that such an outcome should not be included in the program. Some of the suggestions given here will be helpful in both short- and long-range plans.

It may take 3 to 5 years just to establish a drug program that begins to demonstrate consistent degrees of effectiveness in terms of knowledge and attitude purposes. If such a program is ongoing for a number of additional years, if it is a total program as described in this book, if it utilizes personnel who are able to communicate effectively with students, and if sufficient funds and competent teachers are available, perhaps more effective results in the reduction of certain drug use can be achieved despite the difficulties of assessing behavioral changes.

A third problem in evaluation concerns the use of performance objectives that are primarily cognitively oriented. This emphasis is brought on by the need for schools to demonstrate educational accountability. The approach has dangers when applied to the drug problem because schools may again place themselves in the trap of trying to treat the symptom, and of imparting solely subject matter rather than being concerned with students, their feelings, and their attitudes. Although there is no quarrel with the performance objectives concept, the program should not be solely oriented toward knowledge and understanding. The need for an approach emphasizing attitudes and practices will present a challenge to teachers and schools. They will need to establish reasonable, achievable objectives in these categories as defined in Chapter 7 as well as devices to assess these goals. School personnel will therefore need to carefully review the attitudinal and practice inventories presented here and adapt, devise, or create others so these inventories are functional. Thus schools will be better able to provide data that will enable them to demonstrate accountability in the affective and action domains as well as in the cognitive domain.

The conduct of evaluation studies that do not utilize true experimental designs is seen by some experts as a problem. They believe consideration should be given to ascertaining the reliability and validity of instruments and the use of pretest-posttest measures with control groups as part of the procedure.

Kushner[14] has said that the use of loosely defined criteria such as changes in grade point averages, referrals for discipline, absentee rates, and drug usage attitudes toward illicit drug use for evaluation are not acceptable. Randall and Wong[21] claim that the assessment of the frequency of drug-related incidents and arrests as well as the number of calls on hot-lines are sloppy data and inconclusive evidence.

There is no easy solution to the matter of evaluation in the school drug program. It is expected that the material and inventories in this chapter will not only provide assistance but will also motivate school personnel to develop improved assessment procedures.

ILLUSTRATIVE EVALUATION INSTRUMENTS
Total program evaluation instrument

"Criteria for Evaluating the School Drug Program" is a useful instrument that will help in the gross assessment of the total school drug program both from a quantitative and a qualitative standpoint. It seeks primarily subjective evidence but the data could be collected objectively if a sufficient number of individuals take part. This involvement would remove the possibility of bias that may develop from the use of a small number of observers. If the advisory drug committee wishes to authorize this device to be self-administered by a representative committee from each school in the district, the compiled information would provide greater objectivity in the data collected. (See p. 284.)

Education program evaluation instruments

A variety of devices usable in the instructional program are presented in this section. These instruments are listed according to the following categories and subcategories:

1. Objectives
   a. Knowledge instruments
   b. Attitude instruments
      (1) Related to drugs
      (2) Related to youth alienation, unrest, problems, social and psychological needs, and interests
   c. Practices survey form
   d. Knowledge-attitude instrument
2. In-service instruments
3. Resource materials
   a. Films and filmstrips
   b. Materials

Objectives

The instruments to measure objectives will include those to assess knowledge (cognitive domain), attitudes (affective domain), and practices (action domain). They are designed to be used in a variety of ways: (1) to pretest students and utilize the data to determine needs, interests, and problems for curriculum development and course content; (2) to posttest students following instruction to determine behavioral changes; and (3) to serve as self-tests to help initiate discussion. These devices may need modification and adaptation to local situations and communities.

Knowledge instruments. Three knowledge devices will be introduced:

1. The "High School Drug Knowledge Questionnaire" contains 46 multiple-choice questions prepared by the Colorado State Department of Education for high school students. (See p. 288.)
2. The "High School Drug Knowledge Test" includes 74 true-false questions prepared by the Great Falls Public Schools, Montana, for ninth graders. (See p. 294.)
3. The "Revision of the University of Illinois Smoking Knowledge Test" is a set of 44 questions prepared for use in the University of Illinois smoking project for grades 7 to 12. (See p. 297.)

Attitude instruments. There are two groups of attitude instruments. One group contains five techniques related to attitudes about drugs. The second group includes two instruments related to alienation and unrest.

Drug attitudes

1. The "Alcohol and Alcoholism—Attitudinal Measure" presents a series of statements relating to the use of alcohol, teaching about alcohol, the drinking problem in school, and the person with a drinking problem. Weir used this device in a study of high school students in Canada. (See p. 302.)
2. The "Attitude Toward Smoking Marijuana" instrument may be helpful to measure attitudes toward smoking marijuana ranging from favorable to unfavorable. This scale may be used to determine the feelings toward marijuana of one individual or of a group. (See p. 303.)
3. The "Drug Attitude Survey" is a use-

ful self-test to start a classroom discussion. (See p. 304.)
4. The "Evaluating Your Self-Esteem" is a useful instrument for junior and senior high schools. (See p. 305.)
5. "Opinions on the Use and Control of Beverage Alcohol" consists of 33 questions prepared by the Great Falls Public Schools, Great Falls, Montana, for seventh grade students. (See p. 307.)

Alienation and unrest

1. The "Youth Alienation Survey" will help to determine the concerns young people have with individuals and society. It may help to get at the root causes of youth unrest and the drug problem. (See p. 310.)
2. "My Checklist" was prepared by the Oregon State Board of Education to help discover some of the psychological difficulties young children may be experiencing. (See p. 312.)

Practice survey form. The technique identified may be useful in surveying students at the junior and senior high school levels to determine the extent of their use and misuse of drugs. The device also has utility as a pre- and posttest to determine behavioral changes.

1. The "Survey Form Used in 1970" in San Mateo, California, where such surveys have been conducted for the past 4 years on thousands of junior and senior high school students. (See p. 313.)

Knowledge-attitude instrument. The "Alcohol Education Pretest" was prepared by the Michigan Department of Education. It may be useful in gathering information and determining high school students' feelings about alcohol in order to ascertain the nature of the content to be covered. Parts I and II may serve for pretest and posttest purposes. (See p. 314.)

In-service

The instruments provided in this section are illustrative of some of the devices usable in determining the effectiveness of in-service programs. Two very helpful procedures are included. One is a device to measure opinions about the program at weekly intervals, and the second is a procedure to be used as a culminating, or final, program evaluation instrument.

Attitudes instruments

1. The "Weekly Program Opinions" is a type of instrument that may be used where a training session involves one or more weeks. (See p. 317.)
2. The "Final Program Evaluation" is a device to be used as a culminating evaluation measurement. (See p. 318.)

Resource materials

The volume of films, filmstrips, records, books, pamphlets, cassettes, and other resource materials that is being produced demands ways of determining the best ones for the educational program. Evaluation procedures must be available to determine the quality of these items. The following devices will be helpful with the assessment task.

1. The "Film Rating Scale" is a simple device that can help to quickly arrive at a conclusion regarding a film. It may also be used for filmstrips by omitting inappropriate criteria. (See p. 319.)
2. "Materials Evaluation" was prepared by the Mental Health Planning Committee of Milwaukee County, Wisconsin. It is a multi-itemed evaluation procedure that is more complex than the others previously introduced. It may be better suited to the needs of some schools and school districts than the "Evaluation of Materials." (See p. 320.)

Text continued on p. 321.

CRITERIA FOR EVALUATING THE SCHOOL DRUG PROGRAM

Instructions: 1. Place a check (✔) in the appropriate box under "Provision" for each criterion.
2. Place a number in the appropriate box under "Effectiveness" that best illustrates the effectiveness of the criterion.
   Scale: POOR 0 1 2 3 4 5 GOOD
3. Add appropriate comments under "Needed changes."

CRITERIA	PROVISION			EFFECTIVENESS	NEEDED CHANGES
	YES	NO	PARTLY		

BASIC OBJECTIVES
1. Familiarity with nature and extent of drug problem among students
2. Operation of a school drug program
3. Drug program includes more than education
4. Goals are behaviorally centered
5. Treatment of students based on causal relationships rather than symptomatic behavior
6. Focus on improvement of interpersonal relations and helping students find identity
7. Students actively participate in a variety of ways
8. Skills development in values clarification, decision-making, and coping
9. Community involved in the program
10. Related to and coordinated with community efforts

FORMAL EDUCATION
1. Organization of program
   a. Part of health education
   b. Correlated with other subjects
2. Curriculum
   a. Graded program K through 12
   b. Curriculum guide available
      (1) Concept approach used
      (2) Behavioral objectives provided

Continued.

(3) Content includes
   (a) Pharmacological aspects
   (b) Psychological aspects
   (c) Sociological aspects
   (d) Spiritual aspects
(4) Variety of stimulating and interesting methods of teaching
(5) Realistic assessment procedures established
3. Alternative education and activities
4. Teachers
  a. Communicate well with students
  b. Qualified to teach about drugs
5. Resources
  a. Variety of materials available
  b. Resource teacher in each school
  c. Use of community
6. Instructional program for parents

INFORMAL EDUCATION
1. Opportunities through
  a. Rap sessions—one-to-one or small groups
  b. Drop-in centers
  c. Hot-lines
  d. Others
2. Individuals available for "rapping"
  a. Teachers
  b. Counselors
  c. Nurse
  d. Students
  e. Ex-addicts
  f. Physicians
  g. Others
3. Parents
  a. Personnel available and procedures established to help with
    (1) Information

CRITERIA FOR EVALUATING THE SCHOOL DRUG PROGRAM—cont'd

CRITERIA	PROVISION			EFFECTIVENESS	NEEDED CHANGES
	YES	NO	PARTLY		
(2) Guidance and assistance					
4. Use of Community resources					
SERVICES					
1. Identification of drug abusers and users					
a. Procedures established					
b. Personal familiarity with procedures					
2. Handling of drug users and abusers					
a. Procedures established					
b. Personnel roles identified					
c. Availability of teachers, counselors, nurses, or others for help when needed or requested					
d. Rehabilitation and treatment help for students					
3. Personnel familiar with community resources available to help students					
4. Coordination with community resources					
5. Adjustments of school program for drug abusers to help with rehabilitation					
SCHOOL ATMOSPHERE					
1. Personnel awareness of student alienation and unrest					
2. Action to reduce student alienation and unrest					
3. Action to satisfy students' physical and psychological needs					
4. Action to satisfy students' psychological and social needs					
5. Action toward more humaneness in school with attention to					
a. Individualized instruction					
b. Student involvement					
c. Meaningful learning					

d. Success opportunities
e. Performance objectives criteria
f. Freedom of student expression
g. Improved human relationships
h. Listening to students
i. Flexible scheduling of classes
j. Greater teacher involvement in school affairs and decisions
k. Provision for warm, friendly, secure atmosphere

COORDINATION
1. Availability of drug coordinator for school system
2. Drug advisory committee
3. Written policies and procedures that include:
   a. Educational program
   b. Services program
   c. Identification of roles of personnel and students
   d. Handling students using, suspected of using, or under the influence of drugs
   e. Handling law violations and other conditions, including:
      (1) Suspension and expulsion
      (2) Student search rights
      (3) Student questioning rights
      (4) Personnel records
      (5) Readmission
   f. Confidentiality and police relations
   g. Counseling, guidance, and rehabilitation
   h. Possession or sale of drugs
   i. Undercover police on campus
4. Financial support
5. In-service programs for school personnel

HIGH SCHOOL DRUG KNOWLEDGE QUESTIONNAIRE*

1. Drugs that are more likely than others to cause dream images are
   a. stimulants.
   b. depressants.
   c. hallucinogens.
   d. opiates.
   e. none of the above.
2. Physical dependence on drugs is a condition in which
   a. the body needs the drug.
   b. larger doses are required.
   c. a strong desire for the drug has developed.
   d. the body always suffers pain.
   e. none of the above.
3. Tolerance has developed when
   a. the body rejects the drug.
   b. the drug makes the user sick.
   c. the body gets used to the drug.
   d. the drug must be injected into the blood.
   e. withdrawal symptoms set in.
4. Drugs that stimulate the central nervous system and give a feeling of being pepped up are
   a. barbiturates.
   b. amphetamines.
   c. hallucinogens.
   d. opium products.
   e. THC derivatives.
5. A condition that may be caused by misuse of amphetamines is
   a. withdrawal illness.
   b. a depressed feeling.
   c. the need for larger doses.
   d. sleepiness.
   e. all of the above.
6. Amphetamines are used medically for the relief of
   a. drowsiness and mild depression.
   b. fear and excitement.
   c. feelings of restlessness.
   d. nervousness.
   e. none of the above.
7. A person who has taken an amphetamine is likely to be
   a. calm, quiet, and inactive.
   b. unsteady.
   c. talkative and restless.
   d. unable to stay awake.
   e. losing sense of time and space.
8. The most common medical use of barbiturates is
   a. to produce sleep.
   b. to relieve pain.
   c. for weight control.
   d. for research studies.
   e. to combat depression.

*From Measures used in the drug evaluation, Appendix A, unpublished data, Colorado Department of Education.

HIGH SCHOOL DRUG KNOWLEDGE QUESTIONNAIRE—cont'd

9. Continued use of barbiturates over a period of time can cause
   a. tolerance.
   b. physical dependence.
   c. emotional dependence.
   d. none of these.
   e. all of the above.
10. Barbiturate users are likely to
   a. stay awake for long periods.
   b. fall asleep easily.
   c. feel restless and excited.
   d. experience loss of appetite.
   e. none of the above.
11. The effects of marijuana on the body are closely related to those caused by
   a. stimulant drugs.
   b. depressant drugs.
   c. hallucinogenic drugs.
   d. opiate derivatives.
   e. none of the above.
12. The long history and widespread use of marijuana have
   a. established evidence that the drug is harmless.
   b. shown that the drug causes recklessness.
   c. created confusion about the effects of the drug.
   d. shown that it leads to heroin use.
   e. none of the above.
13. Marijuana does not cause
   a. an effect on the central nervous system.
   b. emotional dependence.
   c. physical dependence.
   d. an effect on the sense of time.
   e. occasional fear and anxiety.
14. A dose of cocaine would most likely cause the body to become
   a. depressed.
   b. stimulated.
   c. sleepy.
   d. nauseated.
   e. none of the above.
15. The strongest of the following opium drugs is
   a. morphine.
   b. heroin.
   c. codeine.
   d. cocaine.
   e. all are the same strength.
16. The effects of heroin will most likely cause
   a. a dulling of senses of fear, tension, and anxiety.
   b. excitement and increased energy.
   c. restlessness and oxygen in the blood.
   d. inability to sleep or relax.
   e. mild hallucinations.
17. Some cough medicines can cause drug dependence if misused because they contain
   a. meperidine.
   b. Benzedrine.

Continued.

HIGH SCHOOL DRUG KNOWLEDGE QUESTIONNAIRE—cont'd

    c. codeine.

    d. morphine.

    e. Methedrine.

18. Hallucinogens are sought because they
    a. relax tension, induce elation.
    b. increase alertness, reduce sleepiness.
    c. produce a sense of calm, well-being.
    d. cause exciting visions and increased intelligence.
    e. cause varying illusions and escape from reality.

19. Abuse of airplane glue, gasoline, and other solvents causes
    a. excitement, weightlessness.
    b. depression, laziness, relaxation.
    c. intoxication, confusion, tissue damage, and comas.
    d. hallucination, depression.
    e. feelings of temporary restored alertness and energy.

20. Which of the following drugs causes psychological dependence but not physical dependence?
    a. Seconal
    b. Benzedrine
    c. Morphine
    d. Heroin
    e. Dilaudid

21. There is scientific evidence to indicate that physical dependence can be established with use of marijuana.
    a. Definitely false
    b. Probably false
    c. I do not know
    d. Probably true
    e. Definitely true

22. Most people who use marijuana will also try heroin.
    a. Definitely false
    b. Probably false
    c. I do not know
    d. Probably true
    e. Definitely true

23. Alcoholism is our primary national addiction problem.
    a. Definitely false
    b. Probably false
    c. I do not know
    d. Probably true
    e. Definitely true

24. LSD is addicting in the sense of producing physical dependence.
    a. Definitely false
    b. Probably false
    c. I do not know
    d. Probably true
    e. Definitely true

25. Of the people you know personally, who do you feel is best informed about drugs?
    a. My teachers or counselors
    b. A friend or group of friends
    c. My parents

HIGH SCHOOL DRUG KNOWLEDGE QUESTIONNAIRE—cont'd

    d. My doctor

    e. Other _____

26. If you were having trouble handling drugs (a bad trip, etc.), where would you go for help?

    a. To my parents

    b. To a close friend

    c. To a teacher

    d. To my doctor

    e. To a drug center (assuming one were available)

27. Why do you feel parents and students have trouble communicating about drugs?

    a. Parents are not willing to listen.

    b. Students are not willing to listen.

    c. Parents do not know enough about drugs and drug-related problems.

    d. Parents and students do not have enough common activities.

    e. The value systems of parents are too different from the value systems of students.

28. How comfortable do you feel talking to your parents about drugs?

    a. Extremely uncomfortable

    b. Fairly uncomfortable

    c. Fairly comfortable

    d. Extremely comfortable

29. Who do you talk with most about drugs?

    a. My parents

    b. A certain friend

    c. A group of my friends

    d. My teachers

    e. No one

30. Why do people your age use drugs?

    a. They enjoy drugs.

    b. Drugs help them communicate with people.

    c. Their friends use them.

    d. They help them understand themselves.

    e. They are curious about the effects.

31. Why do people your age not use drugs?

    a. They are afraid of the possible harmful physical consequences (addiction, deformed children, etc.).

    b. They are afraid of the possible harmful psychological consequences (nervous breakdown, hysteria, etc.).

    c. Their parents are against drugs.

    d. Their friends advised against using drugs.

    e. They are afraid of getting arrested and having a legal record.

32. It is possible to identify drug users by their physical appearance.

    a. I strongly disagree.

    b. I disagree but with reservations.

    c. I have no feelings about this issue.

    d. I agree but with reservations.

    e. I strongly agree.

33. The mass media have made the use of illegal drugs appear attractive to youth.

    a. I strongly disagree.

    b. I disagree but with reservations.

    c. I have no feelings about this issue.

Continued.

HIGH SCHOOL DRUG KNOWLEDGE QUESTIONNAIRE—cont'd

    d. I agree but with reservations.

    e. I strongly agree.

34. There can be no single successful method of prevention or treatment of drug abuse for all individuals.

    a. I strongly disagree.

    b. I disagree but with reservations.

    c. I have no feelings about this issue.

    d. I agree but with reservations.

    e. I strongly agree.

35. Drug abuse by an individual is merely a symptom of a deeper underlying personal problem.

    a. I strongly disagree.

    b. I disagree but with reservations.

    c. I have no feelings about this issue.

    d. I agree but with reservations.

    e. I strongly agree.

36. Adults must modify their use of drugs such as tobacco and alcohol before they can expect youth to modify their use of drugs such as marijuana and LSD.

    a. I strongly disagree.

    b. I disagree but with reservations.

    c. I have no feelings about this issue.

    d. I agree but with reservations.

    e. I strongly agree.

37. The great majority of drug abusers are youth under age 21.

    a. I strongly disagree.

    b. I disagree but with reservations.

    c. I have no feelings about this issue.

    d. I agree but with reservations.

    e. I strongly agree.

38. The elimination of dangerous drugs from society would only bring about the abuse of other dangerous substances.

    a. I strongly disagree.

    b. I disagree but with reservations.

    c. I have no feelings about this issue.

    d. I agree but with reservations.

    e. I strongly agree.

39. Every community has a potential drug abuse problem.

    a. I strongly disagree.

    b. I disagree but with reservations.

    c. I have no feelings about this issue.

    d. I agree but with reservations.

    e. I strongly agree.

40. There are as many causes for drug abuse as there are drug abusers.

    a. I strongly disagree.

    b. I disagree but with reservations.

    c. I have no feelings about this issue.

    d. I agree but with reservations.

    e. I strongly agree.

HIGH SCHOOL DRUG KNOWLEDGE QUESTIONNAIRE—cont'd

To what extent do you feel each of the following drugs should be legalized?
41. Narcotics
    a. Totally prohibited
    b. Available only by prescription or for research.
    c. As available as liquor
    d. As available as tobacco
    e. No restrictions
42. Marijuana
    a. Totally prohibited
    b. Available only by prescription or for research.
    c. As available as liquor
    d. As available as tobacco
    e. No restrictions
43. Psychedelics
    a. Totally prohibited .
    b. Available only by prescription or for research.
    c. As available as liquor
    d. As available as tobacco
    e. No restrictions

HIGH SCHOOL DRUG KNOWLEDGE TEST*

TRUE-FALSE QUESTIONS

T F   1. The term "drug" applies only to substances that are used as medicines.

T F   2. The medical meaning of the term "narcotic" differs from the legal meaning of the term.

T F   3. Drug dependence is said to exist only when a person is physically and psychologically dependent on a drug.

T F   4. Psychological dependence on a drug is easier to overcome than physical dependence.

T F   5. When a person has developed tolerance to a drug, he needs increasing amounts of that drug in order to react satisfactorily to its presence.

T F   6. Amphetamine, when self-administered to prevent sleepiness while driving, may cause intoxication which affects the driver's ability to handle his car safely.

T F   7. Barbiturates, taken in excessive amounts, cause a severe depression of the central nervous system, which may result in unconsciousness or death.

T F   8. When alcohol and barbiturates are taken together, the drugs tend to neutralize each other, causing a relatively mild reaction.

T F   9. Barbiturates, if taken repeatedly, may cause total drug dependence comparable in severity to heroin dependence.

T F 10. Amphetamine may be self-administered with relative safety because it does not lead to drug dependence.

T F 11. The dangerous drugs differ from the narcotics in that their excessive use leads only to psychological dependence, whereas narcotic abuse leads to both psychological and physical dependence.

T F 12. The young person who abuses dangerous drugs is likely already to have a history of delinquent behavior.

T F 13. It has been shown through experimentation that the use of amphetamines can substantially improve athletic performance.

T F 14. The organic solvents present in glues and plastic cements are capable of damaging the brain, affecting liver and kidney functions, and interfering with the blood-forming function of the bone marrow.

T F 15. There is no evidence that glue sniffing leads to the development of dependence.

T F 16. It is believed that the abuse of volatile chemicals will soon be solved through the development of nonintoxicating solvents to replace those now present in glues and plastic cements.

T F 17. Marijuana is an important medicinal drug because of its effectiveness as a pain-killer.

T F 18. Marijuana is a contraband drug, and whoever produces or distributes it is guilty of a crime punishable as a felony.

T F 19. Most marijuana entering the United States today comes by way of Mexico.

T F 20. The plant Cannabis sativa, from which marijuana is derived, grows only in warm, humid climates.

T F 21. The plant from which marijuana is derived has been known and used as a drug for several thousand years.

T F 22. A person who feels he must take marijuana (or any other drug) in order to enjoy life or to belong in a group has failed to make a normal, wholesome adjustment to life and has not learned to function as an independent, responsible member of society.

*Adapted from Tobacco, drug, alcohol unit, ninth grade, Great Falls, Mont., 1971, Great Falls Public Schools.

HIGH SCHOOL DRUG KNOWLEDGE TEST—cont'd

T F 23. If other people are using marijuana (or some other drug), it is best for you to use it too, so as not to appear different.

T F 24. If you can not find success or enjoyment in life, it is wise to try to forget your sense of failure by drinking alcohol or taking drugs.

T F 25. Since most marijuana users today do not progress to heroin, there is little reason not to use marijuana.

T F 26. Marijuana contains a powerful chemical that appears to incite its users to commit acts of violence.

T F 27. There is now believed to be little or no relation between the use of marijuana and the commission of acts of violence.

T F 28. A person who forms a **habit** of marijuana use may find it exceedingly difficult to break that habit.

T F 29. The use of marijuana opens the way for many persons to the use of other drugs.

T F 30. When a drug is said to be "nonaddicting" it means that a person using the drug can stop any time he wants to.

T F 31. A person should make decisions in terms of his own standards and convictions rather than in terms of the pressures and practices of other people.

T F 32. Marijuana, while apparently acting as a stimulant, dulls the higher control centers of the brain so that one's conduct may become socially unacceptable, for one's normal inhibitions no longer prevail.

T F 33. A person under the influence of marijuana is able to think more clearly and act more efficiently than he would under normal conditions.

T F 34. When a person has taken marijuana, he is likely to experience a period of stimulation followed by a period of depression.

T F 35. LSD may be used only for purposes approved by the Federal Food and Drug Administration.

T F 36. Any licensed physician can obtain LSD from the Food and Drug Administration for the purpose of conducting scientific investigations.

T F 37. People with stable personalities seldom experience adverse effects after taking LSD.

T F 38. Since the early 1940s, scientists have known that LSD causes hallucinations.

T F 39. LSD is one of the most potent drugs known to man.

T F 40. LSD has an accepted place in medical practice.

T F 41. After a user takes LSD, his mind "expands" and he becomes more aware of his surroundings.

T F 42. Psychological dependence may result from the use of LSD.

T F 43. A user taking the same amount of LSD in the same surroundings a second time will have an experience similar to the one he had the first time.

T F 44. Hallucinations experienced after a person has taken LSD can recur several months later, even though he has not taken any more of the drug.

T F 45. An individual's value system often changes after he has taken LSD.

T F 46. After taking LSD, the user becomes more social; that is, he relates more closely to those around him.

T F 47. A number of persons have committed suicide after taking LSD.

T F 48. Some people use LSD in order to withdraw from reality.

T F 49. A person who has used LSD several times can predict the kind of side effects, if any, that a new user might expect.

T F 50. Persons who use LSD seldom use any other drugs.

T F 51. In Montana it is illegal to have LSD in one's possession.

T F 52. LSD is derived from the sacred mushroom, which has long been used by the Indians in Mexico.

Continued.

T F 53. LSD is a relatively mild drug that can be used safely in large amounts.

T F 54. Once it is brought under medical control, LSD promises to be a "miracle drug" in that it helps people to solve their problems and adjust better to life.

T F 55. LSD and other hallucinogens are now subject to the same federal controls as the dangerous drugs.

T F 56. The use of LSD is frequently accompanied by severe and dangerous side effects.

T F 57. Physicians prescribe LSD for persons who have symptoms of anxiety and depression.

T F 58. LSD has a special attraction for adolescents who are searching for identity.

T F 59. LSD can help adolescents resolve the conflicts of "growing up."

T F 60. Involvement in narcotic use, if it occurs, is likely to take place only after prior experience with other drugs.

T F 61. Heroin is legally used in the United States today as a medicinal drug.

T F 62. The process of injecting heroin (or any other foreign substance) directly into the veins carries serious danger of infection.

T F 63. Since heroin appears not to damage body tissue, its use is not serious from the standpoint of health.

T F 64. The use of heroin leads rapidly and almost inevitably to total drug dependence.

T F 65. The recent increase in sex crimes throughout the United States is attributable, in part, to the increase in narcotic use.

T F 66. Narcotic dependence may be said to be cured when a person has been relieved of the physical aspects of dependence.

T F 67. The narcotic addict in Great Britain, once he has registered with designated authorities, is entitled automatically to receive a supply of drugs to maintain his desired level of dependence.

T F 68. The "clinic plan" of administering sustaining doses of narcotics to addicts was tried in the United States in the 1920s and deemed a success at the time.

T F 69. The American Medical Association has come out in favor of the adoption of the British method of narcotics control in the United States.

T F 70. The United States has made significant progress in international narcotic control.

T F 71. In the United States the dispensing of drugs by a physician to an addict for the gratification of his desire or need for drugs is now considered by the courts to fall within the province of legitimate medical practice.

T F 72. Whereas control of drug abuse in the United States rests largely in the hands of law enforcement personnel, control in Great Britain is vested in the medical profession.

T F 73. Since the drug abuse pattern in the United States differs drastically from that in Great Britain, it is doubtful that this country will ever move toward wholesale adoption of the British method of narcotic control.

T F 74. Under Montana law the mere possession of marijuana or of a narcotic (other than one prescribed by a physician) is illegal.

REVISION OF THE UNIVERSITY OF ILLINOIS SMOKING KNOWLEDGE TEST*

1. A study of the smoking habits of American teen-agers reveals that
   a. more teen-agers than adults smoke cigarettes.
   b. more junior high students smoke than high school students.
   c. approximately 30% of all teen-agers smoke cigarettes.
   d. more teen-age girls than teen-age boys smoke cigarettes.
2. Cigarette commercials no longer show professional athletes smoking. Which of the following is **not** true of cigarette advertisements?
   a. Cigarette advertisers sponsor athletic contests on TV.
   b. Some athletes give testimonials against smoking for poster displays.
   c. Cigarette commercials include the health effects of smoking.
   d. Cigarette smoking is associated with participation in recreational activities.
3. The work load of the heart of a cigarette smoker is increased due to
   a. carbon monoxide reducing the oxygen-carrying capacity of the blood.
   b. the acceleration of the clotting time of blood.
   c. increased thickening of the walls of the arterioles and small arteries.
   d. all of the above.
4. Surveys indicate that most teen-agers smoke because they
   a. like the taste of tobacco.
   b. are rebelling against authority.
   c. want to belong to the group.
   d. say it calms them down.
5. Nicotine, an ingredient in cigarette smoke, is
   a. stimulating to the nervous system.
   b. depressing to the nervous system.
   c. both stimulating and depressing.
   d. neither stimulating nor depressing.
6. The reason most adult smokers would advise teen-agers not to start smoking is that
   a. doctors are against smoking.
   b. it is unlawful for teen-agers to smoke.
   c. cigarette ads to not give the whole truth.
   d. it is easier not to start than to give up smoking.
7. One reason scientists think cigarette smoking is a cause of lung cancer is due to the
   a. increased activity of the cilia of smokers.
   b. thickening of respiratory membranes of smokers.
   c. higher incidence of lung cancer among cigarette smokers.
   d. all of the above.
8. Which of the following is **not** true of coronary heart disease?
   a. Coronary heart disease is the leading cause of death.
   b. It kills 2½ times more smokers than lung cancer each year.
   c. It claims a majority of its victims in the 20 to 30 age group.
   d. It is a greater health hazard for smokers rather than nonsmokers.

Please study the following table concerning the rate of smoking by sex and education. Use this information for answering question 9.

Number of years of education	MALES (100%)			FEMALE (100%)		
	Never smoked regularly	Former smokers	Present smokers	Never smoked regularly	Former smokers	Present smokers
5 to 8	24.3	20.1	55.5	64.8	4.8	30.0
9 to 12	30.1	17.6	52.2	55.9	8.4	35.5
13 and over	36.3	22.6	41.1	53.7	12.0	34.1

*Adapted from Creswell, W. H., Jr., and others: Youth smoking behavior characteristics and their educational implications, Washington, D.C., 1970, U.S. Public Health Service.

Continued.

REVISION OF THE UNIVERSITY OF ILLINOIS SMOKING KNOWLEDGE TEST—cont'd

9. The table given on p. 297 does **not** indicate that
   a. the percentage of female smokers generally increases with an increase in education.
   b. a higher percentage of males than females smoke.
   c. the more highly educated females quit smoking more often than do the highly educated males.
   d. the percentage of male smokers generally decreases with an increase in education.

10. Emphysema in recent years has
    a. increased slightly for both men and women.
    b. increased moderately for men; remained unchanged for women.
    c. increased considerably for men and is increasing for women.
    d. remained the same for both men and women.

11. Metastasis relates to the
    a. thickening of the walls of the arteries.
    b. spreading of cancer cells to other parts of the body.
    c. destruction of the tiny air sacs of the lungs.
    d. result of poor circulation in the body extremities.

12. The percentage of high school girls who now smoke is
    a. shown to be gradually decreasing.
    b. progressively approaching that of high school boys.
    c. greater than that of high schools boys.
    d. greater than that of adult women.

13. A disease characterized by a progressive reduction of blood flow to the extremities has long been recognized as due primarily to the use of tobacco. This disease is called
    a. Buerger's disease.
    b. bronchitis.
    c. coronary heart disease.
    d. emphysema.

14. Most people continue to smoke because of
    a. psychological factors.
    b. addiction to nicotine.
    c. physiological effects.
    d. aesthetic reasons.

15. Cigarette smokers tire easily because
    a. the lungs decrease in size.
    b. dirt and dust cannot be filtered.
    c. of inefficient gas exchange in the lungs.
    d. the membranes lose their elasticity.

16. Which of the following best describes the effect of nicotine?
    a. It dilates the blood vessels.
    b. It constricts the blood vessels.
    c. It has no effect on the blood.
    d. Little is known on the subject.

17. The person **most** likely to get lung cancer is the
    a. pipe smoker.
    b. cigar smoker.
    c. cigarette smoker.
    d. ex-smoker.

REVISION OF THE UNIVERSITY OF ILLINOIS SMOKING KNOWLEDGE TEST—cont'd

18. Which of the following acts directly as a cleaning and filtering system for the lungs?
    a. Bronchi
    b. Cilia
    c. Trachea
    d. Alveoli
19. Approximately how many cigarettes does it take to affect the pulse rate?
    a. One
    b. Five
    c. Ten
    d. Twenty
20. The "smoker's cough," a type of chronic bronchitis, is
    a. the result of constriction of nasal passages of the smoker.
    b. caused by irritation of mucous membranes of the respiratory tract.
    c. due to the chemicals in the cigarette paper.
    d. not really related to smoking.
21. The purpose of studying about smoking is to
    a. create an awareness of health hazards.
    b. present both sides of the issues.
    c. help with individual decision making.
    d. accomplish all of the above.
22. The pattern of cigarette smoking among women reveals that
    a. more women than men smoke.
    b. the number of women smokers has decreased.
    c. approximately 30% of the women smoke.
    d. women start smoking earlier than men.
23. The ingredient in cigarette smoke that is believed to be the cause of lung cancer is
    a. nicotine.
    b. carbon monoxide.
    c. tobacco tars.
    d. charcoal.
24. An immediate effect of cigarette smoking is the
    a. dilation of the pupils.
    b. increase in body temperature.
    c. increase in blood pressure.
    d. slowing down of pulse rate.
25. Smoking affects the diet by
    a. leading to an increase in the appetite.
    b. increasing the sensitivity of the taste buds.
    c. decreasing the flow of gastric juices.
    d. increasing the level of blood sugar.
26. Cancer is generally described as a (an)
    a. inflammation of the membranes in the throat.
    b. irritation of cells in the bronchi.
    c. uncontrollable growth of abnormal cells.
    d. break up of cells within the lungs.

Read the information concerning the following four teen-agers and then answer questions 27 and 28.
    Margaret—majority of her close friends smoke; boyfriend smokes
    Joyce—a few of her friends smoke; boyfriend smokes
    Bill—neither father nor mother smokes; friends mainly nonsmokers
    Donald—both father and mother smoke; friends mainly smokers

Continued.

27. The two teen-agers **most** likely to become smokers are
    a. Joyce and Margaret.
    b. Donald and Margaret.
    c. Bill and Joyce.
    d. Donald and Joyce.
28. The two teen-agers **least** likely to become smokers are
    a. Bill and Donald.
    b. Margaret and Donald.
    c. Donald and Joyce.
    d. Joyce and Bill.
29. A loss of elasticity of the tiny air sacs in the lungs is most characteristic of
    a. Buerger's disease.
    b. cancer.
    c. bronchitis.
    d. emphysema.
30. Cigarette commercials do **not** include appeals to one's
    a. emotional feelings.
    b. smoking pleasures.
    c. rational thought.
    d. sexual awareness.
31. When compared to nonsmokers, cigarette smokers tend to have
    a. a greater life expectancy.
    b. a shorter length of life.
    c. the same mortality rate.
    d. the same morbidity rate.
32. The walls of the blood vessels of cigarette smokers are apt to be
    a. thinner than nonsmokers.
    b. thicker than nonsmokers.
    c. more brittle than nonsmokers.
    d. more elastic than nonsmokers.
33. Unlike the tars in cigarettes, nicotine has the greatest effect on
    a. respiration.
    b. circulation.
    c. digestion.
    d. excretion.
34. In patients with emphysema
    a. there is a paralysis of the alveoli.
    b. cancerous growths appear in the lungs.
    c. there is a decreased blood flow to the extremities.
    d. air cannot flow freely out of the lungs.
35. Through advertising, people are persuaded to buy certain brands of cigarettes because they
    a. are under the subtle influence of suggestion.
    b. identify cigarette smoking with social pleasures.
    c. associate smoking with beautiful, sophisticated people.
    d. are influenced by all of the above.
36. The reason most people fear lung cancer is because it is
    a. the leading cause of death.
    b. a permanent handicap.
    c. nearly always fatal.
    d. difficult to diagnose.

REVISION OF THE UNIVERSITY OF ILLINOIS SMOKING KNOWLEDGE TEST—cont'd

The following boys are on the high school track team:
Rob—distance runner
Bill—discus thrower
Bob—sprinter
Paul—pole vaulter

37. Of the above athletes, the one whose performance will probably be **least** affected by smoking is
    a. Rob.
    b. Bill.
    c. Bob.
    d. Paul.
38. Of the above four trackmen, the one whose performance will probably be **most** affected by smoking is
    a. Rob.
    b. Bill.
    c. Bob.
    d. Paul.
39. One of the first serious effects of smoking is the
    a. paralysis of the cilia.
    b. lowering of the blood pressure.
    c. tar that accumulates on the lips.
    d. heat of the smoke in the lungs.
40. Studies have shown that many high school boys do not smoke because of their
    a. awareness of the health hazards.
    b. inability to afford the expense.
    c. participation in athletics.
    d. aesthetic considerations.
41. Cigarette smoking produces all of the following **except** a (an)
    a. decrease in temperature in the extremities.
    b. reduction of the oxygen in the blood.
    c. rise in the blood sugar level.
    d. increase in body weight.
42. The body part most affected by pipe smoking is the
    a. lungs.
    b. trachea.
    c. lips.
    d. bronchial tubes.
43. As a result of regular cigarette smoking there is
    a. an overall decrease in reaction time.
    b. a slowing of the blood flow through the capillaries.
    c. an increase in the total vital capacity of the lungs.
    d. an overall increase in the body's temperature.
44. The health hazards of cigarette smoking increase with
    a. the number of cigarettes smoked.
    b. the number of years a person smokes.
    c. the amount of smoke inhaled.
    d. all of the above.

ALCOHOL AND ALCOHOLISM—ATTITUDINAL MEASURE*

Instructions: Read the following group of seven statements and mark a 1 in front of the statement you **like** the most. Then mark a T in front of any other statements you agree with. Next mark a 2 in front of the statment you **dislike** the most. Then mark an F in front of any other statements you do not agree with. You need not mark all the statements if you do not want to. Read all seven statements before you mark any of them. There are three groups to be done this way.

1. As far as the use of alcohol is concerned:
   _____ There should be no restrictions as to when and who can use alcohol.
   _____ The present laws should not be as strict as they are toward the use of alcohol.
   _____ People should be able to ignore some of the laws about the use of alcohol at times.
   _____ People should be able to make a free choice as to how they want to use alcohol as long as they don't interfere with the choice of others.
   _____ People who develop a problem because of alcohol should not be allowed use it.
   _____ Strict laws should be enforced as to when and who can use alcohol.
   _____ No one should be allowed to use alcohol in any form.

2. In teaching about alcohol and problem drinking the school should present:
   _____ Any true or false facts that will keep people from drinking.
   _____ Any true facts that will keep people from drinking.
   _____ The true facts but should lean toward convincing people not to drink.
   _____ The true facts so a person can make a choice based on hearing both sides of the story.
   _____ Only facts that the students and parents want to hear.
   _____ Only the bare minimum facts required by state law.
   _____ Absolutely nothing, since this area is not the school's concern.

3. A person who has a drinking problem:
   _____ Is completely incompetent and should be put in an institution for his own good.
   _____ Is such a weakling that he should be forced to accept treatment.
   _____ Is dealing with his own personal problem and society should not interfere.
   _____ Is physically, mentally, socially, and/or spiritually ill and should be treated as any other ill person.
   _____ Should be given a chance to make restitution with the law and to promise that he won't drink anymore.
   _____ Should be held responsible for his actions against the law when drinking, the same as when he is not drinking.
   _____ Is a threat to society and should be treated as any other criminal.

*From Weir, W. R.: J. Alcohol Educ. **15:**1-8, 1969.

ATTITUDE TOWARD SMOKING MARIJUANA*

Recently increasing publicity has been given to smoking marijuana. The following scale is meant to explore some of your **feelings** toward smoking marijuana. It is **not** meant to test what you know about marijuana. Read each item carefully and **circle** the number opposite each statement with which you **agree.** Make **no marks** opposite the statement with which you **disagree.**

(S)

4.9	149.	Smoking marijuana is a requirement for successful living.
4.7	147.	Smoking marijuana is necessary if one is to achieve his potential.
4.5	145.	Smoking marijuana is an excellent way to increase one's understanding of the world about him.
4.3	143.	Smoking marijuana is too good a thing to be given up.
4.1	141.	Smoking marijuana can be a helpful way of adjusting to the world around us.
3.9	139.	A person should be allowed to smoke marijuana if he wants to.
3.7	137.	Smoking marijuana can be justified.
3.5	135.	Smoking marijuana is all right in some cases.
3.3	133.	The benefits of smoking marijuana depend entirely upon the individual.
3.1	131.	Smoking marijuana is not necessarily wrong.
2.9	129.	Smoking marijuana is one way of trying to be different.
2.7	127.	Smoking marijuana is not absolutely bad but it is not good either.
2.5	125.	I question whether or not it is morally right to smoke marijuana.
2.3	123.	Smoking marijuana is not a necessary part of life.
2.1	121.	Smoking marijuana is an emotional "crutch."
1.9	119.	Smoking marijuana is a foolish thing to do.
1.7	117.	Smoking marijuana is wrong.
1.5	115.	Smoking marijuana is bad.
1.3	113.	Smoking marijuana is a foolish way to try and escape reality.
1.1	111.	Smoking marijuana shows an utter lack of self-respect.

SCORING THE SCALE

Each statement has a scale value. These scale values are indicated in column (S). This column is not to be included in the scale given to the student and is shown here only to simplify the explanation of scoring. The scale encompasses statements that reflect a point of view that can be rated on a five-point continuum: 5 = very favorable; 4 = favorable; 3 = neither favorable nor unfavorable; 2 = unfavorable; and 1 = very unfavorable.

The individual "score" or measure of attitude is the scale value of the middle or median value of those statements to which the student responds. For example, if a student agrees with and responds to statements 137, 131, 129, and 117, his median score is 2.9. According to the scoring system, 2.9 indicates that this student's attitude toward smoking marijuana is neither favorable nor unfavorable. Let us further assume that a student agrees with and responds to statements 121, 119, 117, and 115. Here his median or middle "score" would be 1.8, which indicates an unfavorable attitude toward smoking marijuana. Individual "scores" from a class may be averaged to obtain a class mean score toward smoking marijuana. The numerical value of this mean score indicates the class attitude toward smoking marijuana. For example, the scores of 35 students in a classroom average a mean score of 2.23. From our scoring values we may ascertain that the attitude of this class toward smoking marijuana is unfavorable since 2.0 indicates an unfavorable expression of attitude.

*From Vincent, R. J.: J. Sch. Health **40:**454-456, 1970.

DRUG ATTITUDE SURVEY

Directions: Give your feeling about each of the items below by marking in the column to the right the number, 1 to 5, which most accurately expresses your opinion at this time.

1. Strongly agree
2. Agree
3. Neither
4. Disagree
5. Strongly disagree

NUMBERS

1. When in a group, go along with the group view because it is usually right. _____
2. Parents should let kids experiment with drugs if they want to. _____
3. If your friends use marijuana, you should too so that you are not different. _____
4. If you can not succeed in or enjoy life, you have a good reason to want to forget it all by drinking or taking drugs. _____
5. Since marijuana use today does not lead to heroin use, there is little reason against using marijuana. _____
6. The laws against marijuana should be made more lenient. _____
7. There is little or no harm in using marijuana so long as a person does not indulge too frequently. _____
8. A user of LSD experiences mind expansion and greater awareness of his surroundings. _____
9. Taking LSD makes you become more sociable and more closely related to those around you. _____
10. Some people withdraw from reality through the use of drugs. _____
11. The side effects, if any, that a new user might expect can be predicted by a person who has used LSD several times. _____
12. LSD promises to be a "miracle drug," once it is brought under medical control, because it helps people solve problems and adjust to life. _____
13. Adolescents trying to resolve the conflicts of growing up can be helped by LSD. _____
14. People who use drugs are stupid. _____
15. People who use drugs are just trying to find out what it is like. _____
16. The laws about drugs should be more strict and enforced more. _____
17. The laws about drugs should be made more lenient for the first offense. _____
18. The laws about drugs should be eliminated. _____
19. Anybody who gives or sells drugs to kids should not be punished any more than someone who takes it. _____
20. Anybody who furnishes kids with drugs should be severely punished. _____

EVALUATING YOUR SELF-ESTEEM*

Reply to the following statements, using this scale:

0—not true	1—somewhat true
3—largely true	4—true

SCORE   **STATEMENT OF PRESENT CONDITION OR ACTION**

_____ 1. I usually feel inferior to others.

_____ 2. I normally feel warm and happy toward myself.

_____ 3. I often feel inadequate to handle new situations.

_____ 4. I usually feel warm and friendly toward all I contact.

_____ 5. I habitually condemn myself for my mistakes and shortcomings.

_____ 6. I am free of shame, blame, guilt, and remorse.

_____ 7. I have a driving need to prove my worth and excellence.

_____ 8. I have great enjoyment and zest for living.

_____ 9. I am much concerned about what others think and say of me.

_____ 10. I can let others be "wrong" without attempting to correct them.

_____ 11. I have a strong need for recognition and approval.

_____ 12. I am usually free of emotional turmoil, conflict, and frustration.

_____ 13. Losing normally causes me to feel resentful and "less than."

_____ 14. I usually anticipate new endeavors with quiet confidence.

_____ 15. I am prone to condemn others and often wish them punished.

_____ 16. I normally do my own thinking and make my own decisions.

_____ 17. I often defer to others on account of their wealth or prestige.

_____ 18. I willingly take responsibility for the consequences of my actions.

_____ 19. I am inclined to exaggerate and lie to maintain a self-image.

_____ 20. I am free to give precedence to my own needs and desires.

_____ 21. I tend to belittle my own talents, possessions, and achievements.

_____ 22. I am free to speak up for my own opinions and convictions.

_____ 23. I habitually deny, alibi, justify, or rationalize my mistakes and defeats.

_____ 24. I am usually poised and confortable among strangers.

_____ 25. I am very often critical and belittling of others.

_____ 26. I am free to express love, anger, hostility, resentment, joy, etc.

_____ 27. I feel very vulnerable to others' opinions, comments, and attitudes.

_____ 28. I rarely experience jealousy, envy, or suspicion.

_____ 29. I am a "professional people pleaser."

_____ 30. I am not prejudiced toward racial, ethnic, or religious groups.

_____ 31. I am fearful of exposing my "real self."

_____ 32. I am normally friendly, considerate, and generous with others.

_____ 33. I often blame others for my handicaps, problems, and mistakes.

_____ 34. I rarely feel uncomfortable, lonely, and isolated when alone.

_____ 35. I am a compulsive "perfectionist."

_____ 36. I accept compliments and gifts without embarrassment or obligation.

_____ 37. I am often compulsive about eating, smoking, talking, or drinking.

_____ 38. I am appreciative of others' achievements and ideas.

_____ 39. I often shun new endeavors because of fear of mistakes or failure.

_____ 40. I make and keep friends without trying.

_____ 41. I am often embarrassed by the actions of my family or friends.

_____ 42. I readily admit my mistakes, shortcomings, and defeats.

_____ 43. I experience a strong need to defend my acts, opinions, and beliefs.

*Project Promise, Washoe County School District, Reno, Nevada.

Continued.

EVALUATING YOUR SELF-ESTEEM—cont'd

_____ 44. I take disagreement and refusal without feeling "put down" or rejected.
_____ 45. I have an intense need for confirmation and agreement.
_____ 46. I am eagerly open to new ideas and proposals.
_____ 47. I customarily judge my self-worth by comparison with others.
_____ 48. I am free to think any thoughts that come into my mind.
_____ 49. I frequently boast about myself, my possessions, and my achievements.
_____ 50. I accept my own authority and do so as I, myself, see fit.
_____ **SELF-ESTEEM INDEX** (total)

TO OBTAIN YOUR SELF-ESTEEM INDEX

Add the individual scores of all **even** numbered statements (e.g., 2, 4, 6, 8). From this total subtract the sum of the individual scores of all **odd** numbered statements (e.g., 1, 3, 5, 7). This **net score** is your **current** Self-Esteem Index, or SEI. For example: If the sum of all the individual scores of the even numbered statements is 37 and the sum of all the individual scores of the odd numbered statements is 62, your SEI is 37 − 62 or a _minus_ 25. The possible range of one's Self-Esteem Index is from −75 to +75. Yours will fall somewhere in between. Do not be concerned about your SEI, no matter how low, or even _negative_. Remember, your self-esteem simply is what it is, the _automatic_ product of your heritage and total life experience, and thus nothing to be ashamed or embarrassed about. It is important, however, that you be honest with yourself in order to obtain as valid a score as possible. For this score is a beginning reference point in gauging your progress in building self-esteem. Also remember that no matter how low your present SEI may be, you can bring it up to any desired value by conscientious effort.

OPINIONS ON THE USE AND CONTROL OF BEVERAGE ALCOHOL*

Directions: The following statements are concerned with the use and effects of alcohol as a beverage. Some of the statements deal with facts and some reflect opinions. You are asked to consider each of the statements and indicate your choice in the proper column. If you are in agreement with what the statement says, place an "X" opposite the statement in the column headed "agree." If you disagree with the statement, place an "X" in the column headed "disagree." If you do not know whether you agree or disagree with the statement, or if you are doubtful, place an "X" in the column marked "uncertain."

	AGREE	DISAGREE	UNCERTAIN
1. Even among the experts, very little is known of the effects of alcohol upon the human body.	_____	_____	_____
2. Frequent drunkenness and alcoholism means the same thing.	_____	_____	_____
3. Drinking alcoholic beverages, though begun in moderation, will lead eventually to alcoholism.	_____	_____	_____
4. The present trend in the consumption of alcoholic beverages in the United States indicates a decrease in per capita consumption.	_____	_____	_____
5. The increase in alcohol is the fundamental cause of most alcoholism.	_____	_____	_____
6. Most people who drink alcoholic beverages do so moderately.	_____	_____	_____
7. Alcohol is directly responsible for a large proportion of the crimes committed.	_____	_____	_____
8. Alcoholic beverages are a form of poison.	_____	_____	_____
9. Alcohol, in the form of a beverage, is a good stimulant and, therefore, effective in the treatment of snakebite, shock, or a common cold.	_____	_____	_____
10. There are several kinds of alcohol, but ethyl alcohol is the one contained in alcoholic beverages.	_____	_____	_____
11. The alcohol content of alcoholic beverages produced by fermentation is greater than that of beverages produced by distillation.	_____	_____	_____
12. The chemical effect of alcohol on the body is similar to that of ether and acts as an anaesthetic or depressant on the nervous system.	_____	_____	_____
13. Alcohol beverages are a form of food.	_____	_____	_____
14. The same amount of alcohol taken in the form of whiskey is more "potent" than that taken in the form of wine.	_____	_____	_____

*From Tobacco, drug, alcohol unit, seventh grade, Great Falls, Mont., 1971, Great Falls Public Schools.

Continued.

OPINIONS ON THE USE AND CONTROL OF BEVERAGE ALCOHOL—cont'd

	AGREE	DISAGREE	UNCERTAIN
15. Alcohol may, when taken in small amounts, serve a beneficial purpose in bringing about relaxation, lessening body tension, and acting as a "social lubricant."	___	___	___
16. People who drink alcoholic beverages do not make good parents.	___	___	___
17. Excessive drinking produces serious physical and mental diseases.	___	___	___
18. Alcohol in high concentration is known to be irritating to body tissues; therefore, when whiskey, containing 50% alcohol by volume, is taken into the body, it irritates and causes inflammation of the organs of the body, especially the brain.	___	___	___
19. Alcohol taken into the body in beverage form is absorbed from the stomach and taken directly into the bloodstream without change.	___	___	___
20. Most people can drink alcoholic beverages without injury to their health.	___	___	___
21. The habit of excessive drinking puts a great strain upon the heart and is thus responsible for much heart disease.	___	___	___
22. Prohibition of the manufacture, sale, and use of alcoholic beverages prevents people from drinking and thereby solves the problems of excessive drinking and alcoholism.	___	___	___
23. The best known method for measuring the amount of alcohol in the brain is to measure the concentration of alcohol in the blood.	___	___	___
24. Magazines and newspapers containing liquor advertisements should not be patronized.	___	___	___
25. Scenes which show persons drinking alcoholic beverages, with or without ill effects, should not be permitted in the movies.	___	___	___
26. The use of alcoholic beverages has existed for thousands of years in all countries despite all legal and social attempts to prohibit it.	___	___	___
27. Many persons can increase their skill in operating an automobile after taking a little alcohol.	___	___	___
28. Chronic alcoholics are more susceptible to respiratory diseases, especially	___	___	___

OPINIONS ON THE USE AND CONTROL OF BEVERAGE ALCOHOL—cont'd

	AGREE	DISAGREE	UNCERTAIN
pneumonia, and are less able to survive them than nonalcoholics.			
29. Any use of alcoholic beverages by the state encourages drinking by giving it official approval.	_____	_____	_____
30. The use of alcoholic beverages in the home is not necessarily harmful to good family life.	_____	_____	_____
31. Various attitudes toward serving and drinking alcoholic beverages are found among different groups in our society.	_____	_____	_____
32. Judgment, vision, and reaction time in individual performance are frequently impaired by even small amounts of alcohol.	_____	_____	_____
33. The money obtained from taxes on alcoholic beverages should not be used for the support of schools or for the aged.	_____	_____	_____

YOUTH ALIENATION SURVEY

This is a survey to determine your opinions on a few general issues. Since opinions are of a personal nature, there are no right or wrong answers. Please try to answer as honestly as possible. All responses will be kept in the strictest of confidence.

Directions: Indicate in the column on the right the number that best represents your opinion.

1. Disagree strongly
2. Disagree
3. Neutral
4. Agree
5. Agree strongly

NUMBERS

1. Nowadays a person has to live pretty much for today and let tomorrow care of itself. ⎯⎯⎯
2. Religion is playing an important role in solving today's problems. ⎯⎯⎯
3. None of the political candidates running for election ever represents my view. ⎯⎯⎯
4. I usually have the courage of my convictions. ⎯⎯⎯
5. Deep down I know I am not the person I would like to be. ⎯⎯⎯
6. With the advance of science, the world is daily becoming a better place to live. ⎯⎯⎯
7. The best way to get things done is to operate within the channels of the existing political system. ⎯⎯⎯
8. If people are allowed to do whatever they want, they are likely to cause trouble. ⎯⎯⎯
9. The stuff they teach in schools just does not seem useful in the real world. ⎯⎯⎯
10. Having pull is more important than ability in getting a good job. ⎯⎯⎯
11. Parents today are not strict enough with their children. ⎯⎯⎯
12. More and more I feel helpless in the face of what is happening in the world today. ⎯⎯⎯
13. I used to think my prospects for success were pretty good, but now I am beginning to wonder. ⎯⎯⎯
14. Most of the decisions made by the courts are unfair. ⎯⎯⎯
15. Our society may not be ideal, but things are not as bad as most people claim. ⎯⎯⎯
16. You can always find friends if you try. ⎯⎯⎯
17. Most people would not work if they did not have to eat. ⎯⎯⎯
18. Ask not what your country can do for you; ask instead what you can do for your country. ⎯⎯⎯
19. No one has the right to tell me how to run my life. ⎯⎯⎯
20. Despite what others may say, I know I am on the right track in life. ⎯⎯⎯
21. Nobody really cares about anybody's problems but his own. ⎯⎯⎯
22. A factory worker can lead just as full a life as anyone else. ⎯⎯⎯
23. It is important to teach young people strict obedience to their parents. ⎯⎯⎯
24. The future is so unpredictable that there is not much point in making long-range plans. ⎯⎯⎯
25. Active discussion of politics can eventually lead to a better world. ⎯⎯⎯
26. Family responsibilities come first, even at great personal cost. ⎯⎯⎯
27. Other people seem to find it easier to decide what is right than I do. ⎯⎯⎯
28. Everyone is always trying to tell me what to do. ⎯⎯⎯

YOUTH ALIENATION SURVEY—cont'd

29. Most people in public office are genuinely interested in the problems of the average person. _____

30. I would take a boring job if I thought the chances for promotion were good. _____

31. We are just so many cogs in the machinery of the system. _____

32. Young people must be made to realize that there is a lot they can learn from their elders. _____

33. This world is run by only a few people in power. _____

34. It is worthwhile to have friends, no matter how much trouble they may seem to be. _____

35. Most religious leaders are really out of touch with what is happening today. _____

36. You can't fight city hall. _____

37. As long as no one is hurt, the police ought to mind their own business. _____

38. One thing I know I can always fall back on is my religion. _____

39. Marriage is out of date. _____

40. Any job can be interesting if you work hard at it. _____

41. If I had my life to live over, I would probably do the same things. _____

42. Even if the odds seem against you, it is possible to come out on top by persisting. _____

43. When I am really honest with myself I realize that I just do not have what it takes. _____

44. My friends would not let me down if I really needed them. _____

45. It takes a few nonconformists to show the rest of the world how to shape up. _____

46. I think I could make a go of almost anything if I really put my mind to it. _____

MY CHECKLIST*

Name _____ Grade _____ Age _____ Date _____

	MAKES ME HAPPY	MAKES ME UPSET OR ANGRY	DON'T CARE
Accidentally breaking something			
Sleeping late in the morning			
Being scolded, even though I didn't mean to cause trouble			
A quiet, orderly house			
Being called to get up			
Being told I did wrong			
Having to say "sorry," even though I should			
Having to eat what I don't like			
Winning a game			
Being teased or called names			
Going places I want to go			
Being shoved around			
Being told how nice I am			
Having someone take my things without asking			
Doing my lessons well			
Not being allowed to do what I want to do			
Being told that I have done a good job			
Knowing I have made a mistake			
Being told to go to bed			
Being kind to someone			
Being told to "hurry up" when I am already hurrying			
Losing a game			
Brothers and sisters being mean			
Being able to tell my troubles to someone I like			
Someone else being teased or bothered			
Feeling guilty about something			
Other			

This is what I wish:

*Adapted from Toward responsible drug education, grades K-4, Salem, 1970, Oregon State Board of Education.

SURVEY FORM USED IN 1970*

> **Instructions:** This survey is being made in county schools to get some facts. NO ONE IN YOUR SCHOOL WILL SEE THIS REPORT AFTER YOU FILL IT OUT. YOU CANNOT BE IDENTIFIED. Please do not report any drug used because a doctor or dentist prescribed it for you, or gave it to you. We appreciate your help. The only way we can get a fair picture is to come directly to the persons who know.

THIS REPORT WAS MADE BY:

☐ MALE   ☐ FRESHMAN   ☐ SOPHOMORE   ☐ GRADE 7
☐ FEMALE   ☐ JUNIOR   ☐ SENIOR   ☐ GRADE 8

I have used (during the past 12 months)	0	1 to 2	3 to 9	10 to 49	50+
Tobacco					
LSD					
Marijuana					
Alcoholic beverages					
Amphetamines (meth, speed, bennies, pep pills)					
Barbiturates (downers, reds, yellow jackets, blues)					
Heroin					
Cocaine					
Solvents					

*Adapted from Five mind-altering drugs (plus one), San Mateo, Calif., 1970, Department of Public Health and Welfare.

ALCOHOL EDUCATION PRETEST*

General instructions: This booklet contains a collection of statements concerning alcohol and its use. We are going to study this topic, and to insure that our sessions are of maximum value to all members of the class, we must know as much as possible about the needs of our class for knowledge about alcohol. Please answer all questions as frankly and completely as you can. It will not be necessary to sign your name or otherwise identify yourself personally, since it is group rather than individual results we want to consider. Nonetheless, each of your responses will be important in determining what we stress in this series, so please read each item carefully before answering.

Part I. How much do you know about alcohol?

Below are some statements concerning alcohol and its use. If you think that the statement is **True,** encircle the letter **"T"** before the statement. If you think that the statement is **False,** encircle the letter **"F"** before the statement. Be sure to answer every question. If you don't know the answer make a guess.

T F 1. Alcohol, the chemical found in all alcoholic beverages, is a stimulant.
T F 2. Drinking alcohol will warm you up by increasing body temperature.
T F 3. Alcohol in small amounts can increase athletic skill.
T F 4. Two or three drinks can reduce your ability to operate a machine.
T F 5. It's a sign of manliness to be able to drink a lot.
T F 6. Some people are better drivers after a couple of drinks because they purposely drive more carefully.
T F 7. Alcoholic drinks are necessary at a party if people really want to have a good time.
T F 8. Alcohol is good for colds.
T F 9. Excessive drinking of alcohol may injure body organs by "pickling" them.
T F 10. Drunkenness of a person clearly shows he is addicted to alcohol.
T F 11. There are fewer alcoholics among those who stick to beer and wine than among those who drink hard liquor.
T F 12. The earlier the alcoholic patient looks for help, the better are his chances of recovery.

Part II. How do you feel about alcohol?

A number of statements concerning alcohol and its use are listed below. Please indicate your agreement or disagreement with each statement by checking the column to the right of each statement which comes nearer to describing your feeling. There are no right or wrong answers. Your first reaction to the statement is what we are interested in. Make a choice for every statement. Check only one column for each statement.

	AGREE	DISAGREE
1. The general public is already sufficiently informed about the facts of alcoholism.	____	____
2. If an alcoholic wanted to be cured, he could accomplish the matter himself.	____	____
3. The alcoholic suffers from a severe illness and needs treatment to a much greater degree than the usual medical complaints.	____	____
4. Drinking on some social occasions should be done if it helps the individual to fit in with others.	____	____

*Adapted from A curriculum guide for alcohol education for teachers, bulletin no. 371, Lansing, 1970, Michigan Department of Education.

ALCOHOL EDUCATION PRETEST—cont'd

5. Only people like physicians, social workers, and the like should ____ ____
receive information concerning alcoholism.
6. Alcoholism is the direct result of a sick society. ____ ____
7. No one should criticize the alcoholic without knowing why he ____ ____
drinks.
8. General hospitals should not accept alcoholics for treatment. ____ ____
9. More research programs are needed about alcoholism. ____ ____
10. Drinking alcoholic beverages should be classed with the illegal ____ ____
use of dope.
11. The alcoholic has no one to blame for his troubles but himself. ____ ____
12. The facts about alcohol should be taught in every high school in ____ ____
America.
13. The families of alcoholics should encourage them to seek expert ____ ____
treatment for their condition.
14. Alcoholism begins as the sin of drinking and ends as a sinful ____ ____
habit.
15. Information on alcoholism should be available to any citizen who ____ ____
has the interest to write for it.
16. Doctors who spend their time treating alcoholics are wasting ____ ____
their time.
17. Public education concerning alcohol is a waste of time and ____ ____
money.
18. Alcoholic beverages are harmless when used in small amounts. ____ ____

Part III. What would you like to know about alcohol?

Rate the following topics according to their importance to you. Put the number "1" on the blank line in front of the topic you most want to learn about, the number "8" in front of the topic which interests you least and assign numbers "2" to "7" to the balance of the items in order of their importance to you. If two topics are equally important to you, rate them with the same number and omit the next number.

_____ The effects of alcohol on emotions, mental processes, and body organs (including hereditary effects).

_____ The physiological effects of alcohol with emphasis on its effect on behavior.

_____ Knowledge about the symptoms, causes, treatment, and hope for recovery in alcoholism.

_____ Knowledge of drinking customs with emphasis on why people drink, why young people shouldn't drink, and the variations in current drinking patterns and practices.

_____ Legal regulations about alcoholic beverages, and enforcement of these regulations, including justification for sale of such beverages in our society.

_____ The relationship of alcohol use to such areas as driving and social interaction, including its effect on sexual promiscuity.

_____ What is being done and what can be done to help solve school-related alcohol problems.

_____ What is alcohol and what are the differences between alcoholic beverages.

Feel free to comment below about this questionnaire, alcohol education, alcoholism, or anything related to alcohol use. Use the back of this page if you need more space.

Continued.

ALCOHOL EDUCATION PRETEST—cont'd

SCORING AND INTERPRETING THE PRETEST

Part 1. Correct answers are F, F, F, T, F, T, F, F, F, F, F, T.

Score one point for each correct answer. Sum all items for total score. Sum overall total scores and divide by the number of students for the group score. The higher the score, the better informed is the group.

Average score	Interpretation
11-12	Well-informed group
8-10	Somewhat better than chance
5-7	Chance performance. No knowledge
0-4	Misinformed

Part II.

Item	Favorable	Weight	Item	Favorable	Weight
1.	Disagree	3.0	10.	Disagree	3.7
2.	Disagree	2.9	11.	Disagree	2.2
3.	Agree	1.7	12.	Agree	3.1
4.	Agree	1.4	13.	Agree	3.7
5.	Disagree	2.6	14.	Disagree	2.8
6.	Disagree	2.7	15.	Agree	2.7
7.	Agree	2.1	16.	Disagree	3.7
8.	Disagree	2.4	17.	Disagree	3.7
9.	Agree	2.4	18.	Agree	2.1

Score each item answered as above with the weight for that item. Sum all weights for total score. Sum overall total scores and divide by the number of students for the group score. The higher the score, the more favorable the group attitude toward education about alcohol use and treatment of alcoholism as an illness.

Average score	Interpretation
33.8 to 48.6	Highly favorable attitude
22.2 to 33.7	Moderately favorable attitude
11.8 to 22.1	Neutral attitude
5.2 to 11.7	Moderately unfavorable attitude
0.0 to 5.1	Highly unfavorable attitude

Part III. Sum across students for a total score on each topic. Divide the total score for each topic by the number of students rating that topic. Rank order the topics with the lowest score first. The lower the score, the higher the group interest in that topic.

Any remarks made in response to the invitation to "Feel free to comment" in Part III may be interpreted as evidence of strong concern on the part of the respondent about the topic mentioned. Particularly in topic areas suggested spontaneously by two or more students, some opportunity to clarify or discuss these topics should be provided in subsequent class sessions.

WEEKLY PROGRAM OPINIONS

Directions: Please rate the program presentations to the extent they helped achieve the goals of the program by recording the appropriate number in the boxes provided using the following scale:

NOT EFFECTIVE   1   2   3   4   5   6   7   HIGHLY EFFECTIVE

Week no.							PROGRAM						
TRAINING CENTER GOALS	Allure of drugs	Turn on without drugs	Discussion group	Social psychology	Discussion group	Over-the-counter drugs	Predrug users	Discussion group	Field trip	Drug scene 1970	Amphetamines	Marijuana	Youth and the community
Pharmacological effects of drugs													
Psychological effects of drugs													
Sociological effects of drugs													
Community action—resources													
Leadership training													
Laws, police, courts													
Parenting education													
Communication procedures													
Curriculum development													
Teaching strategies													
Resource materials													
Counseling and guidance													
Values clarification													
Alternative education and alternative activities													

FINAL PROGRAM EVALUATION

I. What is your overall rating of the program? (check one item)

_____ Excellent

_____ Very good

_____ Good

_____ Fair

_____ Poor

II. Content and activities of Training Center

Please indicate the degree to which you believe each of the following helped prepare you for participation in a drug education program. Circle the appropriate number from "1" (poor) to "5" (excellent) for each of the six areas. Also, please make any comments or suggestions in the space provided for each area.

	POOR				EXCELLENT
1. Lectures by staff Comments:	1	2	3	4	5
2. Lectures by visiting consultants Comments:	1	2	3	4	5
3. Field trips Comments:	1	2	3	4	5
4. Group discussions Comments:	1	2	3	4	5
5. Films Comments:	1	2	3	4	5
6. Resource/reading material Comments:	1	2	3	4	5

7. If you were planning a training center such as this
   a. what aspects would you retain?
   b. what aspects would you eliminate?
   c. what aspects would you modify, and in what ways?

III. Structure of program

Please judge each of the following and make any comments you feel appropriate.

	POOR				EXCELLENT
1. Living arrangements Comments:	1	2	3	4	5
2. Organization of Training Center Comments:	1	2	3	4	5
3. Tempo or pace of activities Comments:	1	2	3	4	5
4. Physical setting of lectures/meetings Comments:	1	2	3	4	5
5. Psychological climate Comments:	1	2	3	4	5

Additional comments:

FILM RATING SCALE

Scale: 1 = POOR; 2 = FAIR; 3 = AVERAGE; 4 = GOOD; 5 = EXCELLENT

QUALITIES TO BE RATED	1.	2.	3.	4.	5.	6.	7.	8.	9.
FILM TITLES									
Is the content accurate?									
Is the film up to date?									
Is the film well organized?									
Are the objectives clear?									
Is the film a good source of information?									
Rate the following technical qualities:									
Photography									
Sound									
Music									
Voice									
For what grade level is the film suited? (Is this a teacher reference?)									
What overall rating would you give the film?									

MATERIALS EVALUATION*

I. Title _____

II. Subject emphasis _____

III. Understanding—education level:
K-3 _____ 4-6 _____ 7-9 _____ 10-12 _____

IV. Commercial references made—frequency
High _____ Medium _____ Low _____

V. In accordance with the above determinations, rate the material's presentation attributes.

	EXTENT			QUALITY		
	high	medium	low	superior	good	poor
1. Subject coverage						
a. Scientific facts						
b. Objective approach						
c. Judgments made based on scientific validity						
d. Moralizing on the subject						
e. Currency of facts						
f. Stimulation of thought and discussion						
g. Continuity						
h. Relevance to intended audience						
2. Overall subject coverage rating						
3. Multiethnic considerations						
4. Readability (when applicable)						
5. Audio-understandability (when applicable)						
6. Currency of visual appeal						
7. Relevance of visual appeal to intended audience						
8. General value in relation to cost						
9. General value in relation to length						

VI. General recommendations and level of use
Schools only _____ Adults only _____ Schools and adults _____
Reference _____ No possible use _____

VII. Additions or comments on any of the above information _____
_____
_____

*Adapted from Guidelines for the prevention of drug abuse problems through education, interim report, Milwaukee, 1971, Mental Health Planning Committee of Milwaukee County, Wisconsin.

MATERIALS EVALUATION—cont'd

VIII. Evaluation summary

_____ Book	Evaluator _____
_____ Pamphlet	Place of employment _____
_____ Film	Position _____
_____ Slides or transparencies	Evaluation date _____
_____ Film strip	Overall quality of material
_____ Poster	Superior _____ Good _____
_____ Cassette or audiotape	Poor _____ Inadequate _____
_____ Record	

SOURCES AND RESOURCES OF INSTRUMENTS

The sources and resources listed below will provide additional assistance for schools and school districts in search of evaluation instruments.

SOURCES

1. Abrams, L. A., Garfield, E. F., and Swisher, J. D., editors: Accountability in drug education: a model for evaluation, Washington, D.C., 1973, Drug Abuse Council, Inc. (Variety of instruments.)
2. Cassel, R. N., and Zander, G.: Teach me what I want to know about drugs for junior high school students, Internat. J. Addictions 9:541-567, 1974. (Ego development scale, drugs questionnaire.)
3. Drug Abuse Research Instrument Inventory, 133 Mount Auburn St., Cambridge, Mass. 02138. (Attitudes and knowledge instruments.)
4. Duvall County School Board, Research Services, 1450 Flagler Av., Jacksonville, Florida 32207. (Drug, alcohol, and cigarettes use opinion survey form.)
5. ERIC Clearinghouse for Tests, Measurements and Evaluation, Educational Testing Service, Princeton, N.J. 08540. (Annotated bibliographies of a variety of instruments.)
6. Friedman, C. J., and others: Development and application of a drug attitude questionnaire, Drug Forum 3:331-347, 1974. (Attitudes and drug use questionnaires.)
7. Horan, J. J., and Williams, J. M.: The tentative drug use scale: a quick and relatively problem free outcome measure for drug abuse prevention projects, J. Drug Educ. 5:381-384, 1975. (Drug use scale.)
8. Counselor Recording and Tests, Box 6184, Acklen Station, Nashville, Tenn. 37212. (Piers-Harris children's self-concept scale.)

9. The Publications Division, Institute for Social Research, The University of Michigan, P.O. Box 1248, Ann Arbor, Michigan 48106. (Robinson and Shaver, Measures of Social Psychological Attitudes —self-esteem, life satisfaction and happiness, alienation, values.)
10. Reinhardt, R. A.: The family drug awareness group, J. Drug Educ. 4:167-168, 1974. (Evaluation inventory for a community-school relationship.)
11. Samuels, M., and Samuels, D.: The complete handbook of peer counseling, Miami, 1975, Fiesta Publishing Co. (Variety of instruments.)
12. Simpson, M. L., and Koenig, F. W.: The use of the semantic differential technique in drug education research: an example and some suggestions, J. Drug Educ. 5:251-259, 1975.
13. Wright, T. H.: Learning to listen: a teacher's or a student's problem? Phi Delta Kappan 52:625-628, 1971. (Student opinionnaire of teacher.)

RESOURCES

1. Abrams, L. A., Garfield, E. F., and Swisher, J. D., editors: Accountability in drug education: a model for evaluation, Washington, D.C., 1973, Drug Abuse Council, Inc.
2. Bandura, A.: Principles of behavior modification, New York, 1969, Holt, Rinehart and Winston.
3. Buros, O. L.: The seventh mental measurements yearbook, Highland Park, N.J., 1971, Gryphon Press.
4. Division of Resource Development, Preventive Branch: Why evaluate drug education? Rockville, Md., 1975, National Institute on Drug Abuse.
5. Knapp, R. R.: The measurement of self-actualization and its theoretical implications, San Diego, Calif., 1971, Educational and Industrial Testing Service.
6. Lake, D., and others: Measuring human behavior, New York, 1973, Teachers College Press.
7. Robinson, J., and Shaver, P.: Measures of social

psychological attitudes, Ann Arbor, 1970, University of Michigan Press.

8. Swisher, J., and others: Experimental comparison of four approaches to drug abuse prevention among ninth and eleventh graders, J. Counsel. Psychol. **19:**328-332, 1972.

9. Webb, E., and others: Unobtrusive measures: nonreactive research in social sciences, Chicago, 1966, Rand-McNally, Inc.

REFERENCES

1. Blum, R. H., and others: Drug education: results and recommendations, Lexington, Mass., 1976, Lexington, Mass., 1976, Lexington Books.

2. Burkett, S. R.: Some comments on a statewide alcohol-education program, J. Alcohol Drug Educ. **21:**30-33, Winter, 1976.

3. Conceptual guidelines for school health programs in Pennsylvania, Harrisburg, 1970, Division of Health, Physical and Conservation Education, Pennsylvania Department of Education.

4. Cornacchia, H. J., and Staton, W. M.: Health in elementary schools, ed. 4, St. Louis, 1974, The C. V. Mosby Co.

5. Creswell, W. H., Jr., and others: Youth smoking behavior characteristics and their educational implications, Washington, D.C., 1970, U.S. Public Health Service.

6. A curriculum guide for alcohol education for teachers, Bulletin no. 371, Lansing, 1970, Michigan Department of Education.

7. Curriculum guide for drug education, grades K-12, Lovell, Wyoming, 1970, Superintendent of Schools.

8. Drug abuse education curriculum guide and resource materials for grades K-12, Dallas, 1970, Superintendent of Schools, Dallas Independent School District.

9. Drug abuse education, grades 6, 9, 12, Towson, Md., 1969, Baltimore County Board of Education.

10. Educational Research Service Report: Drug education: goals, approaches, evaluation, Arlington, Va., 1975, ERS.

11. Five mind-altering drugs (plus one), San Mateo, Calif., 1970, Department of Public Health and Welfare.

12. Guidelines for the prevention of drug abuse problems through education, interim report, Milwaukee, 1971, Mental Health Planning Committee of Milwaukee County, Wisconsin.

13. Journal of Alcohol and Drug Education **19:**29, Spring, 1974.

14. Kushner, J. N.: Evaluating primary prevention. A speech presented to the National Association of State Drug Abuse Program Coordinators Annual Meeting, June 11, 1976.

15. Louria, D. B.: A critique of some current approaches to the problems of drug abuse, Am. J. Public Health **65:**581-583, June, 1975.

16. Measures used in the drug evaluation, appendix A, Colorado Department of Education.

17. Neeman, R. L., and Neeman, M.: Complexities of smoking education, J. School Health **45:**17-23, January, 1975.

18. Pargman, D.: Teacher evaluation of the school drug education program, Sch. Health Rev. **1:**14, 1970.

19. Peterson, R.: Prevention program launched with little or no evaluation, Addiction Research Foundation of Ontario, Canada, March, 1974.

20. Pollock, M. B.: Mood-altering substances: a behavior inventory, J. Educ. Measurement **7:**211-212, 1970.

21. Randall, D., and Wong, M. R.: Drug education to date: a review, J. Drug Educ. **6:**1-21, 1976.

22. Richards, L. G.: Evaluation in drug education, Sch. Health Rev. **2:**22-27, 1971.

23. Schapps, E., and others: Primary prevention research: a preliminary review of program impact studies, Walnut Creek, Calif., 1976, Pyramid Project.

24. Senior high school health guide, Unit IV, Drug abuse and health, Salt Lake City, 1971, Utah State Board of Education.

25. Smart, R. G., and Fejer, D.: Drug education: current issues, future decisions, Toronto, Canada, 1974, Addiction Research Foundation of Ontario.

26. Survey of drug use among junior and senior high school students in the state of Idaho, Boise, 1970, Idaho State Department of Public Instruction.

27. Tobacco, drug, alcohol unit, seventh grade, Great Falls, Montana, 1971, Great Falls Public Schools.

28. Toward responsible drug education, grades K-4, Salem, 1970, Oregon State Board of Education.

29. Vincent, R. J.: A scale to measure attitude toward smoking marijuana, J. Sch. Health **40:**454-456, 1970.

30. Weir, W. R.: Alcohol and alcoholism education: attitude development and change, J. Alcohol Educ. **15:**1-8, 1969.

Drug abuse in sports

Enough has been written about the unwarranted use of drugs by athletes to consider this an important part of the school drug abuse problem. Yet the actual extent of such drug use by high school players is difficult, if not impossible, to accurately determine. One reason for this is that competition, secrecy, and ethical considerations prevent coaches, players, or team doctors from talking much about such use even when it is discovered. In fact there is an official attitude of negativism against all forms of drug misuse, and also, typically, total denial that drugs are a problem on the playing field.

Perhaps more important than the actual extent of such drug use is a careful definition of just what is meant by "drugging" or "doping," terms that are confusing and frequently misused. In widely varying circumstances the simplistic term "doping" will be used in conjunction with any situation involving drugs and athletes. Doping is typically defined as "the use of *any* chemical substances not normally present in the body, and not essential to a healthy person competing in athletics." Both medical and athletic organizations concerned with regulating competitive sports have officially condemned doping of athletes.

When the issue of such use or abuse is to be considered, several confusing aspects must be separately examined. Are we talking about use by an athlete of a specific drug taken just prior to a game to improve his short-term athletic performance, to relieve pain, or to build up body tissue? Or are we talking about legitimate pharmaceuticals administered to an athlete by a physician to counteract injury or to treat disease? Or perhaps is the real issue illegal drug use or abuse as part of an athlete's personal life-style or of his peer-group associations having no direct relevance to his athletics?

Athletes, just like other students, smoke marijuana, get drunk, smoke cigarettes against the coach's orders, and sometimes even take dangerous drugs like LSD, amphetamines, or heroin. Such drug abuse may be part of a compulsive pattern or merely part of a life-style not at all related to athletics, although it may cause a problem on the playing field. In fact such misuse is typically reflected only in impaired athletic performance and generally deteriorated health.

An athlete may self-medicate with legitimate preparations to deal with real or imagined problems with no intention of directly affecting his performance. For example, he may "snitch" some Darvon Compound from the family medicine cabinet to stop an aching knee, or he may dose himself with vitamin pills.

Yet in another completely different circumstance, the athlete may be examined, diagnosed by a team physician, and legitimately prescribed medicine to combat illness or pain. This is precisely where the most ambivalent "gray area" of medicine and ethics begins. The team physician may also assist the players in coping with pain or injury in a situation where the player should, for his best health interests, not be allowed to continue to participate. Even the coach may provide, or allow to be provided, drugs or substances ill-advised for sports play. Where should these fine distinctions be drawn? For example, exactly how badly should a player be injured before he should stop playing? To what extent should drugs be administered to an injured player so he can continue to play? No one knows exactly, of course, except probably the team physician. Every physician will exercise a slightly differing human judgment but, perhaps at the same time, be subtly influenced by the acute demand that the players be allowed to play and that the team win!

The most dramatic and the most publicized circumstances occur when the players take, with the coach's and team physician's approval, pep pills and other improper substances merely to improve performance. This is usually what is meant by the expression "doping." It would be safe to say that the use of amphetamines, or pep pills, is generally more of a problem on college teams and in professional athletics where the stakes are high and the winning edge narrow. Nevertheless the school must be aware that high school and junior high school students do take stimulants not condoned, and generally unknown, by either the coach or the team physician.

It has been reported, however, that the practice of doping flourishes at all levels of organized sports despite official disapproval. The problem of utilization of drugs to increase an athlete's performance is acknowledged in professional athletics and to a much lesser degree, among high school and college athletes. The high school athlete is not yet owned by the institution but the motivation for optimal performance is perhaps just as strong as at the college or "pro" level. Coaches will obviously go to great lengths to gain a competitive edge. In fact some feel that just to keep up with the competition, the athlete *must* use amphetamines for that extra drive, anabolic steroids for body building, or pain medication to mask the symptoms of a disabling injury. This reputedly happens in high schools and colleges and in international competition, not just in professional sports. The fact that these are potentially dangerous drugs, totally unsuitable for sports, is well known, at least to the medical profes-

sion. Yet it has been suggested that some team physicians are a party to this underground practice; they cannot approve drug use, but by turning their backs on it they are tacitly condoning it.

Baugh[1] has stated that there is a general belief that by taking "dope" athletes improve their playing performance. The accusation has been made, sometimes irresponsibly, that team doctors dope injured players with pain killers to keep them in the game, or at least that these physicians are openly permissive about the use of stimulants—"speedies" or "greenies"—by players who want some quick pep.

One of the largest drug abuse problems among young athletes is not associated with nonprescription drugs, but with the socially acceptable drugs alcohol and tobacco, use of which represents a violation of good training practices. However, Baugh reported that in a survey of high school students, a large number of athletes use drugs but less frequently than nonathletes. He said that 79% claimed they used less alcohol and 92% used less tobacco.

Dr. Robert K. Kerlan,[6] an orthopedic surgeon, team physician for the Los Angeles Lakers and the Los Angeles Kings, and consulting physician for the California Angels and the San Diego Padres, has organized all athlete's medications into three classes. Group one, the harmless and useless group, includes vitamins, dextrose (sugar), or those agents that will not harm unless taken to excess. Excessive use of vitamin B_{12}, for example, should be discouraged unless a rare case of pernicious anemia exists. Group two includes drugs with definite value in the treatment or sequelae of specific injury, such as the anti-inflammatory and pain-killing agents. Phenylbutazone and oxyphenabutazone are used principally for relief of muscular and skeletal problems such as arthritis, gout, and inflamed elbow; indomethacin is an anti-inflammatory agent; hydrocortisone is an anti-inflammatory steroid; and trypsin is an enzyme used to dissolve blood clots. The use of oral muscle relaxants (probably of no value in painful conditions) and local anesthetics or analgesics may lead to further injury. These agents must be administered under the constant supervision of a physician. With phenylbutazone, for example, regular blood checks must be made, and with indomethacin the gastrointestinal tract must be observed. Group three is made up of all the useless and potentially dangerous agents —the stimulants, or pep pills, the depressants, or downers, and the various hormones, including the anabolic steroids (trade names —Dianabol, Deca-Durabolin, Durabolin, Nilevar, Anevar, Anadrol). Anabolic- or metabolic-increasing steroids are male sex hormones that can powerfully affect the physical growth and sexual maturity of the young athlete. Artificial introduction and use of such hormones in excess of normal body production may create abnormal increases in height and body weight with disturbances in the masculinity of the male. Artificial use of such hormones may profoundly disturb the individual's normal growth processes; thus these are considered by most physicians to be totally unsuitable for general use. Michaelson[9] and Novich[11] report that amphetamines do little to improve or may give a false impression of better performance.

Dr. Kerlan believes that drugs in groups one and two may occasionally be necessary adjuncts to treating athletes. However, those drugs in group three are for diseases rarely encountered among healthy male athletes. Their use must be substantially restricted; they have no place in sports.

Unfortunately athletes of any age or level tend to be fetishists, somewhat superstitious, and remarkably given to embracing ritual or any drug or food substance that has the reputation of making athletes excel. For example, the world's best fed athletes consume millions of unnecessary vitamin capsules and tablets each year. Athletes participating in individual sports seem to be more prone to drug fads than team sports members, and so may have to be particularly cautioned concerning the dangers involved. Weight lifters and field event athletes seem especially susceptible in their quest to gain greater body weight and size, which they equate with increased strength. The use of these anabolic steroids is to be particularly condemned because of virilization, liver involvement, and possibly increased incidence of carcinoma of the prostate. Athletes should be made aware of the potential dangers involved in the use of steroids as well as of the doubtful advantages.

Consumption of honey, sugar preparations, and glucose just prior to game time is also typical even on the high school playing field. Use of sugar is perhaps more logical than any other nutritional aid, since there is an increased utilization of carbohydrates during strenous activity. However, there is *no* evidence that sugar as a pre-event supplement increases athletic performance. Nevertheless there is much honey-water sipping, or chocolate-bar eating by athletes during or preceding competition. Such practices, often encouraged by coaches, add credibility to the concept that ergogenic (energy-producing food substances) aids really work. Coaches should encourage athletes to rely only on healthful living and the physiological outcomes of activity for performance rather than on "gimmicks," "fads," or superstition.

REFERENCES

1. Baugh, R. J.: The use and misuse of drugs among high school athletes, Paper presented at the American School Health Association, Chicago, October, 1971.
2. Baugh, R. J.: The use and misuse of drugs among high school athletes, paper presented at the American School Health Association, Denver, October, 1975.
3. Clark, K. S.: Drugs, sports and doping, J. Maine Med. Assoc. **61**:55-58, 1970.
4. Food facts and fallacies, tips on athletic training VII, Chicago, 1965, American Medical Association.
5. Fowler, W. W.: The facts about ergogenic aids and sports performance, J. Health Phys. Educ. Rec. **40**:37-42, 1969.
6. Fulton, G. B.: Personal communication, April 28, 1971.
7. Kerlan, R. K.: Personal communication, Jan. 8, 1973.
8. The Medical Letter on Drugs and Therapeutics, Drugs Ath. Injur. **17:** May 15, 1975.
9. Michaelson, P.: Drugs and sports: athletes rused into dangerous illusions, The Journal (Addiction Research Foundation of Ontario, Canada), Nov. 1, 1973.
10. Murphy, R. J.: The use and abuse of drugs in athletics, Paper presented at the American Medical Association Convention, Chicago, June, 1970.
11. Novish, M. M.: Drug abuse and drugs in sports, N.Y. St. J. Med. **73:**2597-2600, 1973.

Index

A

Abuse
  of alcohol; *see* Alcohol, abuse of
  of drugs; *see also* specific drug
    alternatives to, 59, 62
    conceptual views of, 28-32
    as cop-out from society, 55-56
    council for, coordination of community action by, 128-130
    definition of, 8, 34, 36
    dilemma of, 3-23; *see also* School(s), drug dilemma in
    factors affecting, 32-33
    influence of school environment on, 56-59
    legal-morality model of, 28-30
    medical-psychiatric model of, 30-31
    observable signs and symptoms of, 229-232
    patterns of, 45-48
    pharmacological aspects of, 63-99
    polydrug, 18, 19
    prevention of; *see* Prevention of drug abuse
    problem of, definition of, 28
    programs for, community action in; *see also* Community, drug abuse programs in
    rationale for, 50-51
    sociological-psychological model of, 31
    in sports, 323-325
    treatment of, laws of California and, 118, 127
  of medicines, 32
Abused drugs, 36-43
  central nervous system depressants as, 37-38
  central nervous system stimulants as, 36-37
  identification of, 228-229
  narcotic drugs as, 40-41
  over-the-counter or nonprescription drugs as, 41-43
  psychedelic drugs as, 38-40
Abusers of drugs
  action for, 234-236
  classification and numbers of, 13-18
  clinical tests in detection of, 234
  follow-up procedures for, 136-242
  procedures for, in Newton Public Schools, 262-263
  self-identification of, 233-234
  self-identified, care of, 236

Activities, alternative, for informal drug education, 218-219
ADAMHA, functions of, 254-255
Addiction
  definition of, 34-35, 36
  to heroin, 40-41
  nonchemical treatment approach to, 96
  physical, to opiates, 92-94
Additive effects of drugs, 66
Adjustment, psychological, checklist for, 312
Administration problems in school drug program, 254-256
Administrative organization of school drug program, 256-257
Adolescent
  psychosocial factors in drug abuse and, 45-62
  world of, 48-55
    affluence in, 54-55
    motives for drug use in, 55
    permissiveness in, 54-55
    psychological motivations in, 51-52
    rationales for drug abuse in, 50-51
    rejection of culture in, 53-55
    search for identity in, 52-53
    student needs justifying behavior in, 52
    two views of, 48-50
    values in, 53
Affluence in world of adolescent, 54-55
Aftercare in treatment of drug addiction, 104-111
Alameda County Schools, drug education program in, 219
Alcohol
  abuse of, 37-38
    federal expenditures for, 268-269
    pharmacological aspects of, 82-85
  and Alcoholism—Attitudinal Measures, 302
  Drug Abuse, and Mental Health Administration, functions of, 254-255
  educational fims on, 206
  methods of teaching about, 177-180
  opinions on use and control of, questionnaire on, 307-309
  questions about, 162
  student needs and interests relevant to, 158-159
  use of, incidence of, 48
Alcohol Education Pretest, 314-316

Alcoholics Anonymous, 84
Alienation of students, 245-247
  instruments for evaluation of, 282, 310-312
Alpha School for Drug Abusers, 241
Alternative activities for informal drug education, 218-219
Alternative education in formal drug education for students, 146
Alternative school program, 240-241
Amitryptaline, use and abuse of, 96-97
Amotivational syndrome due to marijuana, 88-89
Amphetamines
  abuse of, 36-37
    by adults, 46
    pharmacological aspects of, 69-71
  for hyperactivity, controversy over, 231-232
  signs and symptoms of, 231
  street use of, 70-71
  use of, by athletes, 324, 325
Anabolic steroids, use of, by athletes, 324,325
Anadrol, use of, in sports, 325
Anevar, use of, in sports, 325
Antabuse, 84
Antagonists, narcotic, 96
Antidepressants, use and abuse of, 96-97
Antihistamines, abuse of, 42
Aspirin, abuse of, 42
Athletes, drug abuse among, 323-325
Atmosphere, school, 244-253
  consideration of, physical and psychological needs in, 247-249
  creating humaneness in, 249-252
  criteria for evaluating, 286-287
  educational films and filmstrips on, 208-209
  student alienation and unrest due to, 245-247
Attitudes
  about drugs
    instruments for evaluation of, 282, 302-312, 314-318
    survey of, 304
  hierarchy of, in drug education curriculum, 154
  toward smoking marijuana, scale for, 303
Audiovisual materials for drug education, 206-210
Autonomic nervous system, functions of, 64

B

Bad trip, crisis intervention for, 102-104, 236
Barbiturates
  abuse of, 38
    by adults, 46
    pharmacological aspects of, 80-82
  crisis intervention for, 235
  signs and symptoms of, 230
  withdrawal from, 80, 82
    dangers of, 40-41
Behavior
  effects of cocaine use on, 72
  effects of drugs on, 229-230, 231
  risk-taking
    as motivation for drug abuse, 52

Behavior—cont'd
  risk-taking—cont'd
    and rewards, inventory of, 202, 203
Behavioral approach to drug education, 21-22
Benjamin Franklin Parkway High School as educational alternative, 251
Biological variability of drug effects, 65-66
Birth defects due to marijuana, 89
Boggs Amendment, 115
Books for drug education, 205-206
Boredom as motivation for drug abuse, 52
Brand names of drugs, 67
Brown School, alternative educational program of, 241

C

Caffeine, abuse of, 37, 42-43
  pharmacological aspects of, 79
California, laws of, drug abuse treatment and, 118, 127
Cannabis sativa, 86-90; see also Marijuana
Central nervous system
  depressants of, 67; see also Sedative-hypnotics
  functions of, 64
  physiological action of drugs on, 63-64
  stimulants of, 67; see also Stimulants of central nervous system
Chemical names of drugs, 67
Chlorpromazine, use and abuse of, 96
Cigarettes; see Nicotine, Tobacco
Classification and numbers of drug users and abusers, 13-18
Clinical tests in detection of drug abusers, 234
Cocaine
  abuse of, 36
    pharmacological aspects of, 71-72
  use of
    incidence of, 10
    signs and symptoms of, 231
Comatose patient, crisis intervention for, 102-103
Commercial exploitation as rationale for drug abuse, 51
Commercial sources of drug education materials, 213-214
Communication, educational films on, 207
Community(ies)
  action on drug problems by, 127-134; see also Community(ies) drug abuse programs in
  drug abuse programs in
    administrative organization of, 256-257
    community facilities in, 132-134
    community programs and facilities in, 130-134
    coordination of, by drug abuse council of, 128-130
    Haight-Ashbury Free Medical Clinic in, 130-132
    objectives of, 128
    problems of, 256
    role of law enforcement in, 130
    teen or drop-in center in, 132

Community(ies)—cont'd
  resource personnel of, role of, in drug education for students, 222
  resources of, use of, in drug counseling and guidance, 239-240
  role of, in drug problem, 100-135
    community action for, 127-134
    government programs and resources for, 111-113
    legal perspective on, 113-127
    state laws on, 118-127
    treatment and rehabilitation for, 100-111
  -school coordination in prevention of drug abuse, 13
  therapeutic, in rehabilitation of drug addict, 108-111
Comprehensive Drug Abuse Prevention and Control Act of 1970, 5, 116-117
Compulsive users of drugs, 16, 18
Concept approach to drug curriculum, 150-162
  definition of health applied to drug education in, 150-152
Conceptual views of drug abuse, 28-32
Confidentiality of drug-related information, establishment of policies on, 261-262
Conflicts, personal, as rationale for drug abuse, 50
Controlled Substances Act, 117
Coordination
  of federal agencies for drug problems, 254-255
  of school drug program, 254-273
    criteria for evaluating, 287
Coordinator of drug education, role of, in drug education for students, 221
Coping, educational films on, 207
"Cop-out" from society, drug abuse as, 55-56
Correlated pattern of formal drug education for students, 146-148
Cough medicine, abuse of, 42
Counseling
  for drug abusers, 236-239
  peer, in drug education, 217
Counselors, role of, in drug education for students, 221-222
Crisis intervention for drug abusers, 102-104, 234-236
Culture
  rejection of, in world of adolescent, 53-55
  school, rejection of, as factor in drug abuse, 57-58
Cumulative effect of drugs, 66
Curiosity as motivation for drug abuse, 51
Curriculum in formal drug education for students, 149-175
  basic concepts in, 156-162
  concept approach in, 150-162
  content of, 162-163, 168-175
  guides for, 206
  key concepts in, 155-156
  objectives of, 162, 163-167
  student needs and interests in, 157-160
  values in, 152-155

Cyclazocine in pharmaceutical approach to drug rehabilitation, 105-106

D

Dade County Public Schools, drug education program in, 219-220
Dangerous drugs, definition of, 36
Daytop Village in rehabilitation of drug addict, 111
Deca-Durabolin, use of, in sports, 325
Decision making, educational films on, 207
Decriminalization
  of drug laws, need for, 61-62
  of marijuana in eight states, 119
Delirium tremens, 37
Demerol, use of, signs and symptoms of, 231
Dependence
  on drugs, definition of, 34-35, 36
  physical, on barbiturates, 80
  psychological
    on amphetamines, 70
    on cocaine, 71, 72
    on glue sniffing, 85
    on nicotine, 72-73
    on opiates, 92
Depressants of central nervous system, 67; see also Sedative-hypnotics
Depression
  following cocaine excitation, 71, 72
  following speed binge, 70
Desire for drugs, definition of, 36
Desoxyn, abuse of, 36-37
Detoxification in treatment of drug addiction, 104
Dianabol, use of, in sports, 325
Diet pills, abuse of, 42
Dilemma of drug abuse, 3-23; see also School(s), drug dilemma in
Direct pattern of formal drug education for students, 146-149
Diuretics, abuse of, 42
Doping of athletes, 323
Dose response, effect of, on drug actions, 65
Drop-in centers for informal drug education, 218
Drug(s); see also Specific drug
  abuse of; see Abuse of drugs
  abused, 36-43; see also Abused drugs
  abusers of; see Abusers of drugs
  addition to
    definition of, 34-35, 36
    nonchemical treatment approach to, 96
  alternatives to, 59-62
  attitudes about
    instruments for evaluation of, 282, 302-312, 314-318
    survey of, 304
  categorizing of, 66-68
    in sports, 324-325
  dangerous, definition of, 36
  definition of, 32-34, 36
  dependence on, definition of, 34-35, 36
  desire for, definition of, 36

Drug(s)—cont'd
  different ways we think about, 28-35
  education about, 144-227; *see also* Education, drug
  educational films on, 207-208
  educational filmstrips on, 209-210
  effects of, 64-66
    on behavior, 229-230, 231
  federal laws on, 113-118, 119
  habituation to, definition, 34-35, 36
  influence of, students under, care of, 236
  knowledge about, instruments for evaluation of, 282, 288-301, 314-316
  laws concerning, decriminalization of, 61-62
  methods of teaching about, 181-192
  misuse of, definition of, 8, 34
  over-the-counter or nonprescription, abuse of, 41-43
  pharmacological classification of, 97-98
  physiological action of, 63-66
  possession of, policies of Los Angeles City Schools on, 264-266
  potency of, 66
  prescribed, taking of, at school, 232-233
  problems with
    community action on, 127-134
    role of community in, 100-135; *see also* Community(ies), drug abuse programs in
    in schools, 6-7
  programs for
    administrative organization of, 256-257
    policies and procedures for, 257-262
    role of school personnel in, 266
    in schools, 137-273; *see also* School(s), drug programs in
  psychedelic, abuse of, 38-40
  questions about, 160-162
  sedative-hypnotic, abuse of, 37-38
  services related to, 228-243
  and society, 27-44
  state laws on, 118-127
  student needs and interests relevant to, 158-159
  tolerance to, 66
    definition of, 36
  use of
    definition of, 8, 34
    factors affecting, 32-33
    illegal, 32-33
    motives for, 55
    in society, nature of, as contributing factor in school dilemma, 8-11
    tell-tale evidence of, 232
  users and abusers of
    classification and numbers of, 13-18
    identification of, 229-234
    peer identification of, 233
    policies of Los Angeles City Schools on, 263-264
    potential personality characteristics of, 230, 232
Drug Abuse Control Amendments, 116
Drug Enforcement Agency, 6

Drug scene, 25-135
Durabolin, use of, in sports, 325

E

Education
  about alcohol, pretest of, 314-316
  alternative, in formal drug education for students, 146
  drug, 144-227
    correlation of, with major subject areas, 147
    definition of health applied to, 150-152
    informal; *see* Informal drug education
    meaning of, 18-22
    for parents, 222-224
    for students, 145-222
      formal education in, 145-218; *see also* Formal drug education for students.
      illustrative program for, 219-220
      informal, 218-219
      resource centers for, 220-221
      roles of school and community resource personnel in, 221-222
Effective dose, 65
Elavil, use and abuse of, 96-97
Emergencies, management of, for drug abusers, 234-235
Emotional needs of students in prevention of drug abuse, 248-249
Encounter therapy in rehabilitation of drug addict, 109
Environment, school, influence of, on drug abuse, 56-59
Escape as motivation for drug abuse, 52
Ethanol; *see* Alcohol
Ethyl alcohol; *see* Alcohol
Evaluation
  of drug programs, need for, 255
  of school drug programs, 277-322
    criteria for, 284-287
    instruments for, 281-321; *see also* Instruments for evaluation of school drug programs
    principles of, 279-281
    problems in, 280-281
    scope of, 278
  of self-esteem, scale for, 305-306
Experimenters with drugs, 16, 18
Exploitation, commercial, as rationale for drug abuse, 51
Expulsion for drug abuse, establishment of policies regarding, 259

F

Fayetteville Public Schools, drug counseling in, 239
Federal Food, Drug, and Cosmetic Act, 114-115, 116
Federal government
  agencies of, for drug problems, coordination of, 254-255
  drug abuse programs of
    administrative organization of, 256
    problems of, 254-255

Federal government—cont'd
  expenditures of, for alcohol abuse, 268-269
  financing by, for drug programs, 266-269
  laws of, on narcotics and drugs, 113-118, 119
  programs of, for drug education, 5-6
Fetal-alcohol syndrome, 83
Films
  for drug education, 206-208
  rating scale for, 319
Filmstrips for drug education, 208-210
Financial support of state drug programs, 255
Financing of school drug programs, 266-269
Flashbacks, crisis intervention for, 236
Formal drug education, 20
  criteria for evaluating, 284-285
  for parents, 223-224
  for students, 145-218
    curriculum in, 149-175; see also Curriculum in
      formal drug education for students
    evaluation of, 217
    methods of teaching for, 163, 176-202
    minicourses in, 217-218
    patterns of instruction in, 146-149
    resource materials for, 202, 204-217
Freaking out, crisis intervention for, 103-104
Functional view of adolescence, 48-49

G

Gasoline, abuse of, pharmacological aspects of, 86
Generic names of drugs, 67
Glue
  abuse of, pharmacological aspects of, 85-86
  sniffing of, questions about, 161
Government agencies involved in drug education, 6
Government programs and resources to fight drug
    abuse, 111-113
Government sources of drug education materials,
    214-215
Group School, Cambridge, Mass., drug education
    program in, 220
Guidance for drug abusers, 236-239
Guidelines for policies and procedures in school drug
    programs, 258-259

H

Habituation to drugs, definition of, 34-35, 36
Haight-Ashbury Free Medical Clinic in treatment of
    drug abuse, 130-132
Hallucinogens
  abuse of, 38-40
    pharmacological aspects of, 90-92
  crisis intervention for, 235-236
  educational filmstrips on, 209
  signs and symptoms of, 230-231
Harrison Narcotic Act, 113
  Amendment to, 115
Health
  definition of, applied to drug education, 150-152
  mental, student needs and interests relevant to,
    158-159

Heroin
  abuse of, 40-41
    pharmacological aspects of, 92-95
  addiction to, 40-41
  and marijuana, relationship between, 89
  questions about, 161-162
  use of
    incidence of, 10
    signs and symptoms of, 231
High School Drug Knowledge Questionnaire, 288-
    293
High School Drug Knowledge Test, 294-296
Hot-lines for informal drug education, 218
Human needs, development of school program re-
    sponsive to, 58-59
Humaneness, creation. of, in schools. 249-252
Humanistic approach to prevention of drug abuse, 141
Hydrocarbons, volatile, abuse of, 38
  pharmacological aspects of, 85-86
Hydrocortisone, use of, in sports, 324
Hyperactivity, amphetamines for, controversy over,
    231-232

I

Identity
  achievement of, 248
  search for, in world of adolescent, 52-53
Illegal use of drugs, 32-33
Indomethacin, use of, in sports, 324-325
Influence of drugs, students under, care of, 236
Informal drug education, 21
  criteria for evaluating, 285-286
  for parents, 224
  for students, 218-219
Inhalants, abuse of, 38
  pharmacological aspects of, 82-85
Innovative Youth Services of Racine, drug counsel-
    ing in, 239
Insecurity as motivation for drug abuse, 51
In-service preparation for drug programs, 269-272
  activities and experiences in, 271-272
  essential program components of, 271
  evaluation of, 272
  objectives of, 269-271
  organizational arrangement of, 272
  for participants, 269
Instruction, patterns of, in formal drug education for
    students, 146-149
Instruments for evaluation of school drug programs
  attitude instruments as, 282, 302-312, 314-318
  knowledge instruments as, 282, 288-301, 314-316
  practice survey forms as, 282, 313
  sources and resources for, 321-322
Intoxication with barbiturates, 80
Intra-psychic conflict as rationale for drug abuse, 50

J

Josephone County Council on Drugs, drug counsel-
    ing in, 239
Journals, professional, for drug education, 211

K

Kitsap County Council on Youth, drug counseling in, 239
Knowledge about drugs, instruments for evaluation of, 282, 288-301, 314-316

L

Law enforcement, role of, in community action on drug problems, 150
Learning, principles of, in drug education, 176
Legal-morality model of drug abuse, 28-30
Legal perspective on drug abuse, 113-127
Lethal dose, 65
Local drug abuse programs
  administrative organization of, 256-257
  problems of, 256
Los Angeles City Schools, drug abuse policies and procedures in, 263-266
LSD; see Lysergic acid diethylamide (LSD)
Lysergic acid diethylamide (LSD)
  abuse of, 38-39
    pharmacological aspects of, 90-92
  questions about, 161
  signs and symptoms of, 230

M

Maladjustments, social and psychological, signs of, 248
Mankato, Wilson School in, as educational alternative, 251-252
Marijuana
  abuse of, 39-40
    pharmacological aspects of, 86-90
  amotivational syndrome due to, 88-89
  birth defects due to, 89
  decriminalization of, in eight states, 119
  educational films on, 208
  educational filmstrips on, 209
  penalties for, federal, 119
  possession of, state penalties for, 120-123
  questions about, 161
  recommendations on, 89-90
  relationship of, to drugs of higher abuse potential, 89
  sale of, state penalties for, 123-127
  smoking of, attitude toward, scale for, 303
  subjective effects of, 86-88
  toxicity of, 86
  use of
    incidence of, 10, 45, 46, 47, 48
    long-term chronic, effects of, 88-89
    patterns of, 86
    signs and symptoms of, 231
Marijuana Tax Act, 113-114
Mass media, influence of, on abuse of over-the-counter drugs, 43
Material, resource, for drug education, 202, 204-217
  instruments for evaluation of, 283, 319-321
Medical-psychiatric model of drug abuse, 30-31

Medicine
  abuse of, 32
  cough, abuse of, 42
  definition of, 33-34
Mental health, student needs and interests relevant to, 158-159
Mercaptopurine in modulation of cell-mediated immunity, 97
Mescaline, signs and symptoms of, 230
Methadone
  for heroin detoxification, 95-96
  in pharmaceutical approach to drug rehabilitation, 106
Methamphetamine; see Amphetamines
Methedrine, abuse of, 36-37
Methotrexate in modulation of cell-mediated immunity, 96
Modulation of cell-mediated immunity, 95-97
Monterey, California, drug counseling in, 239
Morality-legal model of drug abuse, 28-30
Morning glory seeds, signs and symptoms of, 231
Morphine
  questions about, 161-162
  signs and symptoms of, 231
Motivation for learning, factors in, 176
Motives for drug use, 55
Multimodality concept in treatment of drug addiction, 100-102
Mustard, nitrogen, in modulation of cell-mediated immunity, 96-97

N

Nalline as narcotic antagonist, 96
Nalorphine as narcotic antagonist, 96
Narcotic Addict Rehabilitation Act, 116
Narcotic Control Act, 115
Narcotic Drugs Import and Export Act, 113
Narcotics, 68
  abuse of, 40-41
    pharmacological aspects of, 92-96
  addiction to
    nonchemical treatment approaches to, 96
    physical, 92-94
  antagonists of, 96
  educational films on, 208
  educational filmstrips on, 210
  federal laws on, 113-118, 119
  heroin as, 92-95
  methadone as, 95-96
  opium as, 92-95
  questions about, 161
  signs and symptoms of, 231
  state laws on, 118-127
  withdrawal from, 41
Narcotics Manufacturing Act, 115-116
National Coordinating Council on Drug Education, 204
National Institute on Alcohol Abuse and Alcoholism, 6

National Institute on Drug Abuse, 6
  on prevention of drug abuse, 255
National programs to fight drug abuse, 111-112
Needs, human, development of school program responsive to, 58-59
Nembutal, withdrawal from, dangers of, 40-41
Nervous system; *see* Central nervous system
New York City Schools, alternative educational program of, 241
New York street academy as educational alternative, 252
Newsletters for drug education, 210-211
Newton Public Schools, drug abuse policies and procedures in, 262-263
Nicotine; *see also* Tobacco
  abuse of, 37
    effect of, on fetus, 83
    pharmacological aspects of, 72-79
Nilevar, use of, in sports, 325
Nonchemical treatment approaches to addiction, 96
Nonprescription drugs, abuse of, 42-43
Nurses
  role of, in drug education for students, 222
  school, role of, in drug program, 266
Nutmeg, use of, signs and symptoms of, 231

O

Obturators, 209, 214-215, 217
Office of Education, 6
  on drug education, 255
  in financing of drug programs, 267-268
Ombudsman
  in drug counseling, 237-238
  in identification of drug abusers, 233
  role of, in drug education for students, 221-222
Opiates, 68; *see also* Narcotics
Opium, abuse of, 40-41
  pharmacological aspects of, 92-95
Opium Poppy Control Act, 115
Organization, administrative, of school drug programs, 256-257
Over-the-counter drugs, abuse of, 41-43
Oxyphenbutazone, use of, in sports, 324

P

Parents, drug education for, 222-224
Patterns of instruction in formal drug education for students, 146-149
P.C.P., abuse of, 46
Peer counseling in drug education, 217
Peer-group pressure as motivation for drug abuse, 51
Peer identification of drug users, 233
Pentobarbital
  use of, signs and symptoms of, 230
  withdrawal from, dangers of, 40-41
Periodic users of drugs, 16, 18
Permissiveness in world of adolescent, 54-55
Personal conflicts as rationale for drug abuse, 50
Personal records of students, establishment of policies on, 260-261

Personality characteristics of potential drug users, 230, 232
Personnel, school, role of, in drug program, 266
Peyote, use of, signs and symptoms of, 231
Pharmaceutical approaches to rehabilitation of drug addict, 105-106
Pharmacological aspects
  of alcohol abuse, 82-85
  of drug abuse, 63-99
Pharmacology
  of marijuana, 40
  of opium, 40-41
Phencyclidine, abuse of, 46
Phenobarbital
  use of, signs and symptoms of, 230
  for withdrawal from short-acting barbiturate, 80, 82
Phenylbutazone, use of, in sports, 324-325
Physical addiction to opiates, 92-94
Physical dependence on drugs, 35, 36
Physical needs of students in prevention of drug abuse, 247-248
Physicians
  role of, in drug education for students, 222
  school, role of, in drug program, 266
Physiological action of drugs, 63-66
Police
  relations of school with, in drug-related problems, establishment of policies on, 261-262
  undercover, on campus, establishment of policies on, 262
Polydrug abuse, 18, 19
Possession of drugs, policies of Los Angeles City Schools on, 264-266
Potency of drugs, 66
Pregnancy, alcohol abuse during, fetal impairment due to, 83
Pressure, peer-group, as motivation for drug abuse, 51
Prevention
  definition of, 11-12
  of drug abuse
    emphasis on, 255
    phases of, 12-13
    primary, 12
    school-community coordination in, 13
    school programs for, 139-143
    secondary, 12
    tertiary, 12-13
Preventive approach to drug abuse, 11-13
PRIDE as illustrative drug education program, 219-220
Principal, role of, in drug program, 266
Professional journals for drug education, 211
Professional sources of drug education materials, 215
Project Adelante, drug counseling in, 238-239
Psilocybin, signs and symptoms of, 230
Psychedelics, 67; *see also* Hallucinogens
Psychiatric approach to rehabilitation of drug addict, 106-107
Psychiatric-medical model of drug abuse, 30-31

Psychic dependence on drugs, definition of, 36

Psychic dimension of drug abuse, methods of teaching about, 197-202

Psychoactive drug, definition of, 33

Psychological adjustment, checklist for, 312

Psychological dependence on drugs, 35

Psychological dimension of health, 151-152

Psychological motivations for drug abuse, 51-52

Psychological needs of students in prevention of drug abuse, 248-249

Psychological-sociological model of drug abuse, 31

Psychologists, role of, in drug education for students, 222

Psychosis, toxic
crisis intervention for, 236
due to amphetamines, 37, 70

Psychosocial factors in drug abuse and adolescent, 45-62

Psychosociological approaches to rehabilitation of drug addict, 107-111

Psychotropic drug, definition of, 33

Public service sources of drug education materials, 215-217

Q

Questioning, rights of students regarding, establishment of policies on, 260

R

Racine, Innovative Youth Services of, drug counseling in, 239

Rap Place, drug counseling in, 239

Readmission following suspension or expulsion for drug abuse, policies on, 261

Rebelliousness as motivation for drug abuse, 52

Records, personal, of students, establishment of policies on, 260-261

Rehabilitation of drug addict
educational films on, 206-207
pharmaceutical approach to, 105-106
psychiatric approach to, 106-107
psychosociological approaches to, 107-111
religious approach to, 111
role of community in, 100-111

Relapse users of drugs, 16, 18

Religious approaches to rehabilitation of drug addict, 111

Resource centers for drug education for students, 220-221

Resource materials for drug education, 202, 204-217
instruments for evaluation of, 283, 319-321

Rewards and risk-taking behavior, inventory of, 202, 203

Rights of students regarding questioning, establishment of policies on, 260

Risk-taking behavior
as motivation for drug abuse, 52
and rewards, inventory of, 202, 203

S

St. Paul Public Schools, alternative educational program of, 241

SAODAP, functions of, 254

School(s)
alternatives to, 240-241
atmosphere of, 244-253; *see also* Atmosphere, school
-community coordination in prevention, 13
culture of, rejection of, as factor in drug abuse, 57-58
drug dilemma in, contributing factors in, 8-22
classification and numbers of drug users and abusers as, 13-18
meaning of drug education as, 18-20
nature of drug use in society as, 8-11
polydrug abuse as, 18
preventive approach as, 11-13
school-community coordination in prevention as, 13
drug problems in, 6-7
drug programs in, 139-143
administrative problems in, 254-256
coordination of, 254-273
drug education in, 144-227; *see also* Education, drug
drug services in, 228-243
evaluation of, 277-322; *see also* Evaluation of school drug programs
financing of, 266-269
in-service preparation for, 269-272
policies and procedures for, illustrations of, 262-266
recent developments in, 5-6
school atmosphere in, 244-253
environment of, influence of, on drug abuse, 56-59
personnel of, role of, in drug program, 266
programs of
adjustment of, for drug counseling and guidance, 240-241
responsive to human needs, development of, 58-59
resource personnel of, role of, in drug education for students, 221-222
role of, in drug programs, 137-273; *see also* School(s), drug programs in
undercover police in, establishment of policies on, 262

School board, role of, in drug program, 266

Search
for identity in world of adolescent, 52-53
rights of students regarding, establishment of policies on, 260

Secobarbital, withdrawal from, dangers of, 40-41

Seconal
use of, signs and symptoms of, 230
withdrawal from, dangers of, 40-41

Sedative-hypnotics, 67, 80-90
abuse of, 37-38
pharmacological aspects of, 80-90

Sedative-hypnotics—cont'd
  alcohol as, 82-85
  barbiturates as, 80-82
  educational films on, 208
  educational filmstrips on, 209
  inhalants as, 85-86
  marijuana as, 86-90
  questions about, 162
  use of, signs and symptoms of, 230
  withdrawal from, dangers of, 40-41
Sedatives, 67; *see also* Sedative-hypnotics
Segregationist view of adolescence, 49-50
Self-actualization as human need, 248, 249
Self-concept
  educational films on, 208
  educational filmstrips on, 208-209
Self-esteem, evaluation of, scale for, 305-306
Self-identification of drug abusers, 233-234
Services, drug-related, 228-243
  criteria for evaluating, 286
Shalom/Operation Discovery, drug counseling in, 239
Sleeping pills, abuse of, 43
Smoking; *see* Nicotine, Tobacco
Sniffing glue, questions about, 161
Social dimension
  of drug abuse, methods of teaching about, 197-202
  of health, 151-152
Society
  cop-out from, drug abuse as, 55-56
  and drugs, 27-44
Sociological-psychological model of drug abuse, 31
Solvents, use of, signs and symptoms of, 231
SPARK as illustrative drug education program, 219
Special Action Office for Drug Abuse Prevention, functions of, 254
Speed, 70; *see also* Amphetamines
Spiritual dimension
  of drug abuse, methods of teaching about, 197-202
  of health, 151, 152
Sports, drug abuse in, 323-325
State governments
  drug abuse programs of
    administrative organization of, 256
    problems of, 255-256
  financing of drug programs by, 266, 268, 269
  laws of, on narcotics and drugs, 118-127
  programs of, to fight drug abuse, 112-113
Steroids, anabolic, use of, by athletes, 324, 325
Stimulants of central nervous system, 67, 69-79
  abuse of, 36-37
  amphetamines as, 69-71
  caffeine as, 79
  cocaine as, 71-72
  crisis intervention for, 235
  educational films on, 208
  educational filmstrips on, 209
  for hyperactivity, controversy over, 231-232
  minor, abuse of, 37
  nicotine as, 72-79

Stimulants of central nervous system—cont'd
  questions about, 162
  use of, signs and symptoms of, 231
Street academy of New York as educational alternative, 252
Students
  alienation and unrest of, 245-247
    instruments for evaluation of, 282, 310-312
  drug education for, 145-222; *see also* Education, drug, for students
  drug needs and interests of, 157-160
  needs of, as motivation for drug abuse, 52
  personal records of, establishment of policies on, 260-261
  rights of, regarding search, establishment of policies on, 260
  role of, in drug education for students, 222
Summerhill School as educational alternative, 251
Superintendent, role of, in drug program, 266
Surveys on drug abuse, practice forms for, 313
Suspension for drug abuse, establishment of policies on, 260
Synanon in rehabilitation of drug addict, 96, 109-111
Synesthesia due to LSD, 90

T

Teachers, role of
  in drug education for students, 221
  in drug program, 266
Teaching, methods of, for formal drug education for students, 163, 176-202
Teen center as approach to drug problem, 132
Teen Challenge in rehabilitation of drug addict, 111
Teen-Peer Facilitator Program, drug counseling in, 239
Television as rationale for drug abuse, 50-51
Textbooks for drug education, 211-213
Therapeutic communities in rehabilitation of drug addict, 108-111
Therapeutic dose, 65
Thorazine, use and abuse of, 96
Threshold dose, 65
Tobacco; *see also* Nicotine
  abuse of, pharmacological aspects of, 72-79
  educational filmstrips on, 210
  knowledge about, University of Illinois test of, revision of, 297-301
  methods of teaching about, 193-196
  smoking of, effect of, on fetus, 83
  student needs and interests relevant to, 158-159
  use of
    effect of, on fetus, 83
    incidence of, 48
Tolerance
  to drugs, 66
    definition of, 36
  to glue sniffing, 85
  to opiates, 94
Toluene, abuse of, 38
Toxic dose, 65

Toxic psychosis
  crisis intervention for, 236
  due to amphetamines, 37
Toxicity
  alcohol, 83
  barbiturate, 80, 82
  chronic amphetamine, 70
  marijuana, 86
Tranquilizers, 68
  abuse of, by adults, 46
  signs and symptoms of, 230
  use and abuse of, 96-97
Transitional view of adolescence, 48-49
Treatment of drug addiction
  educational films on, 206-207
  role of community in, 100-111
Trypsin, use of, in sports, 324
Tutoring in drug education, 217

U

University of Illinois Smoking Knowledge Test, revision of, 297-301
Unrest of students, instruments for evaluation of, 282, 310-312

V

Values
  in drug education curriculum, 152-155
  educational films on, 208
  in world of adolescent, 53
Variability, biological, of drug effects, 65-66
Volatile hydrocarbons, abuse of, 38
  pharmacological aspects of, 85-86

W

Washoe County Schools, drug education program in, 220
Wilson School in Mankato as educational alternative, 251-252
Withdrawal
  from barbiturates, 80, 82
  from narcotics, 41
  from opiates, 95
  from sedative-hypnotics, dangers of, 40-41

Y

Youth alienation survey, 310-311